W0227767

A. Geibel · H. Just
W. Kasper · S. Konstantinides
Editors

Acute Pulmonary Embolism –

A Challenge
for
Hemostasiology

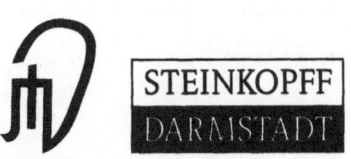 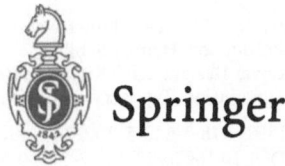

Springer

Editors' addresses:

Dr. A. Geibel · Prof. Dr. H. Just
Universität Freiburg – Med. Klinik III
Abt. Kardiologie und Angiologie
Hugstetter Straße 55
79106 Freiburg

Dr. med. W. Kasper
St. Josefs-Hospital
Medizinische Klinik
Solmsstraße 16
65189 Wiesbaden

Dr. S. Konstantinides
Klinikum der Georg-August-Universität
Zentrum Innere Medizin
Abteilung Kardiologie und Pneumologie
Robert-Koch-Straße 40
37075 Göttingen

Die Deutsche Bibliothek – CIP-Einheitsaufnahme

Ein Titeldatensatz für diese Publikation ist bei
Der Deutschen Bibliothek erhältlich

© by Dr. Dietrich Steinkopff Verlag GmbH & Co. KG, Darmstadt 2000
Softcover reprint of the hardcover 1st edition 2000

The use of general descriptive names, registered names, trademarks, etc. in this publication does not imply, even in the absence of a specific statement, that such names are exempt from the relevant protective laws and regulations and therefore free for general use.

Product liability: The publisher can give no guarantee for information about drug dosage and application thereof contained in this book. In every individual case the respective user must check its accuracy by consulting other pharmaceutical literature.

Medical Editors: Sabine Ibkendanz, Beate Rühlemann – English Editor: Mary Gossen
Production: Heinz J. Schäfer
Cover Design: Erich Kirchner, Heidelberg
Typesetting: Typoservice, Griesheim

ISBN 978-3-642-51192-9   ISBN 978-3-642-51190-5 (eBook)
DOI 10.1007/978-3-642-51190-5

Foreword and Introduction

Inspite of considerable progress in prevention, diagnosis, and treatment, pulmonary embolism has remained a threat to the patient and a challenge for the physician both in conservative, as well as in operative disciplines. Pulmonary embolism is according to pathology observations still the most frequently overlooked clinical diagnosis. In 1–5 per 100 autopsies, clinically unexpected pulmonary emboli are found. In addition, the sequelae of recurrent pulmonary emboli, the syndrome of pulmonary hypertension with or without right heart failure, continues to present a therapeutic dilemma – and no progress is in sight.

In intensive care medicine pulmonary embolism, either acute, massive, and/or recurrent, continues to be both a therapeutic as well as a preventive challenge mobilizing pharmacotherapeutic, catheter-interventional, and operative resources.

Diagnostic, therapeutic, and preventive strategies are currently in use. Their basis, however, seems surprisingly thin, as far as our knowledge on the natural course of this chameleon-like illness with and without fibrinolytic, anticoagulative, catheter or operative treatment is concerned. A large European multicenter register has been initiated by Professors Kasper and Geibel with the help of Boehringer Ingelheim Pharmaceutics, in order to better describe the natural course of pulmonary embolism under current treatment modalities. Furthermore, recently the clinical significance of the valve patent foramen ovale as a source of paradoxical emboli is beginning to be better understood. Many concepts therefore require revision.

In recent years our understanding of the molecular basis of coagulation and fibrinolysis has considerably been expanded. The thrombophilic conditions and their genetic basis are better understood, requiring reassessment of diagnostic and preventive strategies.

Research in intensive care medicine is particularly difficult. There are several reasons:
- The medical personnel in intensive care units is decision-oriented and for the most part under time pressures. In addition there is mostly a shortage of personnel, and research-oriented physicians are seldom found in these units.
- Basic research is today an indispensible part of most projects, even in patient-oriented research. This is notoriously difficult to realize in intensive care units.
- Multicenter trials are the basis for the establishment and validation of new methods and procedures. They are notoriously difficult in intensive care medicine.
- Inspite of the remarkable achievements in intensive care medicine, there are reservations in the public, especially if research is to be carried out.
- Medical ethics as understood today face problems in intensive care. In particular the problem of informed consent or the mere severity of the illness present highly sensitive areas that are not overcome easily.

What can be done? Several recommendations can be given to improve the situation and to allow for better and safer research activities in intensive care units:
- Intensive care units should be an integral part of larger research-oriented clinical institutions. Intensive care medicine as a separate entity does not seem to represent a meaningful solution.
- The medical staff should be exchanged within the rotational schedule and allow research assignments. Appropriate funds need to be allocated.

- Laboratory space in the immediate vicinity of the unit should be supplied. This would enable basic scientists to be harmonically included. At the same time the need for continued availability of the intensive care physician would be possible.
- The nursing staff should be actively involved in the bedside-oriented research projects where-ever possible. Consequently, inclusion in the authorship becomes possible.
- Close contact and exchange with the ethics committee or local IRB, possibly with regular ethics discussions and instructions will solve many problems and pave the way towards the desired partnership and mutual understanding of the significance and importance of research in intensive care medicine.

The public and the medical and the scientific communities are reminded of the particularly difficult situation of clinical research in intensive care medicine in the field of pulmonary embolism.

The Society for Cooperation in Medical Sciences, initiator and organizer of the Gargellen Conferences for many years, traditionally aware of the need for cooperation between basic scientists and clinical researchers, deemed it necessary to assemble an international group of experts, both basic scientists and clinicians, in an attempt to define the current status of our knowledge in the field of pulmonary embolism and hemostaseology. My long-time coworker PD Dr. Annette Geibel has undertaken the difficult task of organization and assembly of the rather heterogeneous group of clinicians and basic scientists. Many of our residents and students have helped with great engagement. Boehringer Ingelheim Pharmaceutics, in particular Dr. Heusel and his coworkers, together with Dr. H.-H. Heinrich from Bayer AG have given us generous financial and logistic support. The publication was expertly and efficiently done by Springer – Dr. D. Steinkopff Verlag Darmstadt. We thank Sabine Ibkendanz for continued help and understanding. My sincere thanks go to the many people who have helped and contributed to the success of this fruitful symposium and the informative and stimulating book.

Freiburg im Breisgau   Prof. Dr. med. Dr. h.c. F. J. G. H. Hansjörg Just

Contents

Foreword and Introduction V

Thrombophilia and thrombogenesis

The molecular mechanisms of inherited thrombophilia
März, W., M. Nauck, H. Wieland 1

Hypercoagulative syndrome: Molecular markers for the identification of
cardiovascular patients at risk
Hoffmeister, H. M., W. Heller, L. Seipel 21

Clinical implications of the new understanding of thrombophilia
Moll, S., D. Gulba 29

The clinical syndrome of acute pulmonary embolism

Mechanisms of ventilation-perfusion mismatch and hemodynamic alterations
in acute and chronic pulmonary embolism
Giuntini, C., A. Santolicandro, R. Prediletto, P. Paoletti, B. Formichi, E. Fornai,
E. Begliomini, R. Puntoni, A. Perissinotto, A. Giannela Neto 43

Clinical course and prognosis of acute pulmonary embolism
Konstantinides S., A. Geibel, W. Kasper 51

Clinical implications of a patent foramen ovale in patients with massive
pulmonary embolism
Geibel, A., S. Konstantinides, W. Kasper 59

The value of echocardiography in the diagnostic work-up of patients with
suspected acute pulmonary embolism
Kasper, W., S. Konstantinides, A. Geibel 67

Scintigraphy-ventilation/perfusion scanning and imaging of the embolus
Stein, P. D. 73

MR-angiography in the diagnosis of pulmonary embolism
Steiner, P., T. H. Hany, G. McKinnon, F. Follath, J. F. Debatin 83

Anticoagulation and fibrinolysis

Anticoagulation

Mechanism of blood coagulation. Newer aspects of anticoagulant and
antithrombotic therapy
Jeske, W., D. A. Hoppenstaedt, R. Pifarre, J. M. Walenga, J. Fareed   95

Low molecular weight heparins – Pharmacological principles and
indications in clinical practice
Harenberg, J.   123

Heparin-induced thrombocytopenia
Cicco, N. A., G. Gerken, M. Frey, H. Just   131

New developments in the thrombolytic therapy of venous thrombosis
Seifried, E., W. Weichert   143

The risk of recurrent venous thromboembolic disease –
implications for treatment
Eichinger, S., P. A. Kyrle, I. Pabinger, K. Lechner   155

A randomized trial of the effect of low molecular weight heparin vs. warfarin
on mortality in the long-term treatment of proximal vein thrombosis
Hull, R. D., G. F. Pineo, R. F. Brant   161

Fibrinolysis

Thrombolytic therapy in pulmonary embolism. Which patients should be
treated, which regimen should be used?
Meyer, G., H. Sors   175

Thrombolytic treatment of pulmonary embolism: Life-saving option or
unacceptable risk?
Konstantinides, S., A. Geibel, W. Kasper   183

Surgical treatment of acute pulmonary embolism
Schlensak, C., T. Doenst, F. Beyersdorf   193

The molecular mechanisms of inherited thrombophilia

W. März, M. Nauck, H. Wieland

Summary Venous thromboembolism is a common acute cardiovascular disease. Thrombotic events develop as the result of multiple interactions between circumstantial and inborn risk factors shifting the delicate balance between pro- and anticoagulant processes towards coagulation. The most important circumstantial risk factors are age, tissue damage, oral contraception, pregnancy, obesity, and sedentary life style. Inborn factors predisposing to thrombosis are present in the majority of patients. These include three groups of defects affecting components of the anticoagulant pathways of blood coagulation, namely antithrombin III, protein C, and protein S. Together these defects are found in 15–20 % of families with thrombophilia. They are extremely heterogeneous at the molecular level which largely precludes their diagnosis by current molecular biology techniques. The relatively rare defects of antithrombin III, protein C, and protein S can be distinguished from two common genetic polymorphisms of procoagulant molecules, factor V-Leiden, the most frequent cause of resistance to activated protein C, and the prothrombin 20210 A allele. Together, these anomalies are detected in almost two thirds of the thrombophilia families. The identification of factor FV-Leiden and prothrombin 20210 A has afforded the scrutinization of interactions between multiple components of genomic matrix and circumstantial factors. These studies indicate that many symptomatic individuals are endowed with more than one genetic and/or environmental risk factor. Thrombophilia thus represents an oligogenetic rather than a monogenetic phenotype, the expression of which is amplified by circumstantial risk factors. As a consequence of the "multiple hit" concept, the laboratory screening of thrombosis patients needs to include all of the known genetic risk factors even if the "clinical" situation seemingly provides sufficient "explanation" for a thrombotic event.

Key words Venous thromboembolism – inherited thrombophilia – protein C, protein S, antithrombin III factor FV-Leiden – Prothrombin 20210A

Venous thromboembolism:
The second most common acute cardiovascular disease

The incidence rate of venous thromboembolism ranges between 1 and 5 per 1000 individuals and year. Following acute myocardial infarction, venous thromboembolism is thus the second most common acute cardiovascular disease, still more frequent than stroke [31] (cf. Fig. 1).

There is little overlap between the classical risk factors for coronary heart and cerebrovascular disease and the risk factors for venous thromboembolism. As already recognized by Virchow, thrombosis occurs when three factors coincide: damage to the vessel wall, decrease in blood flow, and hypercoagulability, i.e., a shift of the balance between pro- and anticoagulant factors towards clot formation. Whereas the first two components of Virchow's triad are mostly due to acquired conditions, hypercoagulability can result from both genetic and acquired (circumstantial) factors.

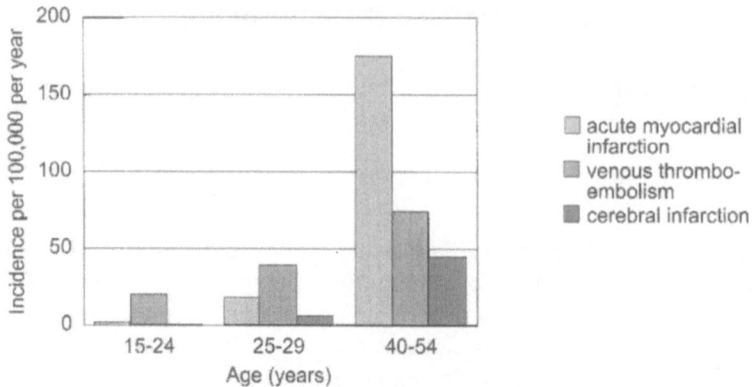

Fig. 1. Incidence rates of acute myocardial infarction, cerebral infarction, and venous thromboembolism in the Netherlands according to hospital discharge diagnoses in 1994 (data adopted from reference 31). Note that the incidence of thrombosis markedly multiplies with age, reflecting that age probably represents one of the strongest circumstantial risk factors for thrombosis.

Inherited factors predisposing to thrombosis are identified in as many as 60 percent of consecutive patients presenting with venous thrombosis and one third of these patients has at least one symptomatic relative. At the time being, the impact of genetics is, thus, more obvious in venous thromboembolism than in atherosclerosis and myocardial infarction.

For almost two decades, inherited antithrombin III (ATIII) deficiency was the only known genetic cause of thrombophilia [9]. At the beginning of the eighties, deficiencies of protein C (PC) and protein S (PS) have been linked to venous thromboembolism [7, 12]. Together, however, these disorders were present in only a few patients with thrombophilia. The situation substantially improved in 1993 when Dahlbäck et al. [8] described resistance to activated PC (APC), caused by a single amino acid substitution in coagulation factor V [5] as a common thrombogenic disorder. Very recently, evidence has accumulated that genetic and non-genetic risk factors act in concert to precipitate thromboembolic events. This suggests that preventive measures aiming at the modification or avoidance of circumstantial risk factors (oral contraceptives, sedentary life-style) will hold promise in the prevention of thromboembolism even in genetically susceptible individuals.

To facilitate the understanding of the molecular mechanisms producing inherited thromboembolism, we will briefly review the physiology of blood coagulation and the anticoagulant system, thereby placing particular emphasis on the structure and function of ATIII, PC and PS, and blood coagulation factor V (FV).

A glance at the blood coagulation system

Upon injury of the vessel wall, hemostasis is initiated by the adhesion and aggregation of *platelets*. Simultaneously, the *blood coagulation cascade* is activated, producing a fibrin network which ultimately stabilizes the platelet thrombus. *Endothelial cells* largely contribute to the control of the blood coagulation cascade. To uphold the patency of intact vessels, the coagulation cascade is restrained by anticoagulant molecules on the surface of the endothelial cells. The luminal membrane of endothelial cells contains thrombo-modulin and glycosaminoglycans which participate as cofactors in the activation of PC and ATIII. Beyond this, the endothelium produces a number of other pro- (tissue factor, von Willebrand factor, plasminogen activator inhibitor-1, platelet-activating factor) and anticoagulant substances (prostacyclin, nitric oxide, tissue factor inhibitor, tissue plasminogen activator, and PS).

The blood coagulation cascade includes two multimolecular complexes of similar organization. The first one, "tenase", proteolytically converts FX to FXa; the second one, "prothrombinase", converts membrane-bound prothrombin to thrombin. Both of these two complexes require calcium and phospholipid surfaces, the latter being provided by the membranes of activated platelets and endothelial cells. The proteolytically active components of the two complexes, the serine proteases FIXa and FXa, require the presence of cofactors. Coagulation factors VIII and V are such cofactors. They are activated by proteolytic cleavage by thrombin or FXa. The active forms of coagulation factors VIII and V (FVIIIa and FVa) bind to negatively charged phospholipids and thus function as receptor sites for the serine proteases FIXa and FXa, respectively. FVIIIa and FVa each accounts for at least a 1000-fold increase of the activity of the tenase and the prothrombinase complex, respectively.

Calcium is required for the co-ordinated assembly of FIXa and FXa on the negatively charged phospholipid surfaces. FIXa and FXa interact with calcium by γ-carboxyglutamic acid residues. These γ-carboxyglutamic acid residues are produced by post-translational carboxylation of glutamic acid located within the so-called Gla domains of FIX and FX. The carboxylation of glutamic acid residues crucially depends on the presence of vitamin K. Gla domains are not only found in FIX and FX, but also in prothrombin, FVII, and in the anticoagulant factors PC and PS. The anticoagulant effects of vitamin K antagonists like warfarin (Wisconsin Alumni Research Foundation) are due to inhibition of γ-carboxylation. In the presence of warfarin, vitamin K-dependent factors are released into the circulation which are deficient in γ-carboxyglutamic acid residues. This markedly reduces their ability to interact with membranes and, thus, down-regulates the entire coagulation cascade (Fig. 2).

The blood coagulation cascade may be initiated by two alternative pathways, conventionally designated the intrinsic and the extrinsic pathway, respectively. Both pathways result in the production of prothrombin from thrombin. The *intrinsic pathway* starts upon exposure of high-molecular weight kininogen, FXII or prekallikrein (contact factors) to negatively charged surfaces (connective tissue and collagen *in vivo*, glass or kaolin *in vitro*), resulting in the activation of FXII. The activation of FXII is followed by sequential activation of FXI, FIX, and FX. Patients with deficiency of FXII, prekallikrein, and high molecular weight kininogen rarely present with bleeding symptoms; patients with FXI deficiency usually have mild bleeding tendency. This suggests that, *in vivo*, the most important trigger for the blood coagulation cascade comes from the extrinsic pathway.

The *extrinsic pathway* is initiated by injuries of the endothelium and the exposure of subendothelial tissue to the blood stream. Thus, tissue factor (TF, an integral membrane glycoprotein in the adventitia) comes into contact with the FVII. In the presence of calcium, FVII binds to the extracellular domain of TF and is activated to FVIIa. The complex of TF and FVIIa then activates both FIX and FX. Under physiological conditions FIX is a better substrate for the TF/FVIIa complex than FX. This directly couples the intrinsic to the extrinsic pathway and explains why bleeding tendency is much more severe in FIX deficiency than in deficiencies of other factors of the extrinsic pathway. With the formation of FXa, the intrinsic and the extrinsic pathway converge. Together with FVa,

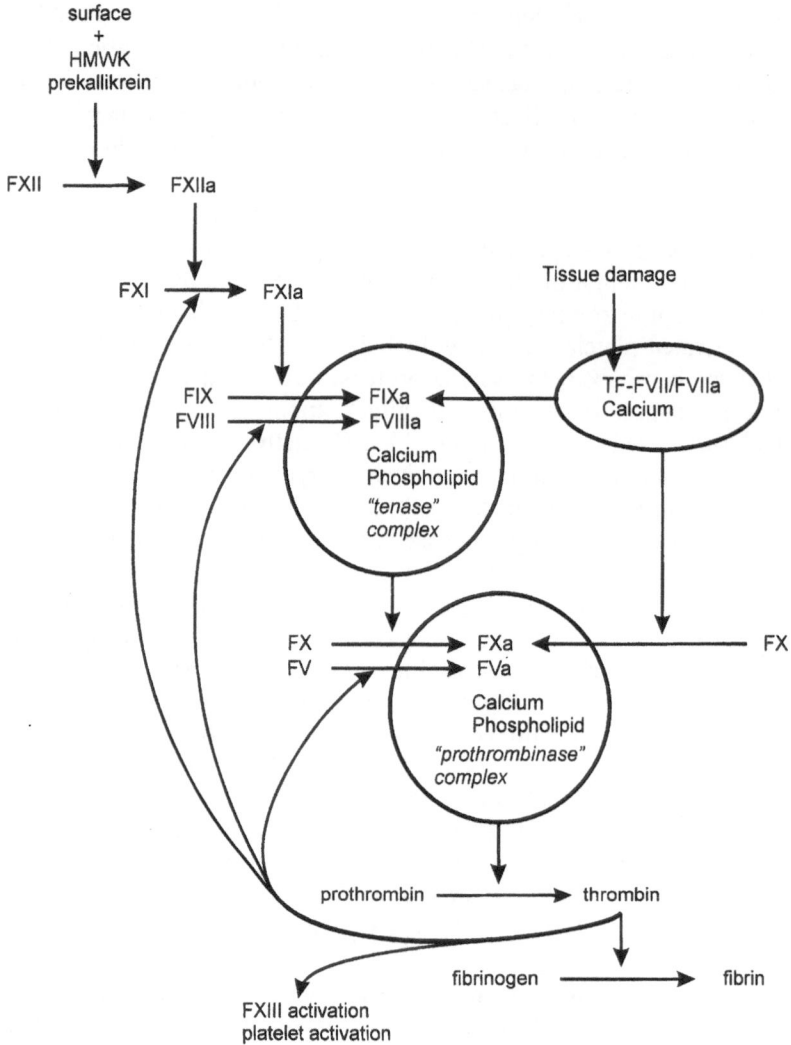

Fig. 2. The coagulation cascade. Under physiological conditions, the most important trigger for the blood coagulation cascade comes from the extrinsic pathway which is started by tissue damage and exposure of tissue factor (TF) to FVII/VIIa. The intrinsic pathway is initiated by exposure of the contact factors (high molecular weight kininogen, FXII, and prekallikrein) to negatively charged surfaces. The complex of FVIIa and tissue factor not only activates FX but also FIX. This connects the extrinsic to the intrinsic pathway. Once small amounts of thrombin are generated, the intrinsic pathway is activated via positive feedback. Thus, the intrinsic pathway is important to amplify rather than to start fibrin formation.

calcium, and phospholipids, FXa builds up the "prothrombinase" complex which produces thrombin from prothrombin. By limited proteolysis, thrombin, in turn, converts soluble fibrinogen into insoluble fibrin. Thrombin has yet other important functions. It catalyses the activation of FXIII to become FXIIIa, a transglutaminase which covalently cross-links fibrin monomers, and, in positive feedback loops, amplifies its own generation by activating FIX, FVIII, and FV.

Thrombophilia – failure to restrain coagulation

A battery of regulatory molecules is present in the plasma and on the surface of endothelial cells to harness the explosive activation of the blood coagulation cascade. These factors ensure that coagulation remains confined to the site of vessel injury rather than becoming generalized. Key components of the anticoagulant system are ATIII, PC, and PS. Deficiencies of these proteins are major inborn risk factors of thromboembolism.

Genetic defects of anticoagulant regulators causing thrombophilia

Together, deficiencies of ATIII, PC, and PS are encountered in approximately 15 percent of the families with inherited thrombophilia. They have in common that they are rare in the general population and extremely heterogeneous at the nucleic acid level, almost completely precluding their diagnosis by current molecular biology techniques.

Two types of deficiencies of ATIII, PC, and PS can be distinguished. Type I deficiencies are characterized by parallel reductions of the biochemical activity and the antigen concentration which means that the expression of the respective factor is reduced. In type II deficiencies, in contrast, antigen concentrations are normal, but biochemical activities are reduced.

Deficiency of antithrombin III

The enzymes of the coagulation cascade are serine proteases. Their inhibitors were hence named serpins (serine protease inhibitors). The most important serpin is ATIII, a single chain glycoprotein of 432 amino acids. ATIII is the main inhibitor of thrombin, but also inhibits the FVIIa-TF complex, FXa, FIXa, FXIa, FXIIa, kallikrein, and plasmin. ATIII inhibits the target proteinase by serving as a pseudo-substrate, forming a one-to-one complex with the proteinase. The formation of this complex is accompanied by cleavage of the peptide bond between Arg^{393} and Ser^{394}. The inhibitory activity of ATIII is significantly enhanced by binding to heparin and heparan sulfate proteoglycans on the surface of endothelial cells. In the plasma, isoforms of ATIII are found which vary by the degree of glycosylation in the vicinity of the heparin binding domain. Interestingly, the isoform lacking an oligosaccharide side chain binds to heparin with a tenfold higher affinity.

Homozygous ATIII deficiency is considered incompatible with life, except for mutations affecting the heparin binding site. Heterozygosity for ATIII deficiency increases the risk of venous thromboembolism fivefold in population based case-control studies and ten- to twentyfold, respectively, in families with thrombophilia. Heterozygous ATIII deficient individuals present with thrombosis at an early age, but rarely in the first decade. By the age of 35 years, two third of ATIII deficient patients experienced venous thromboembolism. Thus, the penetrance of ATIII deficiency is higher than that of PC or PS deficiency. The first event is often precipitated by a circumstantial manifestation factor. For instance, forty percent of pregnancies in ATIII deficient gravidae are complicated by thrombosis.

More than 80 mutations leading to *type I deficiency of ATIII* have been described [2, 22]. These are major gene rearrangements, splice site mutations, missense mutations of the signal peptide (preventing membrane transport or removal of the signal peptide), substitutions of cysteine residues crucial to protein folding, nonsense mutations introducing premature stop codons, and in frame or frameshift insertions and deletions.

Three groups of *type II deficiencies* exist. These are *active site mutations* (substitutions of the active site residues Arg[393] and Ser[394] and mutations generating new cleavage sites for the target protease), *defects of the heparin binding domain* (replacement of arginine residues involved in heparin binding, mutations changing the conformation of the heparin binding domain, one interesting missense mutation, Ile[7] → Asn, producing a new glycosylation site), and more than ten *pleiotropic mutations* which affect both heparin binding and the active site, and, in addition, slightly lower antigen concentrations. In type II ATIII deficiency, the determination of the underlying molecular defect is clinically relevant: heterozygotes for mutations of the heparin binding domain are less prone to thromboembolism than individuals with other defects. Many patients with heparin binding-defective ATIII variants presenting with severe arterial or venous thrombosis have been shown to be homozygotes rather than heterozygotes.

Protein C

PC, a serine protease zymogen, is mainly synthesised in the liver (Fig. 3). The precursor form consists of 461 amino acids, including an 18 amino acids signal peptide (targeting PC for secretion) and a pro-peptide of 24 residues which serves the recognition by γ-carboxylase. Circulating PC consists of 419 amino acids. In the Golgi apparatus, PC is cleaved between Arg[157] and Thr[158], the two chains remaining linked by a disulphide bridge. Prior to secretion the light chain is further truncated by proteolytically removing Arg[157] and Lys[156] to yield mature PC consisting of two chains of 262 and 155 amino acids, respectively.

The gla domain of PC (residues 1–37) is followed by a so-called aromatic stack (residues 38–45), two modules with homology to the epidermal growth factor (EGF) (amino acids 46–91 and 92–136, respectively) and the serine protease domain which encompasses residues 139 through 419. PC is activated on the surface of endothelial cells by thrombin bound to thrombomodulin. Thrombin cleaves the bond between Arg[169] and Leu[170] of PC, thereby releasing an activation peptide from the heavy chain. His[211], Asp[257], and Ser[360] constitute the catalytic triad of activated PC (APC). The only known substrates of APC are membrane bound FVa and FVIIIa. Cleavage of FVa occurs at the arginine residues 506, 306, and 679; cleavage of FVIIIa at arginines 562, 336, and 740. APC requires phospholipids, calcium, and PS as cofactors; inactivation of FVIIIa may in addition depend on intact FV as a cofactor. Once formed, APC is only slowly inhibited by PC inhibitor (PCI), α_1-antitrypsin, and α_2-macroglobulin.

The endothelial PC receptor (EPCR) is a recently identified regulatory component of the PC anticoagulant pathway [10]. It is a transmembrane protein belonging to the major histocompatibility class 1 family of molecules. One function of EPCR is to amplify the conversion of PC to APC by thrombin and thrombomodulin; the second one is to inhibit the anticoagulant activity of APC by shifting the specificity of APC away from FVa and FVIIIa, possibly towards another yet unknown substrate. In this respect, EPCR acts similar to thrombomodulin which directs specificity of thrombin from fibrinogen to PC. EPCR is mainly expressed on large vessels and is virtually absent in the capillaries. This may provide sufficient amounts of APC in the arterial branch of the vessel system in heterozygous PC deficiency, and EPCR deficiency would be anticipated to promote arterial rather than venous thrombosis.

The PC system is probably the most important regulator of blood coagulation (Fig. 4). It is activated when thrombin is generated at intact endothelium. Thrombin instantly binds to thrombomodulin where it looses its procoagulant properties and adopts the ability to activate PC. Activated PC inhibits blood coagulation by limited proteolysis of

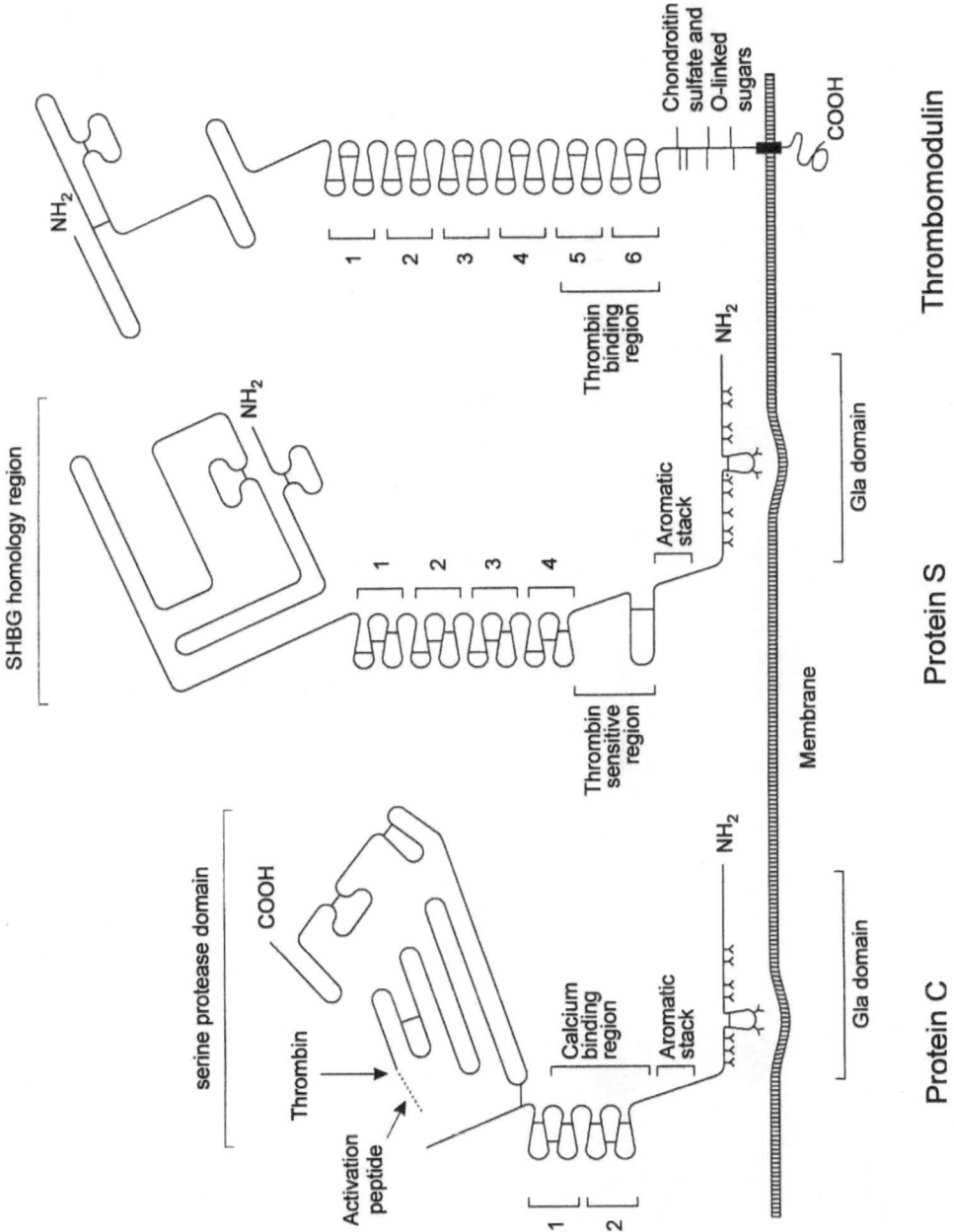

Fig. 3. The domain structures of protein C, protein S, and thrombomodulin. Arabic numbers refers to growth factor domains; Ys indicate γ-carboxyglutamic acid residues of the gla domains. Specific domains of each protein are labeled. For further explanation see text.

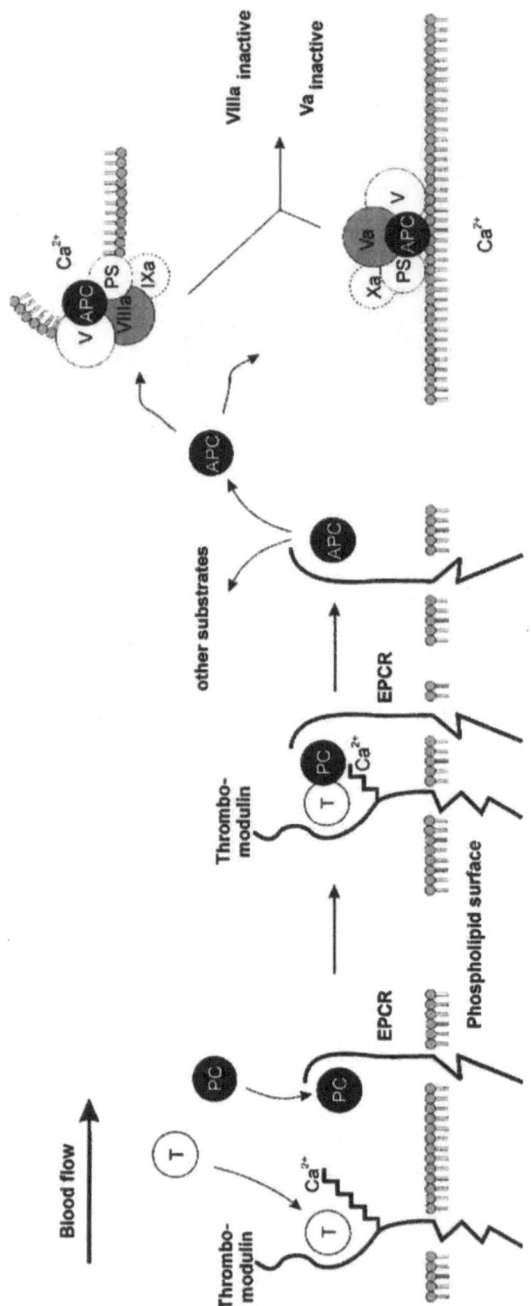

Fig. 4. The protein C anticoagulant pathway. Upon binding to thromboglobulins thrombin loses its procoagulant activity and adopts the ability to activate PC. Activated PC inhibits blood coagulation by limited proteolysis of FVa and FVIIIa. This results in down regulation of the "tenase" and "prothrombinase" complexes and effective inhibition of the coagulation cascade. The endothelial PC receptor (EPCR) on the one hand amplifies the conversion of PC to APC; on the other hand it may inhibit the anticoagulant activity of APC by shifting the specificity of APC away from FVa and FVIIIa towards other yet unknown substrates.

Table 1. Genetic factors producing hypercoagulable states; DVT = Deep vein thrombosis

Disorder	Inheritance	Number of mutations	Prevalence in healthy individuals	Prevalence consecutive patients with DVT	Prevalence in families with thrombophilia
A. Genetic defects					
ATIII deficiency	dominant	> 79	0.2	1	4
PC deficiency	dominant	> 160	0.3	3	6
PS deficiency	dominant	> 69	1.5	1.5	6
Thrombomodulin defects	dominant	?	rare	3	?
Plasminogen deficiency	dominant	?	rare	1	?
Dysfibrinogenemia	dominant	> 15	rare	1	?
Cystathionine β synthase deficiency	dominant	?	rare	?	?
B. Allelic polymorphisms					
Factor V-Leiden	dominant	1	5.0	20	50
Prothrombin $G^{20210} \rightarrow A$	dominant	1	1.5	6	18

FVa and FVIIIa. This results in down regulation of the "tenase" and "prothrombinase" complexes and effective inhibition of the coagulation cascade. The enormous physiological importance of the PC anticoagulant system is underlined by the severe thromboembolic tendency observed in newborns homozygous for PC deficiencies (Table 1).

Inherited deficiency of PC is one of the major genetic causes of familial thrombophilia. Homozygous PC deficiency leads to extensive thrombosis with purpura fulminans shortly after birth. Heterozygous PC deficiency increases the risk of thrombosis in the middle-age by approximately sevenfold in population based case-control studies and approximately tenfold in families with thrombophilia. Until the age of 45 years, approximately 50 percent of the PC deficient individuals have suffered from thrombosis, suggesting an autosomal dominant mode of inheritance. In some families, however, only homozygous or compound heterozygous carriers of PC defects develop thromboses. This lead to the idea that recessive forms of PC deficiency exist. The molecular mechanisms underlying such recessive mode of inheritance are not clear, in particular since the same gene mutations were encountered in families with both modes of transmission.

During the initiation of treatment with vitamin K antagonists, individuals with PC deficiency are at an increased risk of skin necrosis. This is due to the fact that the half life of PC [6 h] is shorter than that of the vitamin K dependent coagulation factors prothrombin [60 h], FIX [25 h], and FX [30 h] which results in a temporal overweight of procoagulant factors in the plasma.

More than 160 mutations have been identified in the PC gene [27, 28]. *Type I deficiencies of PC* were demonstrated to result from frameshift-creating insertions and deletions, from splice-site and promoter mutations, from termination codon mutations and from missense mutations of the signal peptide, the EGF domain, and the catalytic domain. It is not clear why many mutations in the EGF domain and the catalytic domain are associated with type I rather than type II deficiency; most likely these mutants fail to proceed to the cell surface due to improper folding. The mutations causing *type II deficiency of PC* are all missense mutations. They have been found in the propeptide, the gla domain, the activation domain (activation resistant variants), and in the catalytic domain (low proteolytic activity). Three mutations of the pro-peptide and gla domain region create a cysteine residue. This covalently links PC to α_1-microglobulin to yield a high molecular weight non-functional complex circulating in the plasma.

Protein S

PS is a single chain glycoprotein of 75 kD which is expressed in the liver, endothelial cells, in Leydig cells of the testis, in megakaryocytes, and in the central nervous system (Fig. 3). PS is synthesized as a 676 amino acid long precursor protein, containing a signal peptide (residues – 41 through – 18) and a pro-peptide (residues – 17 to – 1) mediating the binding of the vitamin K dependent γ-carboxylases.

Mature PS consists of 635 amino acids. Similar to PC, PS has a gla domain and an aromatic stack. These are followed by a thrombin-sensitive region which is cleaved by thrombin upon inactivation of PS. Binding of PC to PS is mediated by the adjacent four epidermal growth factor domains and by parts of the thrombin-sensitive region. Approximately two thirds of PS circulates in the plasma as a non-covalent heterodimer with the complement 4b-binding protein (C4b-BP), whereas one third of PS is present as a free monomer. Interaction of PS with C4b-BP is mediated by the carboxyterminus of the molecule which is structurally homologous to sex-hormone-binding globulin (SHBG), but does not exhibit steroid hormone binding activity in vivo.

PS has been attributed several functions. It enhances the binding of APC to phospholipids and thus facilitates the cleavage of FVa and FVIIIa at arginine residues 306 and 336, respectively (the second phase of the inactivation process). This function of PS is lost upon thrombin cleavage, suggesting that the thrombin-sensitive region interacts with APC on the phospholipid surface. There is evidence that PS is capable of directly inhibiting thrombin formation by binding to components of the prothrombinase complex (FVa and FXa) and that it co-operates with intact FV (but not FVa) and APC in the inactivation of FVIIIa. In addition, interaction of PS with FVIII in the presence of phospholipids precludes FX activation. Only the free, but not the complexed form of PS is able to act as a cofactor for APC. The role of the PS-C4b-BP complex has not definitely been elucidated so far. It has, however, been speculated that PS directs C4b to negatively charged phospholipid layers to facilitate local down regulation of the complement system.

In families with thrombophilia, deficiency of PS has been found associated with a tenfold risk of thrombosis. In a large case-control study PS deficiency was not found to be a significant risk factor of thrombosis [20], but reduced concentrations of "tree" PS appear to be a risk factor of thrombosis in population-based studies. The first thromboembolic episodes often develop after 50 years of age. Warfarin-induced skin necrosis does occur in PS deficient patients.

Mutations in the PS gene have been found in only 50 percent or less of individuals presenting with PS deficiency. Most PS deficiencies known so far are type I deficiencies. This may be due to the fact that reliable methods to determine the activity of PS have not generally been available. Approximately half of the type I deficiencies are missense mutations of conserved amino acids, the remaining being randomly distributed throughout the coding sequence of the gene. The few known type II deficiencies are due to missense mutations of the pro-peptide and of the EGF homologous region. A particular form of PS deficiency characterized by selective absence of free PS has been referred to as type III deficiency. It appears as if type III deficiency represents a phenotypic variant rather than to represent a distinct genetic entity [41].

Miscellaneous defects

Dysfibrinogenemia is a rare disorder commonly identified by prolonged reptilase time and thrombin time. At least 15 mutations in the genes for the α, β, and γ chain of fibrinogen, respectively, have been identified which result in the phenotype of dysfibrinogene-mia [15]. The strength of the relationship between dysfibrinogenemia and thrombosis is still controversial. Among the individuals with dysfibrinogenemia, only one in four presents with thombosis, one in four presents with haemorrhagic diathesis, and the remaining are asymptomatic.

Thrombomodulin (TM) (Fig. 3) is an integral membrane protein expressed on endothelial cells. It contains a lectin-like module, six EGF-like modules, a serine and threonine-rich region with attached carbohydrate sidechains, a transmembrane region, and a short cytoplasmic tail. The binding of thrombin is mediated by the fifth and the sixth EGF homologous domain. Targeted disruption of the mouse TM gene causes a lethal phenotype [16]. The recent finding that mutations in functionally important elements of the TM promoter are over-represented in survivors of myocardial infarction raises the possibility that there is an association between *genetic variation at the thrombomodulin locus* and inherited thrombophilia as well [18]. Consistently, Ohlin et al. [25] were able to identify eight patients heterozygous for thombomodulin mutations distributed through-out the TM gene. In addition, they demonstrated that the respective mutation co-segregated with thromboembolic disease in four of the families studied.

Other genetically determined conditions like deficiencies of FXII, heparin cofactor II, and of β_2-glycoprotein (apolipoprotein H), have been implicated in the development of venous thrombosis. These conditions are either very rare or their association to thrombo-embolism has not unequivocally been established so far. Disorders of the fibrinolytic system have also been suggested to contribute to the development of thrombosis. There is, however, no firm evidence that deficiencies of plasminogen, tissue-type plasminogen activator (tPA), urokinase-type plasminogen activator (tPA) or increased concentrations of plasminogen activator inhibitor-1 (PAI-1) or plasminogen activator inhibitor-2 (PAI-2) significantly relate to the pathogenesis of thrombosis.

Genetic polymorphisms causing thrombophilia

Associations between the risk of thrombosis and genetic polymorphisms have been established only very recently. Among these polymorphisms are FV (Arg^{506} → Gln), the most frequent cause of resistance to activated PC (APC), and the prothrombin 20210A allele. Both mutations occur at a high frequency in the general population. They are found in approximately two third of thrombophilia families, and interestingly, both involve pro-coagulant rather than anticoagulant factors.

Resistance to activated protein C – a common risk factor of venous thromboembolism

FV and FVIII are high molecular weight glycoproteins with very similar structures and functional properties (Fig. 5). Both FV and FVIII consist of three type A modules and two type C modules which share 40 percent homology between the two factors. The second and the third A modules of FV and FVIII are separated by connecting B domains of 836 and 980 residues, respectively. Unlike the A and C domains, the B domain does not share any homology between the factors with the exception that they have a high content of serine and threonine residues with many potential N-glycosylation sites. The concentra-tion of FV in the circulation is approximately 100-fold higher than that of FVIII. FVIII circulates bound to another plasma protein, the von Willebrand factor (vWF).

FV and FVIII are activated by thrombin or FXa which cleave at least three peptide bonds in either of these molecules. Activation converts FV and FVIII to a heterodimer and heterotrimer, respectively, the subunits of which are held together by divalent cations. FVa and FVIIIa bind to negatively charged phospholipids and serve as enzymatically inactive cofactors of the "prothrombinase" complex and the "tenase" complex, respectively. Inactivation of FVIIIa and FVa is accomplished by APC. APC is highly specific for the membrane-bound activated forms of FV and FVIII, inactive FVIII and FV are only poor substrates. Upon inactivation, three peptide bonds are cleaved in the heavy chains of FVIIIa (Arg^{336}–Met^{337}, Arg^{565}–Gly^{563}, and Arg^{740}–Ser^{741}) and FVa. The inactivation of FVa is biphasic. Arg^{506}–Gly^{507} is cleaved first. This cleavage does not affect cofactor activity itself, but facilitates inactivation by cleavage at positions Arg^{306} (two third reduction in cofactor activity) and Arg^{679} (one third loss in cofactor activity) (Fig. 5).

Dahlbäck and colleges [8] were the first to describe that plasma from thrombosis patients poorly responded to the anticoagulant activity of APC. Shortly thereafter, Bertina et al. [5] identified the molecular mechanism underlying APC resistance as a single point mutation in the FV gene, changing arginine to glutamine at position 506, one of the three sites of FVa cleaved by APC. The mutant FV (also denoted as FV-Leiden) is normally

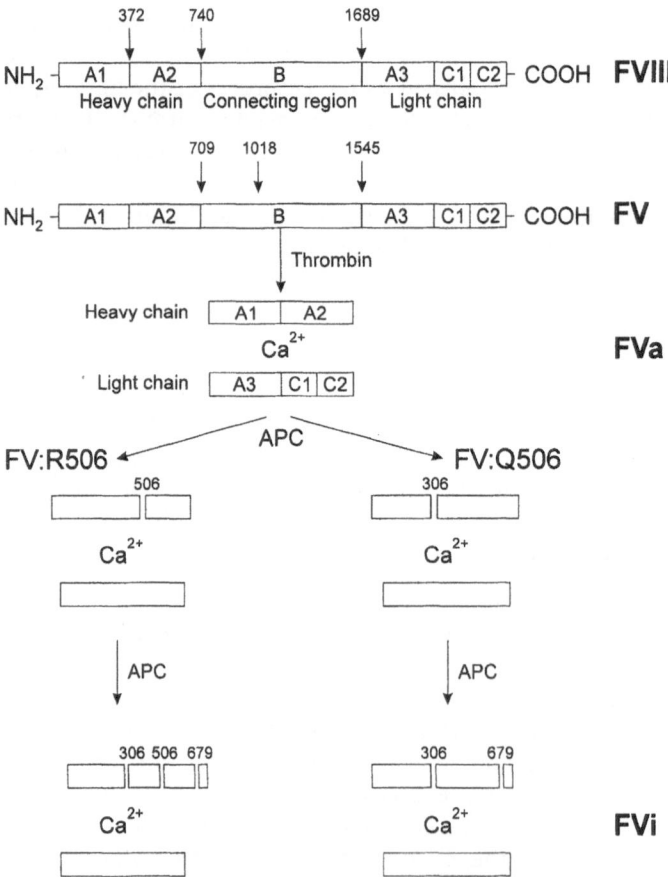

Fig. 5. The domain structures of FV and FVIII and the activation and inactivation of FV. Thrombin cleavage sites are indicated by solid arrows. Both factors VIII and V consist of three homologous A modules, one B module, and two homologous C modules. Upon activation, both factors are cleaved by thrombin at the sites indicated by solid arrows. During inactivation of FVa, activated protein C first cleaves at Arg^{506}. This facilitates subsequent cleavage at arginine residues 306 and 679. Mutated FVa ($Arg^{506} \rightarrow$ Gln) is not cleaved at position 506, resulting in a significantly reduced rate of FVa degradation.

activated by thrombin or FXa, but the rate at which it is inactivated by APC is 10- to 20-fold lower than normal.

APC resistance makes up the most frequent genetic risk factor of thrombosis known to date. In healthy Caucasians, the prevalence of FV-Leiden is between 2 and 10 percent. The mutation is not found in other ethnic groups such as in Japanese, Chinese, and Africans. In Germany, we and others detected heterozygosity for FV-Leiden in approximately 5 percent of healthy individuals [17,24]. This means that at least 4 million or more people with APC resistance live in Germany. In clinical studies, using different selection criteria, resistance to APC was found in 20 percent of all consecutive cases with venous thromboembolism and in 50 percent among selected patients with thrombophilia. This is far more frequent than the sum of inherited deficiencies of ATIII, PC, and PS and indicates that heterozygotes have a 5- to 10-fold increased risk of thrombosis. Homozygous carriers of the mutant are thought to have a 50- to 100-fold risk. The thrombotic risk in individuals with APC resistance may be further increased by other genetic defects such as ATIII, PC or PS deficiency (see below) and by exposure to circumstantial risk factors such as oral contraceptives, pregnancy, immobilization, and surgery.

The most common clinical manifestations of FV-Leiden are venous thrombosis and pulmonary embolism. Some case reports suggested that FV-Leiden, in particular in the homozygous state, increased the risk of arterial thrombosis as well. In Austrian patients with stroke the prevalence of FV-Leiden was increased tenfold compared to healthy controls [14]. We found an approximately twofold higher prevalence of FV-Leiden in patients with coronary heart disease regardless of whether or not they had a history of previous myocardial infarction [24]. Other studies did not confirm these results [29]. Very recently, however, Rosendaal et al. [33] provided evidence for an association between FV-Leiden and myocardial infarction in young women, the effect being most obvious in current smokers. It thus remains unresolved at present to what extent FV-Leiden predisposes to atherosclerosis and/or arterial thrombosis.

Studies validated by FV gene analysis revealed that approximately 10 percent of those individuals exhibiting APC resistance are FV-Leiden negative. This raised the question whether there are genetic causes of APC resistance other than FV-Leiden. Homozygosity for a specific FV gene haplotype (HR2) defined by six polymorphisms was linked to low APC ratios in the absence of FV-Leiden [3], and two mutations altering the codon for Arg^{306} of FVa were identified. For unknown reasons, only one of these two mutations, FV-Cambridge ($Arg^{306} \rightarrow$ Thr) [39], but not FV-Hong Kong ($Arg^{306} \rightarrow$ Gly) [6] resulted in resistance to APC.

The remaining cases with APC resistance, but normal FV genotype are currently considered "acquired" APC resistance. Recent data suggests that this form of APC resistance risk represents a risk factor for venous thrombosis and for cerebral ischemic as important as "classical" APC resistance due to FV-Leiden [30]. The factors causing impaired response to APC in the absence of the FV-Leiden mutation include lupus anticoagulants, high concentrations of the clotting factors VIII, V, IX, X, and of prothrombin, the use of oral contraceptives, and pregnancy. The most frequent among these conditions is obviously elevated FVIII, an acute phase reactant the concentration of which may be elevated up to 800 percent.

Interestingly, thrombosis patients heterozygous for FV-Leiden, but with an APC ratio typical for homozygosity have been observed. The reason for this apparent paradox is that these individuals were compound heterozygotes for FV-Leiden and a type I FV deficiency [13, 35].

Prothrombin 20210A – a polymorphism of the 3' untranslated region of the prothrombin gene

A G to A transition at position 20210 of the prothrombin gene was identified in five out of 28 individuals (18 percent) from families with unexplained thrombophilia, as compared with a frequency of one percent in the general population [26]. In a population-based case-control study, the 20210A allele increased the risk of venous thrombosis almost threefold, regardless of age and sex. The mutation affects the last nucleotide of the 3' untranslated region of the prothrombin gene before the poly A attachment site and may influence prothrombin production. Consistently, almost all individuals with the 20210A allele had prothrombin levels above 115 percent. Elevated prothrombin itself also was found to be a risk factor for venous thrombosis. The 20210A allele strongly interacts with other susceptibility alleles. In two families with both FV-Leiden and the 20210A allele, only those individuals carrying both defects were symptomatic [4].

Abnormal biochemical phenotypes associated with venous thromboembolism

A number of discrete to severe biochemical abnormalities has been linked to the risk of thromboembolism. These biochemical phenotypes may either be brought about by variation at the respective gene loci or relate to non-genetic, i.e. circumstantial factors. Circumstantial risk factors for venous thromboembolism are those relating to tissue damage (injury, immobilisation, surgery), oral contraception, pregnancy and puerperium, obesity, heart failure, varicosis, the antiphospholipid syndrome, and malignancy. Table 2 provides a synopsis of how these factors influence components of the anticoagulant system.

Factor VIII and prothrombin

Soon after the identification of FV-Leiden as being the most frequent cause of APC resistance, it became apparent that as much as one out of ten individuals revealing reduced sensitivity to APC had a normal FV genotype. We now know that many of those APC resistant individuals in whom FV-Leiden is not detected have FVIIIc levels elevated at 150 percent or more. Spiking experiments in normal patient plasma and venous occlusion tests demonstrated that elevation of the FVIIIc resulted in a reduced APC ratio, suggesting that high FVIIIc may largely explain the phenomenon of thrombosis-associ-

Table 2. Non-genetic factors affecting components of the anticoagulant system

Condition	ATIII	PC	PS
Liver cirrhosis	↓	↓	↓
Disseminated intravascular coagulation	↓	↓	↔
L-asparaginase therapy	↓	↓	↓
Bone marrow transplantation	↓	↓	↔
Treatment with vitamin K antagonists	↔	↓	↓
Vitamin K deficiency	↔	↓	↓
Oestrogen replacement	↔	↔	↓
Nephrotic syndrome	↓	↔	↔
Sepsis	↔	↔	↓

ated APC resistance in the absence of FVQ506 [21]. These observations warrant that the determination of FVIIIc be included into thrombophilia screening and future work will have to address the issue whether or not VIIIc represents itself an independent risk factor of thrombosis. The same may hold for prothrombin as recent work indicated that prothrombin concentrations above 115 percent increase the risk of thrombosis approximately twofold, regardless of nucleotide 20210 [26].

Homocysteine – a "new" risk factor for venous thromboembolism?

Along with mental retardation, ectopia lentis, and skeletal abnormalities, venous and arterial thromboembolism are characteristic features of homocystinuria, a very rare autosomal recessive disorder caused by cysthationine β-synthase deficiency. By itself, homozygous cysthationine β-synthase deficiency is too rare to account significantly for the general burden of venous thromboembolism. However, the striking clinical consequences of markedly elevated homocysteine concentrations gave birth to the proposal that moderate hyperhomocysteinemia represented a cardiovascular risk factor as well. Epidemiological evidence suggests that mild hyperhomocysteinemia is associated with increased risk of atherosclerosis and stroke. The relationship between hyperhomocysteinemia and thrombosis has been investigated in 10 studies involving a total of 1200 patients and 1200 controls. Eight of these studies demonstrated positive association with odd ratios that ranged from 2 to 13 [34].

There is substantial evidence that genetic factors contribute to hyperhomocysteinemia [40]. At present, however, the extent to what moderate hyperhomocysteinemia is determined by genetic or circumstantial factors has not been completely elucidated. A slight elevation of homocysteine occurs in heterozygous cysthationine β-synthase deficiency, but may also originate from renal dysfunction and diminished intake of folic acid, vitamin B6, and vitamin B12. Recently, high homocysteine concentrations have been attributed to thermolabile 5,10-methylenetetrahydrofolate reductase (MTHFR). Methylenetetrahydrofolate reductase catalyses the reduction of 5,10-methylenetetrahydrofolate to 5-methyltetrahydrofolate, the main form of circulating folate. 5-Methyltetrahydrofolate serves as a methyl group donor in the conversion of homocysteine to methionine. Frosst et al. [11] identified a common point mutation at nucleotide 677 of a MTHFR cDNA, converting an alanine to a valine residue. This mutation was shown to be correlated with reduced specific MTHFR activity and increased thermolability of the enzyme in lymphocyte extracts. Individuals homozygous for the mutation had significantly elevated plasma homocysteine concentrations [11]. The mutation has a prevalence of 5 to 15 percent in the general population and is thus more frequent than heterozygous cysthationine β-synthase deficiency (1 : 200). Consistent with the association between elevated homocysteine and the MTHFR genotype, evidence has been reported that homozygosity for the MTHFR nucleotide 677 mutation increases the risk of venous thrombosis almost threefold even after individuals with other hereditary causes of thrombophilia were excluded [1].

Thromboemolism is multigenic and multifactorial

It has been known for a long time that the manifestation of thrombophilia varies substantially even within single families with deficiencies in ATIII, PC, and PS. Among

Table 3. Frequency of venous thromboembolism in members of families with combined thrombophilia; DVT = Deep vein thrombosis

Thrombophilia	Associated with FV-Leiden		Sole defect		FV-Leiden only		Neither defect		Reference
	n	DVT (%)	n	DVT (%)	n	DVT (%)	n	DVT (%)	
PC deficiency (6 families)	23	70	34	35	20	10	30	7	(19)
PS deficiency (7 families)	18	72	21	19	21	19	44	2	(42)
ATIII deficiency (6 families)	12	92	7	57	5	20	11	0	(38)

individuals carrying genotypically identical deficiencies of ATIII, PC, and PS, only 50 percent develop thrombosis below the age of 45 years. This has lead to the suggestion that other genetic risk factors modify the expression of these genotypes. The identification of frequent genetic polymorphisms like FV-Leiden the prothrombin 202101 allele, and the MTHFR nucleotide 677 polymorphism has now opened up the opportunity to examine possible interactions between multiple thrombophilia-associated factors. In symptomatic individuals with deficiencies of ATIII, PC, and PS, the prevalence of FV-Leiden is increased 20 to 50 percent, supporting the view that the precipitation of thrombosis is controlled by several genes in heterozygous patients. As shown in Table 3, coexistence of deficiencies of ATIII, PC, and PS with FV-Leiden substantially augments the risk of thrombosis compared to the presence of either of these defects alone.

Very similar risk amplification has been seen in homozygous homocystinuria. In seven families with homocystinuria, each of six homozygotes presenting with thromboses below the age of eight years bore FV-Leiden. In contrast, each of four individuals homozygous for homocystinuria not developing thrombosis below 17 years of age had a normal FV genotype [23]. These findings suggest that hyperhomocysteinemia and APC resistance have synergistic effects on the onset of thrombotic disease. Controversial observations, however, have been reported as to whether or not the coexistence of FV-Leiden, mild hyperhomocystinemia, and (or) MTHFR thermolability amplifies the thrombotic risk as well.

Beyond the complex tangle of genes, circumstantial risk factors govern the precipitation of thrombotic events. Obviously, the most important non-genetic risk factor is age. The number of circumstantial risk factors required to precipitate thrombosis is significantly lower at high age (Table 4), indicating that more thrombogenic factors are

Table 4. Number of thrombosis risk factors in different age categories. Risk factors are: surgery, hospital admission, FV-Leiden, prothrombin 20210A, deficiencies of PC, PS or ATIII, elevated FVIII, oral contraceptive use (dates adopted from reference 31).

Risk factors	< 40 years		> 55 years	
	Cases (%)	Controls (%)	Cases (%)	Controls (%)
n =	160	161	127	124
None	16.9	47.8	22.8	54.8
1	31.9	37.3	37.8	38.7
2	35.6	13.0	33.9	4.8
3	11.9	1.2	3.9	1.6
4	3.8	0.6	1.6	0

required to precipitate thrombosis the younger an individual is. A further important circumstantial risk factor is the use of oral contraceptives. Estrogens in oral contraceptives decrease PS, ATIII, and fibrinolytic activity and increase the concentration of a number of coagulation factors. Women heterozygous for FV-Leiden are at 35-fold greater risk of developing thrombosis if they take oral contraceptives; homozygous women are at several hundredfold risk [32]. However, because the absolute risk of venous thrombosis in oral contraceptive users heterozygous for FV-Leiden is still low (around 30 events per 10,000 women-years) screening for FV-Leiden or APC resistance prior to prescribing oral contraceptives is not generally recommended unless the clinical or family history is significant for thromboembolism.

The diagnosis of thrombophilia in the clinical laboratory

Patients (and their first-degree relatives) should be investigated for genetic risk factors of thrombosis when presenting with thromboembolism below 45 years of age, a positive family history, recurrent thrombosis, warfarin-induced skin necrosis, and thrombosis at unusual sites (cerebral, mesenteric, splenic, portal, hepatic veins). Individuals with single inherited thrombophilic defects are not uncommon and are frequently asymptomatic, whereas many of the symptomatic patients have more than one genetic risk factor. Thrombophilia thus represents an oligogenetic rather than monogenetic phenotype, the expression of which is amplified by circumstantial risk factors. As a consequence, the laboratory screening of thrombosis patients needs to include all of the known genetic risk factors even if the "clinical" situation seemingly provides sufficient "explanation" for a thrombotic event.

The defects of the anticoagulant pathway are too heterogeneous to allow detection by genetic testing. The diagnosis of deficiencies of ATIII, PC, and PS, therefore, still relies on functional and immunological testing. Functional assays for ATIII discriminate well between heterozygous ATIII deficient and normal individuals. In contrast to this, there is considerable overlap of PC activities in heterozygous carriers and normal controls. Coagulant assays for PC may be preferred over the measurement of the activity of the catalytic domain with synthetic substrates as type II PC deficiencies exist in which the interaction of PC with Ca^{2+} is impaired, a type of deficiency which would be overlooked if the activity of the catalytic domain was solely measured. PC and PS levels are low as a consequence of oral anticoagulation and attempts to adjust for effects of vitamin K antagonists by comparing PC and PS with VII or prothrombin have not been satisfactory. Most of the PC and PS clotting assays produce false positive results in APC resistant, but not PC or PS deficient individuals. Some APC resistant patients may, therefore, have been misclassified as type II PC or PS deficiency.

Three strategies are available to screen patients for APC resistance. In the first one, resistance to APC is detected by performing a modified activated partial thromboplastin time (APTT) with or without adding APC to the patient plasma. The result is expressed as the ratio of the clotting time in the presence of APC divided by the clotting time in the absence of APC (normally greater than 2). This type of assay is biased by numerous factors. Significant contamination of the plasma with platelets results in falsely low APC response. As low concentrations of prothrombin and FX produce falsely high sensitivity to APC, it is also not suitable for the analysis of samples from patients taking oral anticoagulants; heparin containing samples should also not be analyzed. In unselected outpatients with clinically suspected acute deep venous thrombosis, the specificities of the original APC-resistance test for the FV-Leiden mutation were only 54 and 28 percent in those patients negative and positive for thrombosis, respectively, on phlebography compared to 85 percent in healthy controls [36], possibly due to the fact that FVIIIc increases during acute phase. Finally, there is ample evidence that the conventional assay for APC resistance become falsely positive in acquired pro-thrombotic conditions like the use of oral contraceptives, lupus anticoagulants, and increased in FVIII (see above).

The second strategy to test for resistance to APC includes dilution of samples with FV-deficient plasma before analysis, a measure which adjusts for variations in the contents of other coagulation factors in the patient sample. The influence of preanalytical variables in this assay is minor; it works well in samples from patients receiving oral anticoagulants and heparin. Pre-dilution with FV-deficient plasma increases the capacity to discriminate between carriers and non-carriers of FV-Leiden to 100 % [37]. However, when selecting a test it should be borne in mind that absolute specificity may not always be desirable. Decreased sensitivity to APC may occur in the absence of the FV-Leiden mutation and this situation may also be indicative of an increased risk of thrombosis.

The third approach is of course to test for FV-Leiden on the nucleic acid level. The most common method includes the amplification of a short segment of the FV gene using polymerase chain reaction and to digest the product with a restriction enzyme (for instance *MnlI*).

So far, no direct functional method is available to screen for the presence of the prothrombin 20210A allele. This implies that the identification of individuals with this abnormality will completely rely on DNA analysis.

Three of the five established genetic risk factors of thrombosis involve the PC system. Hence, attempts have been made to design screening assays capable of detecting all of the genetically determined and acquired disorders of this pathway including FV-Leiden. Future evaluations of these global tests will have to demonstrate that they are sufficiently sensitive to warrant their broad application in the assessment of thromboembolic risk. The high prevalence of disorders of the PC system raises the issue whether it would be cost-beneficial to perform global testing in connection with surgery, pregnancy, and the prescription of oral contraceptives. Prospective studies will be necessary to clarify under which circumstances this might be appropriate.

From genetics to practice

In general, the management of a patient identified as having a laboratory abnormality associated with thrombophilia will depend on a variety of factors such as the patient's individual and family history, the site of the thrombosis, and the presence of other pro-thrombotic risk factors. Thrombophilic women should avoid oral contraceptives. The use of prophylactic anticoagulation with dose-adjusted heparin during pregnancy and the puerperium requires particularly careful consideration. Longterm prophylactic administration of vitamin K antagonists may have to be considered for symptomatic patients with proven abnormalities, especially if thrombosis is recurrent.

In asymptomatic persons with a genetic risk factor, the use of prophylactic anticoagulation should be considered for trauma, surgery, pregnancy, or other high-risk situations. As future research will shed more light on the role of gene with gene and gene with environment interactions in thrombophilia it will become possible to establish more exact guidelines translating the results of basic research into cost-effective therapeutic and prophylactic regimens.

References

1. Arruda VR, von Zuben PM, Chiaparini LC, Annichino-Bizzacchi JM, Costa FF (1997) The mutation Ala677 - Val in the methylene tetrahydrofolate reductase gene: A risk factor for arterial disease and venous thrombosis. Thromb Haemost 77: 818–821
2. Bayston TA, Lane DA (1997) Antithrombin: Molecular basis of deficiency. Thromb Haemost 78: 339–343
3. Bernardi F, Faioni EM, Castoldi E, Lunghi B, Castaman G, Sacchi E, Mannucci PM (1997) A factor V genetic component differing from factor V R506Q contributes to the activated protein C resistance phenotype. Blood 90: 1552–1557
4. Bertina RM (1997) Factor V Leiden and other coagulation factor mutations affecting thrombotic risk. Clin Chem 43: 1678–1683
5. Bertina RM, Koeleman BPC, Koster T, Rosendaal FR, Dirven RJ, de Ronde H, van der Velden PA, Reitsma PH (1994) Mutation in blood coagulation factor V associated with resistance to activated protein C. Nature 369: 64–67
6. Chan WP, Lee CK, Kwong YL, Lam CK, Liang R (1998) A novel mutation of Arg306 of factor V gene in Hong Kong Chinese. Blood 91: 1135–1139
7. Comp PC, Esmon CT (1984) Recurrent thromboembolism in patients with a partial deficiency of protein S. N Engl J Med 311: 1525–1528
8. Dahlbäck B, Carlsson M, Svensson PJ (1993) Familial thrombophilia due to a previously unrecognised mechanism characterised by poor anticoagulant response to activated protein C. Proc Natl Acad Sci USA 90: 1004–1008
9. Egeberg O (1965) Inherited antithrombin deficiency causing thrombophilia. Thrombosis et Diathesis Haemorrhagica 13: 516–530
10. Esmon CT, Ding W, Yasuhiro K, Gu JM, Ferrell G, Regan LM, Stearns-Kurosawa DJ, Kurosawa S, Mather T, Laszik Z, Esmon NL (1997) The protein C pathway: New insights. Thromb Haemostas 78: 70–74
11. Frosst P, Blom HJ, Milos R, Goyette P, Sheppard CA, Matthews RG, Boers GJH, den Heijer M, Kluijtmans LAJ, van den Heuvel LP, Rozen R (1995) A candidate genetic risk factor for vascular disease: A common mutation in methylenetetrahydrofolate reductase. Nature Genetics 10: 111–113
12. Griffin JH, Evatt BL, Zimmermann TS, Kleiss AJ, Widemann C (1981) Deficiency of protein C in congenital thrombotic disease. J Clin Invest 68: 1370–1373
13. Guasch JF, Lensen RP, Bertina RM (1997) Molecular characterisation of a type I quantitative factor V deficiency in a thrombosis patient that is "pseudo homozygous" for activated protein C resistance. Thromb Haemost 77: 252–257
14. Halbmayer WM, Haushofer A, Schön R, Fischer M(1994) The prevalence of poor anticoagulant response to activated protein C (APC resistance) among patients suffering from stroke or venous thrombosis and among healthy subjects. Blood Coagul Fibrinol 5: 51–57
15. Haverkate F, Samama M (1995) Familial dysfibrinogenemia and thrombophilia. Report on a study of the SSC subcommittee on fibrinogen. Thromb Haemost 73: 151–161
16. Healy AM, Rayburn HB, Rosenberg RD, Weiler H (1995) Absence of the blood-clotting regulator thrombomodulin causes embryonic lethality in mice before development of a functional cardiovascular system. Proc Natl Acad Sci USA 92: 850–854
17. Heinrich J, Schulte H, Funke H, Schönfeld R, Köhler E, Assmann G (1995) Frequency of point mutation in factor V gene (1691 G/A), which is associated with resistance to activated protein C, in coronary artery disease patients. Thromb Haemostas 73: 1125 (Abstract)
18. Ireland H, Kunz G, Kyriakoulis K, Stubbs PJ, Lane DA (1997) Thrombomodulin gene mutations associated with myocardial infarction. Circulation 96: 15–18
19. Koeleman BPC, Reitsma PH, Allaart CF, Bertina RM (1994) Activated protein C resistance as an additional risk factor for thrombosis in protein C deficient families. Blood 84: 1031–1035
20. Koster T, Rodendaal FR, Briet E, Van der Meer FJM, Colly LP, Trienekens PH, Poort SR, Reitsma PH, Vandenbroucke JP (1995) Protein C deficiency in a controlled series of unselected outpatients: An infrequent, but clear risk factor for venous thromboembolism (Leiden thrombophilia study). Blood 85: 2756–2761
21. Laffan MA, Manning R (1996) The influence of factor VIII on measurement of activated protein C resistance. Blood Coagul Fibrinolysis 7: 761–765
22. Lane DA, Bayston T, Olds RJ, Fitches AC, Cooper DN, Millar DS, Jochmans K, Perry DJ, Okajima K, Emmerich J, Thein SL (1997) Antithrombin mutation database: 2nd (1997) update. Thromb Haemost 77: 197–211
23. Mandel H, Brenner B, Berant M, Rosenberg N, Lanir N, Jakobs C, Fowler B, Seligsohn U (1996) Coexistence of hereditary homocystinuria and factor V Leiden – Effect on thrombosis. N Engl J Med 334: 763–768
24. März W, Seydewitz H, Winkelmann B, Chen M, Nauck M, Witt I (1995) Mutation in coagulation factor V associated with resistance to activated protein C in patients with coronary artery disease. Lancet 345: 526–527
25. Ohlin AK, Norlund L, Marlar RA (1997) Thrombomodulin gene variations and thromboembolic disease. Thromb Haemost 78: 396–400
26. Poort SR, Rosendaal FR, Reitsma PH, Bertina RM (1996) A common genetic variation in the 3'-untranslated region of the prothrombin gene is associated with elevated plasma prothrombin levels and an increase in venous thrombosis. Blood 88: 3698–3703

27. Reitsma PH (1997) Protein C deficiency: from gene defects to disease. Thromb Haemost 78: 344–350
28. Reitsma PH, Bernardi F, Doig RG, Gandrille S, Greengard JS, Ireland H, Krawczak M, Lind B, Long GL, Poort SR, Saito H, Sala N, Witt I, Cooper DN (1995) Protein C deficiency: A database of mutations, 1995 uptdate. Thromb Haemost 73: 876–889
29. Ridker PM, Hennekens CH, Lindpaintner K, Stampfer MJ, Eisenberg PR, Miletich JP (1995) Mutation in the gene coding for coagulation factor V and the risk of myocardial infarction, stroke, and venous thrombosis in apparently healthy men. N Engl J Med 332: 912–917
30. Rosen SB, Sturk A (1997) Activated protein C resistance-a major risk factor for thrombosis. Eur J Clin Chem Clin Biochem 35: 501–516
31. Rosendaal FR (1997) Thrombosis in the young: Epidemiology and risk factors. A focus on venous thrombosis. Thromb Haemostas 78: 1–6
32. Rosendaal FR, Koster T, Vandenbroucke JP, Reitsma PH (1995) High risk of thrombosis in patients homozygous for factor V Leiden (activated protein C resistance). Blood 85: 1504–1508
33. Rosendaal FR, Siscovick DS, Schwartz SM, Beverly RK, Psaty BM, Longstreth WT, Jr., Raghunathan TE, Koepsell TD, Reitsma PH (1997) Factor V Leiden (resistance to activated protein C) increases the risk of myocardial infarction in young women. Blood 89: 2817–2821
34. Selhub J, D'Angelo A (1997) Hyperhomocysteinemia and thrombosis: Acquired conditions. Thromb Haemost 78: 527–531
35. Simioni P, Scudeller A, Radossi P, Gavasso S, Girolami B, Tormene D, Girolami A (1996) "Pseudohomozygous" activated protein C resistance due to double heterozygous factor V defects (factor V-Leiden mutation and type I quantitative factor V defect) associated with thrombosis. Report of two cases belonging to two unrelated kindreds. Thromb. Haemostas 75: 422–426
36. Svensson PJ, Zoller B, Dahlback B (1997) Evaluation of original and modified APC-resistance tests in unselected outpatients with clinically suspected thrombosis and in healthy controls. Thromb Haemost 77: 332–335
37. Tripodi A, Negri B, Bertina RM, Mannucci PM (1997) Screening for the FV: Q506 mutation evaluation of thirteen plasma-based methods for their diagnostic efficacy in comparison with DNA analysis. Thromb Haemost 77: 436–439
38. van Boven HH, Reitsma PH, Rosendaal FR, Bayston TA, Chowdhury V, Bauer KA, Scharrer I, Conrad J, Lane DA (1996) Factor V Leiden (FV R506Q) in families with inherited antithrombin deficiency. Thromb Haemostas 1996: 417–421
39. Williamson D, Brown K, Luddington R, Baglin C, Baglin T (1998) Factor V Cambridge: A new mutation (Arg[305] → Thr) associated with resistance to activated protein C. Blood 91: 1140–1144
40. Wu LL, Wu J, Hunt SC, James BC, Vincent GM, Williams RR, Hopkins PN (1994) Plasma homocyst(e)ine as a risk factor for early familial coronary artery disease. Clin Chem 40: 552–561
41. Zöller B (1996) Familial thrombophilia: Clinical and molecular analysis of Swedish families with inherited resistance to activated protein C or protein S deficiency. Scand J Clin Lab Invest (Suppl) 226: 19–46
42. Zöller B, Berntsdotter A, de Frutos PG, Dahlbäck B (1995) Resistance to activated protein C as an additional genetic risk factor in hereditary deficiency of protein S. Blood 85: 3518–3523

This article is dedicated to Prof. Dr. H. Just on the occasion of his 65th birthday.

N. W. März (✉) · M. Nauck · H. Wieland
Division of Clinical Chemistry
Department of Medicine
Albert Ludwigs-University
Hugstetter Straße 55
79106 Freiburg im Breisgau, Germany
E-mail: maerz@mz1200.ukl-freiburg.de

Hypercoagulative syndrome: Molecular markers for the identification of cardiovascular patients at risk

H. M. Hoffmeister, W. Heller, L. Seipel

Summary   In many cardiovascular diseases thromb-embolic events play a key role. Especially in patients with acute coronary syndromes a hypercoagulative state is known. Information, however, whether such alterations do exist prior to the clinical event is limited. Recent progress in the development of sensitive and specific tests to determine molecular markers of (re)activation of several pathways of the coagulation and of the fibrinolytic system is evident. The possible impact of such molecular markers for the identification of cardiovascular patients at risk as well as the meaning of such markers to prognosticate future cardiovascular events is summarized.

Key words   Molecular markers – coagulation – fibrinolysis – inflammation – tissue injury

Activity of the coagulation and of the fibrinolysis have been assessed in the past by use of global functional tests. The results of such tests often covered several steps of an activation cascade and failed more or less to localize alterations of the involved systems exactly. Direct determination of activity of a certain protein in plasma is limited due to the fact that high levels of inhibitors cause an inactivation within a very short time. Therefore, ex vivo determination of activities is always limited by some uncertainty, whether the results are representative for the in vivo activity. To overcome these problems a number of new tests, which are designed to measure molecular markers of activation, have been developed in recent years. In general besides the direct measurements of the activity several, other measures can be used to assess the activity of a pathway: i) a precursor can be measured (whether it decreases during enhanced activation); ii) a split product of the activation step can be determined as marker for the activation of a reaction; iii) an end product can be measured directly; iv) a split product of the effect of the activated protein can be assessed; v) the inhibitor level can be determined; vi) the complex of the activated protein with its inhibitor can be measured. The usefulness of each of these approaches to judge the activation of a certain reaction in plasma is highly dependent on factors like the size of the pool of a certain precursor or inhibitor in plasma and the half-life of split or reaction products in the blood.

Several measures were examined and established in the last years to judge the activation of the most interesting pathways in detail. The majority of these tests are based on enzyme-linked-immuno-assays (ELISA) for practical reasons, but other methods as radio-immuno-assays (RIA) could also be applied. In the following sections several molecular markers of the coagulation, the fibrinolysis, the inflammation, and tissue injury will be introduced and their prognostic relevance will be discussed for some cardiovascular diseases associated with intravascular thrombus formation.

Activation markers of the coagulation

In the classical model the beginning of the coagulation cascade is divided into two systems: the intrinsic and extrinsic pathway. Both pathways then result in the activation of thrombin from prothrombin (Fig. 1). This amount of thrombin *generation* can be determined by measuring the prothrombin fragment 1 + 2, which is split from prothrombin during conversion to thrombin. Several tests, which are commercially available, have been developed to detect this marker [12, 21]. The half-life in the circulation of this thrombin generation marker is about 90 minutes.

Active thrombin is acting on fibrinogen and inhibited by antithrombin III. The complex of thrombin with antithrombin III can also be detected and serves as a marker of thrombin *activity*. Determination of the thrombin/antithrombin III has widely been used to assess thrombin activity during various conditions [6, 10].

The *action* of thrombin, e.g., the effect on fibrinogen to convert this to fibrin, can be assessed by measuring the split product fibrinopeptide A [4, 17–19]. A disadvantage of this marker is its short half-life of about 3–5 minutes in the circulation. Therefore, several authors have determined this marker not in plasma, but measured also the urinary excretion [3, 15]. Using these markers, exact characterization of the activation of the coagulation including thrombin generation, activity and action on fibrinogen is feasible.

In cardiovascular diseases, many investigators have focused on acute coronary syndromes and the associated activation of thrombin. In patients with unstable angina pectoris, our group has demonstrated not only an elevated thrombin activity initially during the acute phase, but also during a follow-up over at least 5 days [10]. A stratification between patients, who needed an acute interventional revascularization procedure (PTCA) and those who could be successfully stabilized medically, was not possible [9]. Preliminary reports also indicated that there is some relation between the activation of the coagulation in acute coronary syndromes and the occurrence of myocardial injury [11]. Regarding the outcome of patients with acute coronary syndromes Merlini et al. described that the elevation of the prothrombin fragment 1 + 2 persists, while FPA decreases in patients with favorable outcome [15]. The authors concluded that the latter group of patients could better handle the elevated thrombin generation. From the same

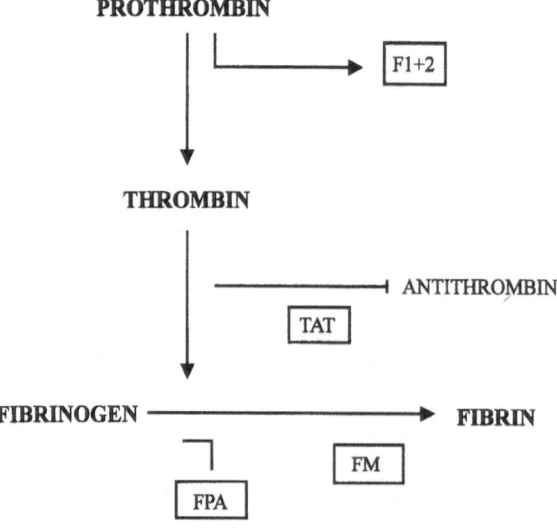

Fig. 1. Activation of the coagulation. F1 + 2 = prothrombin fragment 1 + 2 (marker of thrombin generation); TAT = thrombin-antithrombin III complex (marker of thrombin activity); FPA = fibrinopeptide A and FM = fibrin monomers result from the action of thrombin.

group [3] in another study the early outcome in unstable angina pectoris patients was less favorable, if plasma fibrinopeptide A levels were elevated, while the fibrinopeptide A urinary excretion did not reveal significant results. In acute myocardial infarction, Gulba and coworkers described that the thrombin/antithrombin levels were increased in patients with unsuccessful thrombolysis or reocclusion in contrast to patients with a successful thrombolytic therapy [6]. However, while there is a good overall correlation in these groups, there is wide overlap between patients with favorable and unfavorable outcome in unstable angina pectoris; therefore, markers of the activation of the coagulation seem not to be useful for the acute stratification of individual patient management on the coronary care unit.

Markers of the fibrinolytic system

The fibrinolytic system, e.g., the generation of plasmin from plasminogen and the generation of fibrin is a permanently ongoing process in the blood counterbalancing the tendency for clotting. Besides several functional tests, as mentioned above, certain ELISA tests are available to measure plasma markers of the fibrinolytic system (Fig. 2). One of the best investigated markers is the tissue-type plasminogen activator (antigen). The test to examine this marker, which was frequently used in patients with coronary heart disease [5, 10], determines the mass concentration of the tissue-type plasminogen activator using an ELISA technique. The measurement includes active and inactive tissue-type plasminogen activator, mainly those inactivated by plasminogen activator inhibitor. The measurement of both compounds explains why there is a strong association with the plasminogen activator inhibitor levels and why in patients with coronary heart disease and a risk constellation this marker is increased, while the *activity* of tissue-type plasminogen activator was found to be normal or even decreased [5, 16, 23, 26]. This observation underscores that determination of tissue-type plasminogen activator mass concentration is markedly dependent on the plasminogen activator inhibitor in plasma. The latter is known as a risk marker for coronary syndromes and its diurnal variance is associated with the diurnal variance in the incidence of acute myocardial infarctions [1].

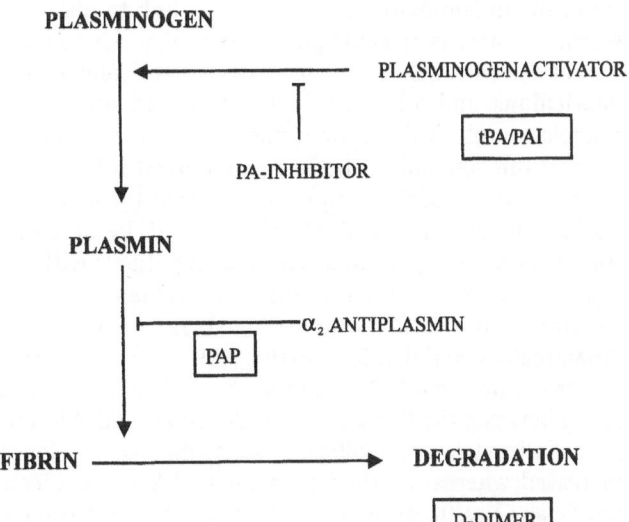

Fig. 2. The fibrinolysis. PA-inhibitor = plasminogen activator inhibitor; tPA/PAI = tissue-type plasminogen activator (tPA) mass concentration (antigen measurement) includes active and inactivated tPA (bound to PAI = plasminogen activator inhibitor); PAP = plasmin-α_2 antiplasmin complex.

To assess plasmin activity, plasminogen as a precursor or antiplasmin as the main inhibitor can be determined and the reduction in these measures could be interpreted as an actually increased activity of the fibrinolytic system (typical finding during thrombolytic therapy). However, for minor changes such tests, which are usually based on chromogenic substrate methods, are not preferable but more sensitive and specific ELISA tests like determination of the plasmin/antiplasmin complex are. Similarly as the thrombin/antithrombin complex for thrombin activity the plasmin/antiplasmin complex is related to the activity of this pathway and has a higher sensitivity than can be expected from measurements of precursors.

As a further measure, split products of fibrin can be assessed as d-dimers. Such split products stem from fibrin; however, it cannot conclusively derived from elevated d-dimer levels that a larger thrombus is present in a patient's circulation. It might also be that a considerable part of elevated d-dimers stems from degradation of soluble fibrin and not from a fixed thrombus [14]. Therefore, the combination of elevated markers of the coagulation and elevated levels of fibrin degradation products means a procoagulant or hypercoagulative state with an increased risk for thrombus formation or an increased turnover in the coagulation/fibrinolytic system. A thrombus formation, however, need not be present as the increased coagulation can be balanced by an increased fibrinolysis in this condition. Such a state was described in patients with unstable angina pectoris for up to 10 days follow-up [10] and in patients with increased risk for future coronary events after admission to a hospital because of thoracic discomfort [7, 16, 24]. It seems to be questionable whether elevated levels of d-dimers are indicative of intracoronary thrombus formation, since – as outlined above – this very small thrombus does not have to necessarily be the source of the degradation products. On the other hand, there is no doubt that a larger thrombosis as deep vein thrombosis causes an increase in fibrin degradation products. Furthermore, measurements of tPA has some importance as prognostic marker for coronary heart disease [22] and for the development of significant coronary artery stenosis [5].

Markers of inflammation

Recently a large number of tests have been reported for the measurement of several markers of the inflammatory processes. One link to the inflammatory system is fibrinogen, which also acts as an acute phase reactant and is a known risk marker for acute atherosclerotic events. Other possible markers are soluble adhesion molecules (e.g., sICAM), interleukins, and other mediators. A second system which constitutes a link between coagulation/fibrinolysis and inflammation is the complement cascade. There are several interactions, including the use of identical inhibitors (C_1-esterase inhibitor). Of the various markers of the complement cascade the membrane attack complex (MAC) sensu "lytic complex" or "terminal complex" can be determined as SC5b-9 in plasma. This complex was described to be elevated in patients with acute coronary syndromes [25].

Recent papers focused on the measurement of the C-reactive protein and of serum amyloid A as two acute phase markers which could indicate already low levels of inflammatory activity, if sensitive ELISA test systems were used. Despite the various reasons, which could cause an increase in these markers, there seems to be a good correlation between the C-reactive protein levels and the future risk of patients with angina pectoris. In a two years follow-up study the risk was doubled if the C-reactive protein was increased, whereas for the serum amyloid A no significant result was observed [8]. In the physicians health study an increased C-reactive protein level was associated with an elevated risk for acute myocardial infarction in stroke, but not for venous thrombosis [22]. It has to be examined in further studies, however, how predictive an elevation of these markers is for the individual patient and whether the prognostic accuracy is well enough to derive diagnostic and therapeutical strategies for patient management from elevated levels of these markers.

Injury marker

For coronary heart disease, there are markers available to assess injury of the heart muscle. This includes measurement of troponin T or troponin I for which test systems for determination of cardiac specific injury markers are available [13]. Furthermore, determination of the creatine kinase mass also is a marker with certain advantages compared with the conventional measurement of creatine kinase activity in plasma. For troponin T it was shown that besides its usefulness in acute myocardial infarction or perioperative infarction, a risk stratification of patients with unstable angina pectoris is possible by determination of the initial level of this marker [2, 20]. A close relation of such a marker to the short- or mid-term outcome is evident, as such a marker describes the tissue injury being the endpoint of the multitude of factors involved in the pathogenesis of acute coronary syndromes. Therefore, while even a thrombotic coronary occlusion could be compensated by a collateralization, the tissue injury as evidence for the severity of an acute coronary syndrome includes all involved factors.

Comparing intravascular thrombosis in the arterial and the venous system, it is evident that the mass of a thrombus in the venous system is usually much larger before it becomes clinically obvious compared with a very small thrombus in the arterial system located at a strategically critical localization as, e.g., the coronary vessels. Therefore, a large number of venous thrombosis is not detected clinically on one hand and on the other hand determination of markers of the coagulation and fibrinolysis in the acute stage of a venous thrombosis is not useful, as such markers have to be elevated. Furthermore, the size of thrombus in venous disease is not closely related to the occurrence of severe clinically events like pulmonary embolism. Therefore, no convincing studies which could describe the usefulness of determination of markers of the coagulation and fibrinolysis for the prognostication of a pulmonary embolism are available today. Furthermore, very small pulmonary emboli are often not detected clinically, and no markers of tissue injury of the lung vessel with the comparative sensitivity as that of troponin T for cardiac tissue are available. Therefore, determination of markers of the coagulation, fibrinolysis, and tissue injury plays no role in the clinical situation of deep vein thrombosis today. For prognostic reasons, determination of risk factors of the coagulation (which plays a more important role in venous versus arterial thrombosis due to the less important sheer stress on the platelets in venous thrombosis) are meaningful. Such risk factors, which have to be determined in patients with venous thrombosis, include deficiency of protein C and protein S, a pathologically activated protein C resistance, a lupus anticoagulant, and other more rare risk conditions.

Conclusion

A large number of molecular markers of hemostasis, fibrinolysis, inflammation and tissue injury can be determined at present with a high sensitivity and specificity. Such measurements are meaningful to investigate pathophysiological mechanisms in patients with thrombus associated vascular diseases. Identification of patients at high risk is possible at an epidemiological level, whereas for the different markers it has to be examined whether they will have a prognostic impact also in the acute setting of the intensive care unit. For most of these markers at the acute stage, the risk stratification of patients using molecular markers of hemostasis and fibrinolysis with respect to acute or subacute clinical events is limited due to the large intra- and interindividual variability and the multitude of systems involved in the pathogenesis of these diseases. In contrast, molecular markers of tissue injury seem to be superior for acute risk stratification in high risk patient populations as they represent the summary of involved systems resulting in the tissue damage and clinical event.

References

1. Angleton P, Chandler WL, Schmer G (1989) Diurnal variation of tissue-type plasminogen activator and its rapid inhibitor (PAI-1). Circulation 79: 101–106
2. Antman EM, Tanasijevic MJ, Thompson B, Schactman M, McCabe CH, Cannon CP, Fischer GA, Fung AY, Thompson C, Wybenga D, Braunwald E (1996) Cardiac-specific troponin I levels to predict the risk of mortality in patients with acute coronary syndromes. N Engl J Med 335: 1342–1349
3. Ardissino D, Merlini PA, Gambo G, Barberis P, Demichelli G, Testa S, Colombi E, Poli A, Fetiveau R, Montemartini C (1996) Thrombin activity and early outcome in unstable angina pectoris. Circulation 93: 1634–1639
4. Cronlund M, Hardin J, Burton J, Lee L, Haber E, Bloch KJ (1979) Fibrinopeptide A in plasma of normal subjects and patients with disseminated intravascular coagulation and systemic lupus erythematosus. J Clin Invest 58: 142–151
5. ECAT angina pectoris study group (1993) ECAT angina pectoris study: baseline associations of haemostatic factor with extent of coronary arteriosclerosis and other coronary risk factors in 3000 patients with angina pectoris undergoing coronary angiography. Europ Heart J 14: 8–17
6. Gulba DC, Westhoff-Bleck M, Jost S, Rafflenbeul W, Daniel WG, Hecker H, Lichtlen PR (1991) Increased thrombin levels during thrombolytic therapy in acute myocardial infarction. Circulation 83: 937–944
7. Hamsten A, Walldius G, Szamosi A, Blombäck M, De Faire U, Dahlen G, Landou C, Wiman B (1987) Plasminogen activator inhibitor in plasma: Risk factor for recurrent myocardial infarction. Lancet 2: 3–9
8. Haverkate F, Thompson SG, Pyke SDM, Gallimore JR, Pepys MB (1997) Production of C-reactive protein and risk of coronary events in stable and unstable angina. Lancet 349: 462–466
9. Hoffmeister HM, Jur M, Heller W, Seipel L (1995) Hyperkoagulabilität bei akutem koronaren Syndrom: Beeinflussung durch eine PTCA als Akutintervention. In: Heinle H, Schulte H, Kaffernik H: Arteriosklerose; W. Kohlhammer, Stuttgart, pp 141–145
10. Hoffmeister HM, Jur M, Wendel HP, Heller W, Seipel L (1995) Alterations of the coagulation, the fibrinolytic and the kallikrein-kinin system in the acute and post-acute phase in patients with unstable angina pectoris. Circulation 91: 2520–2527
11. Hoffmeister HM, Jur M, Heller W, Seipel L (1997) Korrelation zwischen molekularen Schädigungsmarkern und der Gerinnung bei Patienten mit instabiler Angina pectoris. Z Kardiol 86: 68
12. Hursting MJ, Butman BT, Steiner JP et al. (1993) Monoclonal antibodies specific for prothrombin fragment 1, 2 and their use in a quantitative enzyme-linked immunosorbent assay. Clin Chem 39: 583–591
13. Katus HA, Loser S, Hallermayer K et al. (1992) Development and in vitro characterization of a new immunoassay of cardiac troponin T. Clin Chem 38: 386–393
14. Marder VJ (1990) What does the "dimer test" test? Circulation 82: 1514–1515
15. Merlini PA, Bauer KA, Oltrona L, Ardissino D, Cattaneo M, Belli C, Mannucci PM, Rosenberg RD (1994) Persistent activation of coagulation mechanism in unstable angina and myocardial infarction. Circulation 90: 61–68
16. Munkvad S, Gram J, Jespersen J (1990) A depression of active tissue plasminogen activator in plasma characterizes patients with unstable angina pectoris who develop myocardial infarction. Eur Heart J 11: 525–528
17. Nossel HL, Younger LR, Wilner GD, Procupez T, Canfield RE, Butler VP Jr (1971) Radioimmunoassay of human fibrinopeptide A. Proc Natl Acad Sci USA 68: 2350–2353
18. Nossel HL, Yudelman I, Canfield RE et al. (1974) Measurement of fibrinopeptide A in human blood. J Clin Invest 54: 43–53
19. Nossel HL, Ti M, Kaplan KL, Spanondis K, Soland T, Butler VP Jr (1976) The generation of fibrinopeptide A in clinical blood samples: Evidence for thrombin activity. J Clin Invest 58: 1136–1144
20. Ohman EM, Armstron PW, Christenson RH, Granger CB, Katus HA, Hamm CW, O'Hanesian MA, Wagner GS, Kleiman NS, Harrell FE, Califf RM, Topol EJ (1996) Cardiac troponin T levels for risk stratification in acute myocardial ischemia. N Engl J Med 335: 1333–1341

21. Pelzer H, Schwart A, Stuber W (1991) Determination of human prothrombin activation fragment 1 + 2 in plasma with an antibody against a synthetic peptide. Thromb Haemostas 65: 153–159
22. Ridker PM, Cushman M, Stampfer MJ, Tracy RP, Hennekens CH (1997) Inflammation, aspirin, and the risk of cardiovascular disease in apparently healthy men. New Engl J Med 336: 973–979
23. Vaziri ND, Kennedy SC, Kennedy D, Gonzales E (1992) Coagulation, fibrinolytic, and inhibitory proteins in acute myocardial infarction and angina pectoris. Am J Med 93: 651–657
24. Wiman B, Hamsten A (1990) Correlations between fibrinolytic function and acute myocardial infarction. Am J Cardiol 66: 54G–56G
25. Yasuda M, Takeuchi K, Hiruma M, Iida H, Tahara A, Itagane H, Toda I, Akioka K, Teragaki M, Oku H, Kanayama Y, Takeda T, Kolb WP, Tamerius JD (1990) The complement system in ischemic heart disease. Circulation 81: 156–163
26. Zalewski A, Shi Y, Nardone D, Bravette B, Weinstock P, Fischmann D, Wilson P, Goldberg S, Levin DC, Bjornsson TD (1991) Evidence for reduced fibrinolytic activity in unstable angina at rest. Circulation 83: 1685–1691

Prof. Dr. Hans Martin Hoffmeister (✉) · W. Heller · L. Seipel
Medizinische Universitätsklinik
Abteilung Innere Medizin III
Otfried-Müller-Straße 10
72076 Tübingen, Germany

Clinical implications of the new understanding of thrombophilia

S. Moll, D. Gulba

Summary Thrombophilia used to be viewed as a disorder caused by a single congenital thrombophilic abnormality with thrombosis often triggered by an exogenous risk situation. It is becoming clear, however, that it is often a compound state with several congenital and acquired thrombophilic abnormalities. Activated protein C resistance is the most commonly found congenital abnormality. Protein C-, protein S-, and antithrombin III-deficiency continue to play an important role. Hyperhomocysteinemia as a risk factor for arterial and venous thrombosis is being recognized more frequently and is of particular interest, since elevated homocysteine levels can be decreased by simple means: treatment with folic acid and vitamin B_6. However, whether this decreases the risk of thrombosis is not known. Antiphospholipid antibodies are also being recognized more frequently. The special treatment considerations in these patients will be discussed. Polymorphisms of proteins involved in coagulation, such as prothrombin and thrombomodulin, leading to an increased risk of thrombosis are increasingly being discovered. Several well performed clinical studies exist which allow recommendations for the length and intensity of anticoagulation for patients who have suffered a thromboembolic event. However, these studies have grouped together patients with different risk factor profiles and, therefore, only lead to generalized recommendations. By discovering more thrombophilic abnormalities and testing patients for these, a more individual risk stratification will be possible. This will eventually lead to more individual treatment recommendations.

Key words Thrombophilia – thrombosis – APC-resistance – protein C – protein S – antithrombin III – deficiency – homocysteinemia – antiphospholipid antibodies – thrombomodulin – prothrombin

Introduction

Thrombophilia is a tendency to thrombosis. The term is often used to indicate unusual features of the thrombosis and of the patient suffering the thrombosis: 1) early age of onset, 2) several recurrences, 3) strong family history, 4) unusual anatomical location or widespread extent, and 5) spontaneous occurrence without obvious predisposing factors, or severity out of proportion to the recognized stimulus. For such an "atypical" thrombosis the term "idiopathic" thrombosis is often used. In some patients laboratory work-up reveals abnormalities that may explain the occurrence of "idiopathic" thrombosis. These abnormalities can either be congenital, such as for example protein C- or protein S deficiency, or acquired, such as for example antiphospholipid antibodies (even though some of these may also be secondary to a congenital, familial predisposition).

Prior to 1993 the number of known hemostatic disorders predisposing to thrombosis explained only approximately 15–25 % of all idiopathic thromboses (Table 1). With the discovery of activated protein C resistance (APC-resistance) [26] the percentage of

Table 1. Prevalence of thrombophilic abnormalities

	Consecutive (unselected) patients with thrombosis	Thrombophilic (selected) patients with thrombosis
Protein C deficiency (5, 15, 48, 61, 96, 106)	3 %	1–9 %
Protein S deficiency (5, 15, 48, 61, 96, 106)	1–2 %	1–13 %
AT III deficiency (5, 15, 48, 61, 96, 106)	1 %	0.5–7 %
APC resistance (47, 62, 90, 93)	12–21 %	52 %
Homocysteinemia (19, 30, 37)	10–14 %	18.8 %
Antiphospholipid antibodies (43,103)	8.5–14 %	no studies available

idiopathic thromboses that can be explained by hemostatic defects has increased to approximately 50 to 75 % (Table 1). Homocysteine as a risk for venous thrombosis has, as of yet, not received very much attention [19, 30, 37, 75, 91]. If patients were more systematically screened for impairment of their homocysteine metabolism, more of the idiopathic thromboses may be explainable. The same is true for antiphospholipid antibodies. If the prevalence of 14 % in unselected patients presenting with venous thrombosis reported by Ginsberg et al. [43] is confirmed, then antiphospholipid antibodies may explain a significant number of the yet unexplainable idiopathic thromboses. With more frequent application of molecular genetic testing, new risk factors for venous thrombosis are being discovered. One such mutation is the prothrombin G20210A gene mutation, which has been found in 18 % of selected patients with venous thrombosis compared to 1 % of controls [84]. Thrombomodulin mutations have also recently been described [36, 80].

The more congenital risk factors we discover, the more it is becoming apparent that the development of venous thrombosis is multifactorial and often due to a combination of one or several cogenital risk factors and additional acquired influences, such as trauma, pregnancy, intake of oral contraceptives, malignancy, and immobility. Alone, many factors carry only a mild or modest risk for thrombosis. Together, they often exponentially increase the probability of thrombosis [14, 17, 23, 27, 29, 108, 112]. Two or multiple congenital risk factors may be present in one patient, presenting a "compound thrombophilia" [59, 70, 110, 114]. Such a combination often potentiates the risk for thrombosis. Due to the inheritance pattern of these risk factors, individual members of families with two or more risk factors will have different combinations of these risk factors; this could explain the varying clinical phenotype of thrombosis in individuals within one family.

By screening a patient and a patient's family members for the known risk factors, an individualized risk profiles may be determined. An eventual goal of the clinician will be to use these risk profiles to individualize anticoagulant treatment in respect to length and intensity of anticoagulation.

Prevalence of thrombophilic abnormalities

Among unselected, consecutive patients with objectively confirmed deep vein thrombosis, deficiencies of protein C, protein S, and antithrombin III combined account for approximately 5 % (Table 1) [48, 61]. APC-resistance is present in 20 % of consecutive patients with deep-vein thrombosis [62, 93]. Among selected thrombophilic patient groups reported prevalences are difficult to compare, because different inclusion critieria have been used. However, protein C, protein S, and antithrombin III deficiencies combined account for roughly 5 to 10 % in these patient groups and APC-resistance for approximately 50 % [5, 15, 47, 96, 106].

Hyperhomocysteinemia has been found to be present in 10–13.5 % of consecutive patients with venous thromboembolic disease [19, 30], and 18.8 % of young thrombophilic patients [37]. Only few studies exist on the prevalence of antiphospholipid antibodies in patients with venous thromboembolic disease. Antiphospholipid antibodies are of such heterogeneity that prevalence data are difficult to obtain. Two prospective studies found a prevalence of 8.5 % and 14 %, respectively, in unselected patients with venous thrombosis [43, 103].

Clinical aspects of individual disorders causing thrombophilia

Protein C-, protein S-, and antithrombin III-deficiency

Protein C-, protein S-, and antithrombin III-deficiency are the better known coagulation factor deficiencies that have been associated with venous thrombosis.

Protein C- and antithrombin III-deficiencies are classified into type I (reduction of both protein activity and antigen level, i.e., quantitative deficiency) and type II (reduced protein activity but normal antigen level, i.e., qualitative deficiency). Protein S circulates in plasma complexed with C4b-binding protein (~ 60 %) and as free protein S (~ 40 %) (Fig. 1). Only the free protein S has cofactor activity for activated protein C [24]. Protein S deficiencies are classified into three types (Fig. 1). The mutations leading to Protein C, protein S-, and antithrombin III-deficiency have been collected in data bases [40, 64, 89].

In family studies it has been shown that family members who are heterozygous for protein C deficiency have an increased risk of venous thrombosis (approximately 8 to 10-fold) and that by the age of 40 about half of them will have experienced at least one thrombotic event [3, 11]. For protein S deficiency it is very difficult to arrive at risk estimates since the prevalence in the general population is unknown and since there are no reports from family studies formally assessing the relative risk. While family-based studies have clearly shown that protein S is a risk factor for thrombosis [16, 21, 100], a large population-based case-control study did not find protein S deficiency to be a risk factor for thrombosis [61]. It has been speculated that this discrepancy might have arisen because

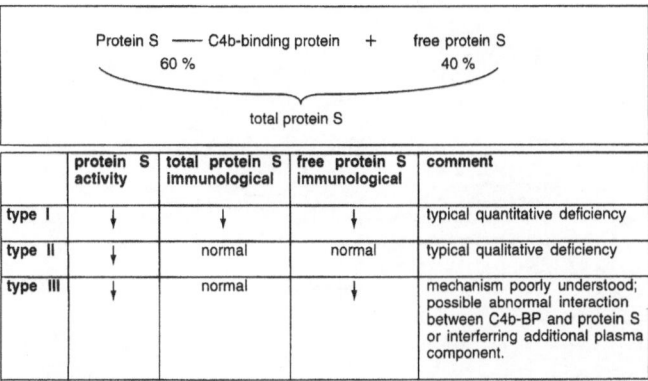

	protein S activity	total protein S immunological	free protein S immunological	comment
type I	↓	↓	↓	typical quantitative deficiency
type II	↓	normal	normal	typical qualitative deficiency
type III	↓	normal	↓	mechanism poorly understood; possible abnormal interaction between C4b-BP and protein S or interferring additional plasma component.

Fig. 1. Protein S in plasma and classification of protein S defficiencies.

of the low prevalence of protein S deficiency studied in that particular population [40] and also that the evidence that protein S deficiency causes thrombosis is much less solid than that for protein C deficiency [65]. Antithrombin III deficiency seems to confer a higher risk of thrombosis than deficiencies of protein C and S. Thrombosis often occurs at a young age and about half of the patients from reported families with antithrombin III deficiency experienced a thrombotic episode before the age of 25 [49, 109]. Antithrombin III deficiency especially has a much higher risk of thrombosis in pregnancy than deficiencies of protein C or S [22]. The fifty-fold difference in the prevalence of antithrombin deficiency in patients with a first episode of thrombosis and a healthy population [48, 107] also suggests a higher thrombotic risk in antithrombin III deficiency than in protein C deficiency although such a difference could not be substantiated in a population-based study [61].

Activated Protein C resistance

Activated protein C resistance (APC resistance) is caused by the inability of activated protein C to inactivate factor Va (Fig. 2) [51]. This may cause a thrombophilic state [26, 62, 105]. In more than 90 % of cases, APC resistance is caused by a single point mutation in the factor V gene, referred to as Factor V Leiden [6, 46, 113]. This mutation prevents activated protein C from binding to factor Va at aminoacid 506, the major cleavage site for the inactivation of factor Va [25]. Factor V Leiden is a very common mutation. Approximately 4 to 5 % of Caucasians are heterozygous and < 0.1 % are homozygous for this mutation, with some known racial and ethnic differences [88, 92]. In a population-based case-control study, APC-resistance was found in 21 % of patients with a first episode of deep vein thrombosis and in five percent of controls, which led to an estimated relative risk associated with APC-resistance of 7 [62]. Homozygous APC-resistance appears to be much less severe than homozygous protein C deficiency, since many homozygous individuals have remained free of thrombosis well into adult life [45, 93]. Still, the risk for thrombosis for those individuals homozygous for the mutation is approximately 10-fold higher than for those heterozygous, estimated to be increased 90-fold compared to individuals without the mutation [93]. There is no association with myocardial infarction or stroke [34, 35, 76, 90].

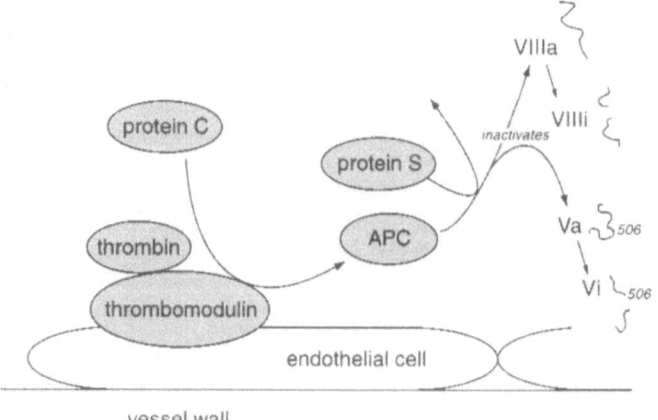

Fig. 2. Activation of protein C and function of activated protein C. APC = activated protein C; Va and VIIIa = activated factor V and VIII; Vi and VIIIi = inactivated factor V and VIII.

The observation that heterozygosity for factor V Leiden is very common but the relative risk of thrombosis it confers is modest infers that there must be additional factors contributing to the development of thrombosis. In keeping with this concept of multiple risk factors working in concert to lead to thrombosis ("compound thrombophilia"), Vandenbroucke et al. found that for women taking oral contraceptives the risk for venous thrombosis increased from 4-fold to 30-fold if they also had the factor V Leiden mutation [112]. Similarly, APC resistance magnifies the risk of thrombosis in patients with protein C deficiency [41,59], protein S deficiency [60,114], and antithrombin III deficiency [110]. Preliminary data show that the combination of factor V Leiden and the T677 allele of the methylenetetrahydrofolate reductase gene may be associated with a higher risk of venous thromboembolism [66], as may the combination of factor V Leiden and the prothrombin allele 20210A [71].

In protein C-, protein S-, and antithrombin-deficiency 32 % to 50 % of the venous thrombotic episodes occur when other risk factors are concomitantly present (surgery, immobilization, pregnancy) [14, 17, 27, 29]. In individuals with APC-resistance, the need for the existence of such risk factors appears to be greater (approximately 60 %) than for other thrombophilic syndromes [36, 115].

Patients who are heterozygous for factor V Leiden have the same risk for recurrent venous thromboembolism after discontinuation of anticoagulation as other patients with idiopathic thrombosis [33]. Of 380 patients with venous thromboembolism studied by Eichinger et al., 29.5 % were carriers of factor V Leiden. After a median observation time of 19 months the patients with factor V Leiden had the same recurrence rate as the patient group without factor V Leiden [33].

Antiphospholipid antibodies

Antiphospholipid antibodies are acquired antibodies directed against phospholipids or phospholipid-binding proteins [95]. They are risk factors for venous [43, 56, 94, 103] and arterial [1, 57, 68] thrombosis. The term "lupus anticoagulant" refers to the subgroup of antiphospholipid antibodies in which one or several of the coagulation screening tests (prothrombin time, activated prothrombin time, dilute Russell viper venom time) are prolonged and where the prolongation can be overcome by the addition of extra phospholipids. The term "anticardiolipin antibodies" refers to the subgroup of antiphospholipid antibodies that are detected with a cardiolipin-coated ELISA plate.

Antiphospholipid antibodies are of particular clinical importance, firstly, because patients with these antibodies have a high rate of recurrence of thrombosis when anticoagulation is discontinued [31, 56, 68, 85, 86] and, secondly, because some of these patients have recurrent thromboses inspite of what is considered "therapeutic" anticoagulation in patients with venous thrombosis who do not have antiphospholipid antibodies, i.e., an international normalized ratio of 2–3 [56].

The risk of recurrence of venous thromboembolism after discontinuation of oral anticoagulation in patients with antiphospholipid antibodies is much higher than in patients without these antibodies. Prandoni et al. found a recurrence rate of 45 % in 20 patients over a period of slightly more than 6 years [85], Rosove and Brewer a recurrence rate of 53 % in a five-year follow-up of 70 patients [94], Derksen et al. [31] in a study of 19 patients a 50 % probability of recurrent venous thromboembolism at two years, and a 78 % probability of recurrence at eight years, and Khamashta et al. [56] a recurrence rate of approximately 80 % at 8 years.

This high rate of recurrence warrants long-term and possibly indefinite anticoagulants treatment in many of these patients. The optimal level of anticoagulation for patients with antiphospholipid antibodies who have sustained a venous thromboembolic event is controversial [43, 56, 77, 87, 94]. Rosove and Brewer recommended that the INR be maintained at 2.6 [94], Ginsberg et al. [43] recommended an INR of 2.0 to 3.0, and Khamastha an INR of 3.0 or above [56]. Moll et al. showed, however, that the INR is invalid for patients with lupus anticoagulants: some lupus anticoagulants lead to a prolongation of the prothrombin time and, in the anticoagulated patient, lead to INRs that do not reflect the true level of anticoagulation [77]. The authors conclude that all previous therapeutic recommendations based on the INR needed to be reconsidered and that patients with lupus anticoagulants need to be monitored with tests insensitive to lupus anticoagulants, for example, chromogenic factor X levels or the Prothrombin-Proconvertin time.

Homocysteinemia

It has been known for several years that elevated plasma homocysteine levels are a risk factor for coronary [20, 32, 42, 81, 83, 104], cerebrovascular [4, 9, 13, 101], and peripheral [9, 20, 73] arteriosclerosis. Boers et al. pooled data up to 1994 from a total of 750 vascular patients and 200 control subjects; hyperhomocysteinemia was detected in 21 % of patients with coronary artery disease, 24 % of patients with cerebrovascular disease, 32 % of patients with peripheral artery disease, and 2 % of the control subjects [8].

That homocysteinemia is also a risk factor for venous thromboembolism has only emerged in the last few years [19, 30, 37, 75, 91]. Falcon et al. compared a group of 80 young patients with venous thromboembolic disease with 51 controls and found a positive association between elevated homocysteine levels and venous thrombosis [37]. Similar results were found by den Heijer et al., comparing 269 patients with deep vein thrombosis with 269 controls [30], and by Cattaneo et al., comparing 89 patients with deep vein thrombosis with 89 controls [19]. Mandel et al. found that patients with concurrent homocystinuria and factor V Leiden have an increased risk of thrombosis [75]. Ridker et al. observed that men with hyperhomocysteinemia who also have factor V Leiden are at significantly increased risk for developing future venous thromboembolic events compared with men with neither or only one of these abnormalities [91].

Plasma homocysteine levels are influenced by the activity levels of several enzymes and cofactors involved in its metabolism (Fig. 3). It has been known for many years that homocystinuria in children is caused by a congenital deficiency of cystathionine-β-synthase [78]. Known reasons for less severely elevated levels of homocysteine are dietary deficiencies of folic acid [18, 32, 53, 102], vitamin B_6 [102], and vitamin B_{12} [12, 102], enzymatic deficiency of cystathionine-β-synthase [9, 20, 32], and decreased activity of methylenetetrahydrofolate reductase (MTHFR) [28, 39, 52, 69, 99]. The latter is frequently caused by a polymorphism of the MTHFR enzyme, the C677T allele, which renders the enzyme thermolabile and decreased in its activity [39, 54, 55]. Five to seventeen percent of the normal population are homozygous for this polymorphism [28, 39, 58, 69, 99]. While several studies have shown an association of this polymorphism with arteriosclerotic disease [54, 58, 99], others have not been able to corroborate these findings [7, 28, 69].

The finding that elevated homocysteine levels are a risk factor for arteriosclerosis and clinical events caused by arteriosclerosis (myocardial infarction, death, ischemic stroke), and also for venous thromboembolism is of utmost interest for the clinician, since elevated homocysteine levels can be lowered and even normalized in a large proportion of patients through treatment with folic acid, vitamin B_6, and betaine [13, 38, 44, 63, 72, 74]. Whether such lowering slows the rate of progression of arteriosclerosis or decreases thromboembolic events is not known yet. It is exciting to speculate that it may. In a study

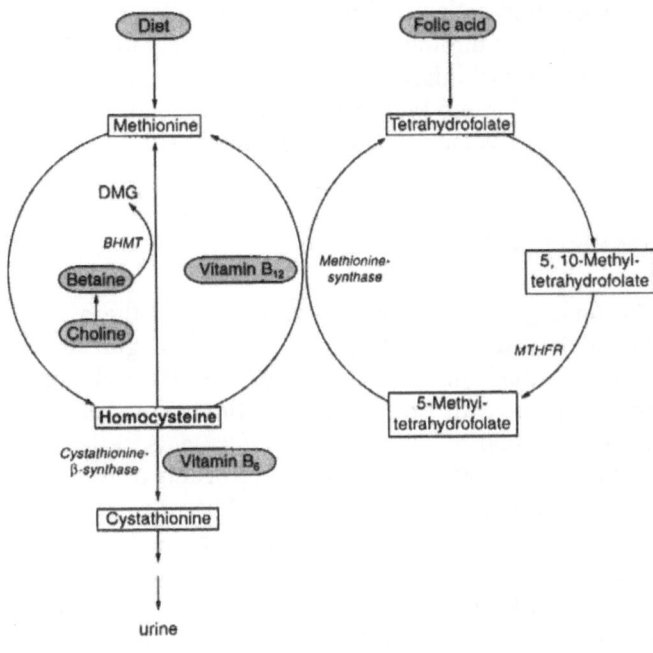

Fig. 3. Homocysteine metabolism and points of action of vitamins. MTHR = methylenetetrahydrofolate reductase; BHMT = betaine homocysteine-methyltransferase; DMG = dimethylglycine.

by Graham et al. on plasma homocysteine as a risk factor for vascular disease, a small group of individuals taking vitamin supplements had a substantially lower risk of vascular disease than a group of individuals not taking such vitamins [44]. Prospective, randomized studies with homocysteine-lowering therapy will have to be awaited. One such study, in which the benefit of therapy with folic acid, vitamin B_6, and vitamin B_{12} on stroke recurrence rate is being assessed, is presently being performed [2].

Thrombomodulin abnormalities

Thrombomodulin is a component of the anticoagulant pathway (Fig. 2). It is a transmembrane protein synthesized by endothelial cells which acts as a receptor for thrombin and as a cofactor of thrombin in the activation of protein C. Plasma is not an abundant source of thrombomodulin, except at times of endothelial cell damage [10]. Activity assays, such as used to diagnose protein C-, protein S-, or antithrombin III-deficiency, can therefore not be used to diagnose thrombomodulin defects.

Van der Velden et al. did not find an association between the common C/T thrombomodulin dimorphism at nucleotide 1418, which predicts an Ala or Val in position 455, and venous thrombosis [111]. The first mutation in the thrombomodulin gene associated with venous thromboembolic disease was reported by Ohlin et al. in 1995 [82]: a patient with pulmonary embolism was found to have a G1456T thrombomodulin gene mutation. Faioni et al. did not find the G1456T mutation in any of 100 Italian patients with venous thromboembolic disease [36]. Norlund et al. described another patient with venous thromboembolic disease with a thrombomodulin mutation (G127A) [80].

In regard to arterial events, Norlund et al. found that the C allele of the C/T dimorphism of the thrombomodulin gene at nucleotide 1418, leading to Ala/Val[455], was associated with premature myocardial infarction [79]. However, Ireland et al. did not find such an association in patients with myocardial infarction [50]. The latter authors also found three different thrombomodulin mutations in five patients of the group of 104 patients with myocardial infarction. Only one of these mutations was present in one patient of their control group [50], suggesting that mutations in the thrombomodulin gene may constitute a risk factor for arterial thrombosis.

Treatment issues

The findings of three important studies within the last two years provide some guidance in the decision on the length of oral anticoagulant therapy in patients with venous thromboembolism. In the first study, Schulman et al. compared six weeks with six months of treatment with oral anticoagulation in patients with a first episode of venous thromboembolism [98]. The group of patients treated for six months had a lower rate of recurrence of venous thromboembolism at two years (9. 5 % versus 18. 1 %). The difference between the two groups occurred between 6 weeks and 6 months after the start of treatment, and the rates of recurrence remained nearly parallel for 1 1/2 years thereafter. In the second study, Levine et al. found that patients with venous thromboembolism after transient risk factors (surgery) had only a very small risk of recurrent disease after discontinuation of a four week treatment period with oral anticoagulants, whereas patients with persisting risk factors had a significantly higher recurrence rate even after three months of treatment [67]. In the third study, Schulman et al. examined the length of time of oral anticoagulation in patients with recurrent venous thromboembolism and compared six months of treatment with indefinite treatment [97]. The latter group had a significantly lower rethrombosis rate than the six months therapy group (2.6 % versus 20.7 % after 4 years). The special considerations necessary in treating patients with antiphospholipid antibodies have been mentioned above.

The studies allow the following conclusions:

1. Patients with venous thromboembolism with transient risk factors, such as surgery, only require short-term anticoagulation. Four weeks may possibly be sufficient.
2. Most patients with permanent risk factors (idiopathic thrombosis, positive family history, protein deficiencies or dysfunctions) should be anticoagulated for six months after a venous thromboembolic event. Longer treatment may be necessary for some patients with multiple risk factors.
3. Patients with permanent risk factors who have already had two or more episodes of venous thromboembolism should be treated long-term with anticoagulation and possibly indefinitely. It is possible that a lower target INR than 2–3 may be sufficient to prevent recurrence of thromboembolism after six months of full anticoagulation. However, studies examining this approach have not been reported yet.
4. An international normalized ratio (INR) of 2–3 is the target INR range in most patients.
5. Patients with antiphospholipid antibodies need to be treated for prolonged periods of time. Their INR may not be an accurate measure of their level of anticoagulation and they may have to be followed by a test insensitive to antiphospholipid antibodies.

In spite of the results of the quoted studies, the choice on the length and intensity of treatment will remain a decision that has to be tailored to the individual patient, the patient's individual congenital and acquired risk factors, the circumstances of the thromboembolic event, the patient's lifestyle, the accompanying diseases, and the patient's individual bleeding risk. More individual risk stratification based on a patient's individual risk profile may in the future allow less generalized, but more individual recommendations on the length and intensity of treatment with anticoagulants.

Appendix

A paper published since submission of this manuscript describes a significantly higher rate of recurrence of deep vein thrombosis in patients with APC-resistance compared to patients without it, once oral anticoagulation has been discontinued [116]. A study is clearly needed to evaluate whether patients with APC resistance and venous thrombosis should receive anticoagulant treatment for a longer period of time than patiens without APC resistance.

References

1. The antiphospholipid antibodies in stroke study group (1990) Clinical and laboratory findings in patients with antiphospholipid antibodies and cerebral ischemia. Stroke 21: 1268–1273
2. Vitamin intervention study for stroke prevention (VISP) (1997) (study announcement). Stroke 28: 1304
3. Alaart CF, Poort SR, Rosendaal FR, Reitsma PH, Bertina RM, Briët E (1993) Increased risk of venous thrombosis in carriers of hereditary protein C deficiency defect. Lancet 341: 134–138
4. Araki A, Sako Y, Fukushima Y, Matsumoto M, Asada T, Kita T (1989) Plasma sulfhydryl-containing amino acids in patients with cerebral infarction and in hypertensive subjects. Atherosclerosis 79: 139–146
5. Ben Tal O, Zivelin A, Seligsohn U (1989) The relative frequency of hereditary thrombotic disorders among 107 patients with thrombophilia in Israel. Thromb Haemost 61: 50–54
6. Bertina RM, Koelemann BPC, Koster T, Rosendaal FR, Dirven, RJ, de Ronde H, van der Velden PA, Reitsma PH (1994) Mutation in blood coagulation factor V associated with resistance to activated protein C. Nature 369: 64
7. Bockxmeer FM, Mamotte CDS, Vasikaran SD, Taylor RR (1997) Methylentetrahydrofolate reductase gene and coronary artery disease. Circulation 95: 21–23
8. Boers GHJ (1994) Hyperhomocysteinemia: a newly recognized risk factor for vascular disease. Neth J Med 45: 34–41
9. Boers GHJ, Smals AGH, Trijbels FJM, Fowler B, Bakkeren JAJM, Schoonderwaldt HC, Kleijer WJ, Kloppenborg PWC (1985) Heterozygosity for homocysteinuria in premature peripheral and cerebral occlusive arterial disease. N Engl J Med 313: 709–715
10. Boffa MC, Karochkine M, Berard M (1991) Plasma thrombomodulin as a marker of endothelium damage. Nouv Rev Fr Hematol 33: 529–530
11. Bovill EG, Bauer KA, Dickerman JD, Callas P, West B (1989) The clinical spectrum of heterozygous protein C deficiency in a large New England kindred. Blood 73: 712–717
12. Brattström L, Israelsson B, Lindegarde F, Hultberg B (1988) Higher total plasma homocysteine in vitamin B12 deficiency than in heterozygosity for homocysteinuria due to cystathionine β-synthase. Metabolism 37: 175–178
13. Brattström L, Israelsson B, Norrving B, Berqvist D, Thörne J, Hultberg B, Hamfelt A (1990) Impaired homocysteine metabolism in early-onset cerebral and peripheral occlusive arterial disease: effects of pyridoxine and folic acid treatment. Atherosclerosis 81: 51–60
14. Briët E, Broekmans AW (1988) Hereditary protein S deficiency. In: Bertina RM (ed) Protein C and Related Proteins. Edinburgh, Churchill Livingstone, pp 203
15. Briët E, Engesser L, Brommer EJP, Broekmans AW, Bertina RM (1987) Thrombophilia: Its causes and a rough estimate of its prevalence. Thromb Haemost 58: 39
16. Broekmans AW, Bertina RM, Reinalda Poot J, Engesser L, Muller HP, Leeuw JA, Michiels JJ, Brommer EJ, Briët E (1985) Hereditary protein S deficiency and venous thrombo-embolism. A study in three Dutch families. Thromb Haemost 53: 273–277
17. Broekmans AW, Conrad J (1988) Hereditary protein C deficiency. In: Bertina RM (ed) Protein C and Related proteins. Edinburgh, Churchill Livingstone, pp 160
18. Carey MC, Fennelly JJ, Fitzgerald O (1968) Homocysteinuria. II. Subnormal serum folate levels, increased folate clearance and effects of folic acid therapy. Am J Med 45: 26–31
19. Cattaneo M, Martinelli I, Mannucci PM (1996) Hyperhomocysteinemia as a risk factor for deep vein thrombosis. N Engl J Med 335: 974 –975
20. Clarke R, Daly L, Robinson K, Naughten E, Cahalane S, Fowler B, Graham I (1991) Hyperhomocysteinemia: An independent risk factor for vascular disease. N Engl J Med 324: 1149–55

21. Comp PC, Esmon CT (1984) Recurrent thromboembolism in patients with a partial deficiency of protein S. N Engl J Med 311: 1525–1528
22. Conrad J, Horellou MH, Van Dreden P, Lecompte T, Samama M (1990) Thrombosis and pregnancy in congenital deficiencies in ATIII, protein C, or protein S: Study of 78 women. Thromb Haemost 63: 319–320
23. Daeninck PJ, Johnston JB, Carson N, Israels SJ (1997) Coexistence of antiphospholipid syndrome and hyperhomocysteinemia in a family with thrombosis. Thromb Haemost: p 337; PS-1384
24. Dahlbäck B (1986) Inhibition of protein Ca cofactor function of human and bovine protein S by C4b-binding protein. J Biol Chem 261: 12022–12027
25. Dahlbäck B (1995) Inherited thrombophilia: Resistance to activated protein C as a pathogenic factor of venous thromboembolism. Blood 85: 607–614
26. Dahlbäck B, Carlsson M, Svensson PJ (1993) Familial thrombophilia due to a previously unrecognized mechanism characterized by poor anticoagulant response to activated protein C: Prediction of a cofactor to activated protein C. Proc Natl Acad Sci USA 90: 1004 –1008
27. de Stefano V, Leone G, Mastrangelo S, Tripodi A, Rodeghiero F, Castaman G, Barbui T, Finazzi G, Bizzi B, Mannucci PM (1994) Clinical manifestations and management of inherited thromobophilia: Retrospective analysis and follow-up after diagnosis of 238 patients with congenital deficiency of antithrombin-III, protein C, protein S. Thromb Haemost 72: 352–358
28. Delougherty TG, Evans A, Sadeghi A, McWilliams J, Henner WD, Taylor LM Jr., Press RD (1996) Common mutation in methylenetetrahydrofolate reductase. Correlation with homocysteine metabolism and late-onset vascular disease. Circulation 94: 3074–8
29. Demers C, Ginsberg JS, Hirsh J, Henderson P, Blajchman MA (1992) Thrombosis in antithrombi-III-deficient persons. Report of a large kindred and literature review. Ann Intern Med 116: 754 –761
30. den Heijer M, Koster T, Blom HJ, Bos GM, Briët E, Reitsma PH, Vandenbroucke JP, Rosendaal FR (1996) Hyperhomocysteinemia as a risk factor for deep-vein thrombosis. N Engl J Med 334: 759– 62
31. Derksen RHWM, de Groot PG, Kater L, Nieuwenhuis HK (1993) Patients with antiphospholipid antibodies and venous thrombosis should receive long term anticoagulant treatment. Ann Rheum Dis 52: 689–692
32. Dudman NPB, Wilcken DEL, Wang J, Lynch JF, Macey D, Lundberg P (1993) Disordered methionine/homocysteine metabolism in premature vascular disease. Its occurrence, cofactor therapy, and enzymology. Arterioscler Thromb 13: 1253–1260
33. Eichinger S, Pabinger I, Stümpflen A, Hirschl M, Bialonczyk C, Schneider B, Mannhalter C, Minar E, Lechner K, Kyrle PA (1997) The risk of recurrent venous thromboembolism in patients with and without factor V Leiden. Thromb Haemost 77: 624–628
34. Emmerich J, Alhenc-Gelas M, Aillaud MF et al. (1997) Clinical features in 36 patients homozygous for the Arg 506-Gln factor V mutation. Thromb Haemost 77: 620–623
35. Emmerich J, Poirier O, Evans A et al. (1995) Myocardial infarction, Arg506 to Gln factor V mutation, and activated protein C resistance. Lancet 345: 321
36. Faioni EM, Merati G, Peyvandi F, Bettini PM, Mannucci PM (1997) The G(1456) to T mutation in the thrombomodulin gene is not frequent in patients with venous thrombosis. Blood 89: 1467
37. Falcon CR, Cattaneo M, Panzeri D, Martinelli I, Mannucci PM (1994) High prevalence of hyperhomocyst(e)inemia in patients with juvenile venous thrombosis. Arterioscler Thromb 14: 1080–1083
38. Franken DG, Boers GHJ, Blom HJ, Trijbels FJM, Kloppenborg PWC (1994) Treatment of mild hyperhomocysteinemia in vascular disease patients. Arterioscler Thromb 14: 465–470
39. Frosst P, Blom HJ, Milos R, Goyette P, Sheppard CA, Matthews RG, Boers GJ, den Heijer M, Kluijtmans LA, van den Heuvel LP, Rozen R (1995) A candidate genetic risk factor for vascular disease: a common mutation in methylenetetrahydrofolate reductase [letter]. Nat Genet 10: 111–3
40. Gandrille S, Borgel D, Ireland H, Lane DA, Simmonds R, Reitsma PH, Mannhalter C, Pabinger I, Saito H, Suzuki K, Formstone C, Copper DN, Espinosa Y, Sala N, Bernardi F, Aiach M (1997) Protein S deficiency: A database of mutations. Thromb Haemost 77: 1201–1214
41. Gandrille S, Greengard JS, Alhenc-Gelas M, Juhan-Vague M, Abgrall JF, Jude B, Griffin JH, Aiach M (1995) Incidence of activated protein C resistance caused by the Arg 506 Gln mutation in factor V in 113 unrelated symptomatic protein C-deficient patients. Blood 86: 219–224
42. Genest JJ Jr., McNamara JR, Salem DN, Wilson PW, Schaefer EJ, Malinow MR (1990) Plasma homocyst(e)ine levels in men with premature coronary artery disease. J Am Coll Cardiol 16: 1114–9
43. Ginsberg JS, Wells PS, Brill Edwards P, Donovan D, Moffatt K, Johnston M, Stevens P, Hirsh J (1995) Antiphospholipid antibodies and venous thromboembolism. Blood 86: 3685–91
44. Graham IM, Daly LE, Refsum HM, Robinson K, Brattström LE, Ueland PM, Palma-Reis RJ, Boers GHJ, Sheahan RG, Israelsson B, Uiterwaal CS, Meleady R, McMaster D, Verhoef P et al. (1997) Plasma Homocysteine as a risk factor for vascular disease. JAMA 277: 1775–1781
45. Greengard JS, Eichinger S, Griffin JH, Bauer KA (1994) Variability of thrombosis among homozygous siblings with resistance to activated protein C due to Arg-Gln mutation in the gene for factor V. N Engl J Med 331: 1559–1562
46. Greengard JS, Sun X, Xu X, Fernandez JA, Griffin JH, Evatt B (1994) Activated protein C resistance caused by Arg506Gln mutation in factor Va. Lancet 343: 1361
47. Griffin JH, Evatt B, Wideman C, A. FJ (1993) Antocoagulant protein C pathway defective in majority of thrombophilic patients. Blood 82: 1989–1993
48. Heijboer H, Brandjes DP, Buller HR, Sturk A, ten Cate JW (1990) Deficiencies of coagulation-inhibiting and fibrinolytic proteins in outpatients with deep vein thrombosis. N Engl Med 323: 1512–1516

49. Hirsh J, Piovella F, Pini M(1989) Congenital antithrombin III deficiency. Incidence and clinical features. Am J Med 87: 34S-38S
50. Ireland H, Kunz G, Kyriakoulis K, Stubbs PJ, Lane DA (1997) Thrombomodulin gene mutations associated with myocardial infarction. Circulation 96: 15-18
51. Kalafatis M, Haley PE, Lu D, Bertina RM, Long GL, Mann KG (1996) Proteolytic events that regulate factor V activity in whole plasma from normal and activated protein C(APC)-resistant individuals during clotting: an insight into the APC-resistance assay. Blood 87: 4695-4707
52. Kang SS, Passen EL, Ruggie N, Wong PWK, Sora H (1993) Thermolabile defect of methylenetetrahydrofolate reductase in coronary artery disease. Circulation 88: 1463-1469
53. Kang SS, Wong PW, Norusis M (1987) Homocysteinemia due to folate deficiency. Metabolism 36: 458-462
54. Kang SS, Wong PWK, Bock HG, Horwitz A, Grix A (1993) Intermediate homocyst(e)inemia resulting from compound heterozygosity of methylentetrahydrofolate reductase mutations. Am J Hum Genet 53: 899
55. Kang SS, Wong PWK, Susmano A, Sora J, Norusis M, Ruggie N (1991) Thermolabile methylenetetrahydrofolate reductase: an inherited risk factor for coronary artery disease. Am J Human Genet 48: 536-545
56. Khamashta MA, Cuadrado MJ, Mujic F, Taub NA, Hunt BJ, Hughes GRV (1995) The management of thrombosis in the antiphospholipid-antibody syndrome. N Engl J Med 332: 993-7
57. Kittner SJ, Gorelick PB (1992) Antiphospholipid antibodies and stroke: An epidemiological perspective. Stroke 23: 119-122
58. Kluijtmans LAJ, van de Heuvel LPWJ, Boers GHJ, Frosst P, Stevens EMB, van Oost BA, Den Heijer M, Trijbels JMF, Rosen R, Blom HJ (1996) Molecular genetic analysis in mild hyperhomocysteinemia.
59. Koeleman BP, Reitsma PH, Allaart CF, Bertina RM (1994) Activated protein C resistance as an additional risk factor for thrombosis in protein C-deficient families. Blood 84: 1031-1035
60. Koeleman BPC, van Rumpf D, Hamulyak K, Reitsma PH, Bertina RM (1995) Factor V Leiden: an additional risk factor for thrombosis in protein S deficient families? Thromb Haemost 74: 580-583
61. Koster T, Rosendaal FR, Briët E et al. (1995) Protein C deficiency in a controlled series of unselected outpatients: an infrequent but clear risk factor for venous thrombosis (Leiden Thrombophilia Study). Blood 85: 2756-61
62. Koster T, Rosendaal FR, de Ronde H, Briët E, Vandenbroucke JP, Bertina RM (1993) Venous thrombosis due to poor anticoagulant response to activated protein C: Leiden Thrombophilia Study. Lancet 342
63. Landgren F, B.I, Lindgren A, Hultberg B (1995) Plasma homocysteine in acute myocardial infarction: Homocysteinelowering effect of folic acid. J Intern Med 237: 381-388
64. Lane DA, Bayston T, Olds RJ, Fitches AC, Cooper DN, Millar DS, Jochmans K, Perry DJ, Okajima K, Thein SL, Emmerich J (1997) Antithrombin mutation database: 2nd (1997) update. For the Plasma Coagulation Inhibitors Subcommittee of the Scientific and Standardization Committee of the International Society of Thrombosis and Haemostasis. Thromb Haemost 77: 197-211
65. Lane DA, Mannucci PM, Bauer KA, Betina RM, Bochkov NP, Boulyjenkov V, Chandy M, Dahlback B, Ginter EK, Miletich JP, Rosendaal FR, Seligsohn U (1996) Inherited thrombophilia: Part 1. Thromb Haemost 76: 651-662
66. Le Cam-Duchez V, Gandrille S, Alhenc-Gelas M, Emmerich J, Borg JY, Aiach M (1997) Additional genetic risk factors for thrombosis in 21 families carrying the factor V Arg 506 Gln mutation (abstract). Thromb Haemost: p165; SC-671
67. Levine MN, Hirsh J, Gent M, Turpie AG, Weitz J, Ginsberg J, Geerts W, LeClerc J, Neemeh J, Powers P et al. (1995) Optimal duration of oral anticoagulant therapy: A randomized trial comparing four weeks with three months of warfarin in patients with proximal deep vein thrombosis. Thromb Haemost 74: 606-11
68. Levine SR, Brey RL, Joseph CLM, Havstad S (1992) Risk of recurrent thrombocembolic events in patients with focal cerebral ischemia and antiphospholipid antibodies. Stroke 23: I29-I32
69. Ma J, Stampfer MJ, Hennekens CH, Frosst P, Selhub J, Horsford J, Malinow MR, Willett WC, Rozen R (1996) Methylenetetrahydrofolate reductase polymorphism, plasma folate, homocysteine, and risk of myocardial infarction in US physicians. Circulation 94: 2410-6
70. Makris M, Preston FE, Beauchamp NJ, Hampton KK, Daly ME, Cooper P, Bayliss P, Peake IR (1997) Conheritance of the 20210A allele of the prothrombin gene increases the thrombotic risk in subjects with familial thrombophilia. Thromb Haemost: p165; SC-672
71. Makris M, Preston FE, Beauchamp NJ, Hampton KK, Daly ME, Cooper P, Bayliss P, Peake IR (1997) Co-inheritance of the 20210A allele of the prothrombin gene increases the thrombotic risk in subjects with familial thrombophilia (abstract). Thromb Haemost: p165; SC-672
72. Malinow MR(1990) Hyperhomocyst(e)inemia. A common and easily reversible risk factor for occlusive atherosclerosis. Circulation 81: 2004-6
73. Malinow MR, Kang SS, Taylor LM, Wong PW, Coull B, Inahara T, Mukerjee D, Sexton G, Upson B (1989) Prevalence of hyperhomocyst(e)inemia in patients with peripheral arterial occlusive disease. Circulation 79: 1180-8
74. Malinow MR, Nieto FJ, Kruger WD, Duell PB, Hess DL, Gluckman RA, Block PC, Holzgang CR, Anderson PH, Seltzer D, Upson B, Lin QR (1997) The effects of folic acid supplementation on plasma total homocysteine are modulated by multivitamin use and methylenetetrahydrofolate reductase genotypes. Arterioscler Thromb Vasc Biol 17: 1157-1162
75. Mandel H, Brenner B, Berant M, Rosenberg N, Lanir N, Jakobs C, Fowler B, Seligsohn U (1996) Coexistence of hereditary homocystinuria and factor V Leiden-effect on thrombosis. N Engl J Med 334: 763-8

76. März W, Seydewitz H, Winkelmann B, Chen M, Nauck M, Witt I (1995) Mutation in coagulation factor V associated with resistance to activated protein C in patients with coronary artery disease. Lancet 345: 526–527
77. Moll S, Ortel TL (1997) Monitoring warfarin therapy in patients with lupus anticoagulants. Ann Intern Med 127: 177–185
78. Mudd SH, Levy HL, Skovby F (1989) Disorders of transsulfuration. In: Scriver CR, Beadet AL, Sly WS, Valle D (eds) The metabolic basis of inherited disease. New York, N.Y.: McGraw-Hill Publishing Co., pp 693–734
79. Norlund L, Holm J, Zöller B, Öhlin AK (1997) A common thrombomodulin amino acid dimorphism is associated with myocardial infarction. Thromb Haemost 77: 248–251
80. Norlund L, Holm J, Zöller B, Öhlin AK (1997) A novel thrombomodulin gene mutation in a patient suffering from severe venous thrombosis (abstract). Thromb Haemost: p549; PS-2248
81. Nygard O, Nordrehaug JE, Refsum H, Ueland PM, Farstad M, Vollset SE (1997) Plasma homocysteine levels and mortality in patients with coronary artery disease. N Engl J Med 337: 230–236
82. Ohlin AK, Marlar RA (1995) The first thrombomodulin mutation identified in the thrombomodulin gene in a 45 year old man presenting with thromboembolic disease. Blood 85: 330–336
83. Pels K, Schoebel FC, Stein D, Jax TW, Heins M, Behnke R, Reinauer H, Strauer BE, Leschke M (1997) Homocystein. Bedeutung für Schweregrad und Ausmass der Koronarsklerose bei angiographisch definierter koronarer Herzkrankheit. Münch med Wschr 139: 149–153
84. Poort SR, Rosendaal FR, Reitsma PH, Bertina RM (1996) A common genetic variation in the 3'-untranslated region of the prothrombin gene is associated with elevated plasma prothrombin levels and an increase in venous thrombosis. Blood 88: 3698–3703
85. Prandoni P, Simioni P, Girolami A (1996) Antiphospholipid antibodies, recurrent thromboembolism, and intensity of warfarin anticoagulation [letter]. Thromb Haemost 75: 859
86. Rance A, Emmerich J, Fiessinger JN (1997) Anticardiolipin antibodies and recurrent thromboembolism. Thromb Haemost 77: 212–224
87. Rapaport SI, Le DT (1995) Thrombosis in the antiphospholipid syndrome (letter). N Engl J Med 333: 993
88. Rees DC, Cox M, Clegg JB (1995) World distribution of factor V Leiden. Lancet 346: 1133–1134
89. Reitsma PH, Bernadi F, Doig RG, Gandrille S, Greengard JS, Ireland H, Krawczak M, Lind B, Long GL, Poort SR, Saito H, Sala N, Witt I, Cooper D (1995) Protein C deficiency: A database of mutations, 1995 update. Thromb Haemost 73: 876–889
90. Ridker PM, Hennekens CH, Lindpaintner K, Stampfer MJ, Eisenberg PR, Miletich JP (1995) Mutation in the gene coding for factor V and the risk of myocardial infarction, stroke, venous thrombosis in apparently healthy men. N Engl J Med 332: 912–917
91. Ridker PM, Hennekens CH, Selhub J, Miletich JP, Malinow MR, Stampfer MJ (1997) Interrelation of hyperhomocyst(e)inemia, factor V Leiden, and risk of future venous thromboembolism. Circulation 95: 1777–1782
92. Ridker PM, Miletich JP, Hennekens CH, Buring JE (1997) Ethnic distribution of factor V Leiden in 4047 men and women: Implications for venous thromboembolism screening. JAMA 277: 1305–1307
93. Rosendaal FR, Koster T, Vandenbroucke JP, Reitsma PH (1995) High risk of thrombosis in patients homozygous for factor V Leiden (activated protein C resistance). Blood 85: 1504–8
94. Rosove MH, Brewer PMC (1992) Antiphospholipid thrombosis: clinical course after the first thrombotic event in 70 patients. Ann Int Med 117: 303–308
95. Roubey R (1994) Autoantibodies to phospholipid-binding plasma proteins: a new view of lupus anticoagulants and other "antiphospholipid" autoantibodies. Blood 84: 2854–2867
96. Scharrer I, Hach-Wunderle V, Heyland H, Kuhn C (1987) Incidence of defective tPA release in 158 unrelated young patients with venous thrombosis in comparison to PC-, PS-, ATIII-, fibrinogen-, and plasminogen deficiency. Thromb Haemost 58: 72
97. Schulman S, Granqvist S, Holmstrom M, Carlsson A, Lindmarker P, Nicol P, Eklund SG, Nordlander S, Larfars G, Leijd B, Linder O, Loogna E (1997) The duration of oral anticoagulant therapy after a second episode of venous thromboembolism. The Duration of Anticoagulation Trial Study Group. N Engl J Med 336: 393–8
98. Schulman S, Rhedin AS, Lindmarker P, Carlsson A, Larfars G, Nicol P, Loogna E, Svensson E, Ljungberg B, Walter H et al. (1995) A comparison of six weeks with six months of oral anticoagulant therapy after a first episode of venous thromboembolism. Duration of Anticoagulation Trial Study Group. N Engl J Med 332: 1661–5
99. Schwartz SM, Siscovick DS, Malinow R, Rosendaal FR, Beverly RK, Hess DL, Psaty BM, Longstreth WT, Koepsell TD, Raghunathan TE, Reitsma PH (1997) Myocardial infarction in young women in relation to plasma total homocysteine, folate, and a common variant in the methylenetetrahydrofolate reductase gene. Circulation 96: 412–417
100. Schwarz HP, Fischer M, Hopmeier P, Batard MA, Griffin JH (1984) Plasma protein S deficiency in familial thrombotic disease. Blood 64: 1297–1300
101. Selhub J, Jacques PF, Bostom AG, D'Agostino RB, Wilson PW, Belanger AJ, O'Leary DH, Wolf PA, Schaefer EJ, Rosenberg IH (1995) Association between plasma homocysteine concentrations and extracranial carotid-artery stenosis. N Engl J Med 332: 286–91
102. Selhub J, Jacques PF, Wilson PW, Rush D, Rosenberg IH (1993) Vitamin status and intake as primary determinants of homocysteinemia in an elderly population [see comments]. JAMA 270: 2693–8

103. Simioni P, Prandoni P, Zanon E, Saracino MA, Scudeller A, Villalta S, Scarano L, Girolami B, Benedetti L, Girolami A (1996) Deep venous thrombosis and lupus anticoagulant. A casecontrol study. Thromb Haemost 76: 187–9

104. Stampfer MJ, Malinow MR, Willett WC, Newcomer LM, Upson B, Ullmann D, Tishler PV, Hennekens CH (1992) A prospective study of plasma homocyst(e)ine and risk of myocardial infarction in US Physicians. JAMA 268: 877–81

105. Svensson PJ, Dahlbäck B (1994) Resistance to activated protein C as a basis for venous thrombosis. N Engl J Med 330: 517–522

106. Tabernero MD, Tomas JF, Alberca I, Orfao A, Lopez Borrasca A, Vicente V (1991) Incidence and clinical characteristics of hereditary disorders associated with venous thrombosis. Am J Hematol 36: 249–254

107. Tait RC, Walker ID, Perry DJ, Carrell RW, Islam SIA, McCall F, Mitchell R, Davidson JF (1991) Prevalence of antithrombin III deficiency subtypes in 4000 healthy blood donors. Thromb Haemost 65: 839

108. Tanis BC, Rosendaal FR, Koster T, Vandenbroucke JP (1997) Combined effect of immobilization and haemostatic risk factors on deep venous thrombosis (abstract). Thromb Haemost: p181; OC–732

109. Thaler E, Lechner K (1981) Antithrombin III deficiency and thromboembolism. Clin Haematol 10: 369–390

110. van Boven HH, Teitsma PH, Rosendaal FR, Bayston TA, Chowdhury V, Bauer KA, Scharrer I, Conrad J, Lane DA (1996) Factor V Leiden (FVR506Q) in families with inherited antithrombin deficiency. Thromb Haemost 75: 417–421

111. van der Velden PA, Krommenhoek-Van Es T, Allaart CF, Bertina RM, Reitsma PH (1991) A frequent thrombomodulin amino acid dimorphism is not associated with thrombophilia. Thromb Haemost 65: 511–513

112. Vandenbroucke JP, Koster T, Briët E, Reitsma PH, Bertina RM, Rosendaal FR (1994) Increased risk of venous thrombosis in oral-contraceptive users who are carriers of factor V Leiden mutation. Lancet 344: 1453–7

113. Voorberg J, Roelse J, Koopmann R, Büller H, Behrends F, ten Cate JW, Mertens K, van Mourik JA (1994) Association of idiopathic venous thromboembolism with single pointmutation at Arg506 of factor V. Lancet 343: 1535

114. Zöller B, Berntsdotter A, Garcia de Frutos P, Dahlbäck B (1995) Resistance to activated protein C as an additional genetic risk factor in hereditary deficiency of protein S. Blood 85: 3518–3523

115. Zöller B, Svensson PJ, He X, Dahlbäck B (1995) Identification of the same factor V gene mutation in 47 out of 50 thrombosis-prone families with inherited resistance to activated protein C. J Clin Invest 94: 2521–2524

116. Simioni P, Prandoni P, Lensing AW, Scudeller A, Sardella C, Prins MH, Villalta S, Dazzi F, Girolami A (1997) The risk of recurrent venous thromboembolism in patients with an Arg506Gln mutation in the gene for factor V (factor V Leiden). N Engl J Med 336: 399–403

S. Moll (✉) · D. Gulba
Franz Volhard Klinik
Humboldt Universität Charité
13122 Berlin, Germany

Mechanisms of ventilation-perfusion mismatch and hemodynamic alterations in acute and chronic pulmonary embolism

C. Giuntini, A. Santolicandro, R. Prediletto, P. Paoletti, B. Formichi, E. Fornai,
E. Begliomini, R. Puntoni, A. Perissinotto, A. Giannella Neto

Summary Studies on gas exchange in pulmonary embolism are not numerous. A few of them have been performed in experimental animals [4]. The methods employed comprise the determination of gas exchange parameters [14], including the physiologic dead space [1], and the multiple inert gas elimination technique [2, 8, 10].

Furthermore, not much effort has been made to relate topographical alterations of ventilation and blood flow, detected by external counting of radioactive tracers, to ventilation/perfusion ($\dot{V}A/\dot{Q}$) disturbances responsible for impaired gas exchange in pulmonary embolism.

This paper reports data on pulmonary gas exchange, $\dot{V}A/\dot{Q}$ distribution by inert gas elimination, and regional lung function by ventilation and perfusion scan in human pulmonary embolism.

Changes of gas exchange parameters

The main parameters of pulmonary gas exchange are shown in Fig. 1, which reports the results of 33 patients with pulmonary embolism [15]. Data have been obtained at the moment of diagnosis, one week, one month, and 6 months later following therapy. The number of unperfused lung segments (embolized segments) at perfusion lung scan is reported as an index of the severity of the pulmonary embolization. This number of ULS is estimated on the lateral views of perfusion lung scan [6]. It is seen that in the acute phase of pulmonary embolization, the fraction of the pulmonary arterial tree obstructed by emboli is 63 % on the average. At this stage, the physiologic dead space (VDphy) is just 45 % of the tidal volume (VT). Also the alveolar dead space, computed according to Robin et al. [17], i.e., applying a correction for the effect of reinspiration of anatomic dead space gas (VDalv), is just 32 %. Thus, it appears that even the largest estimate of the alveolar dead space (VDalv(Ro)) underestimates the percent of the unperfused alveoli as assessed by lung perfusion scintigraphy.

The level of hypoxemia is rather marked. The arterial oxygen tension standardized to a $PaCO_2$ of 40 mmHg, i.e., corrected for the effect of hyperventilation, is 52 mmHg. Correspondingly, we observe a remarkable increase of the alveolar-arterial oxygen gradient ($AaDO_2$) that amounts to 59 mmHg. The arterial-alveolar gradient of carbon dioxide ($aADCO_2$) appears also increased (9.6 mmHg).

In order to explain these findings, it may be helpful to examine the $\dot{V}A/\dot{Q}$ distribution by inert gas elimination and regional lung function by ventilation and perfusion scintigraphy in acute pulmonary embolism [18].

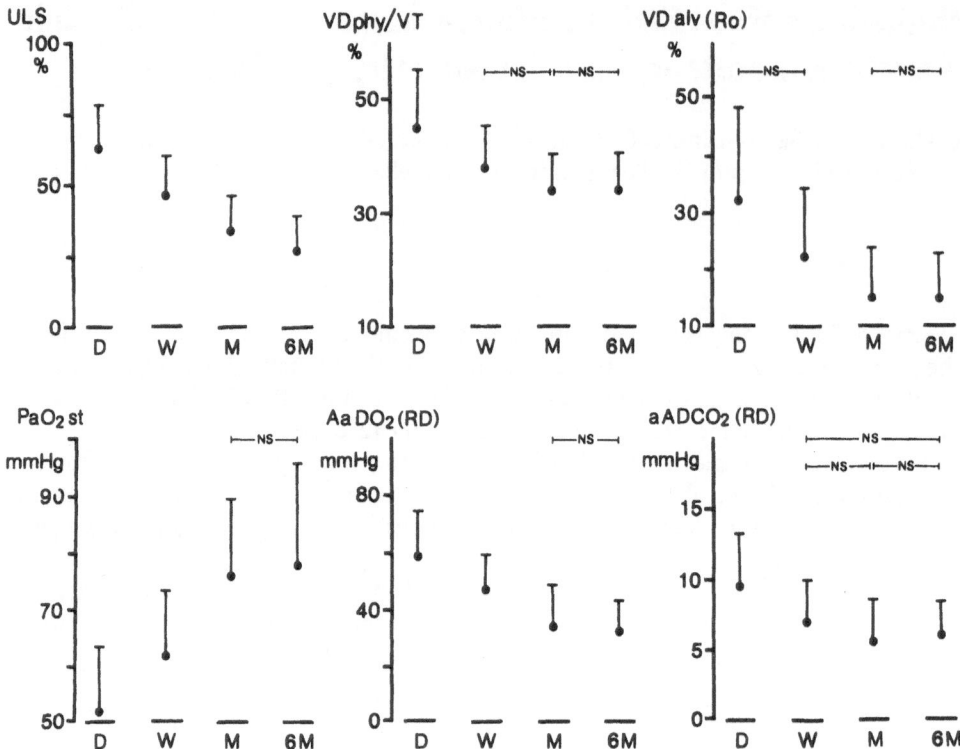

Fig. 1. Changes in number of unperfused lung segments at scintigraphy (ULS) and gas exchange parameters as function of time from diagnosis to 180 days later in 33 patients with pulmonary embolism; see reference (7). D: at time of diagnosis of acute pulmonary embolism; W: after 1 week therapy; M: after 1 month therapy; 6M: after 6 months therapy. PaO_2st: arterial oxygen tension standardized to a $PaCO_2$ of 40 mmHg; VD alv (Ro) : alveolar dead space according to Robin et al. (17). Statistical significance is $p < 0.05$ by Duncan test.

Findings at inert gas elimination

Very few observations are reported in the literature on the $\dot{V}A/\dot{Q}$ distribution in the very acute phase of human embolism. Out of 10 patients, in whom pulmonary embolism was acute or severe (the number of unperfused lung segments averaged 68.9 %), we found redistribution of pulmonary blood flow with development of high and low $\dot{V}A/\dot{Q}$ units in seven instances. In one case, we observed that $\dot{V}A/\dot{Q}$ relationships were only minimally abnormal. Our findings are somewhere at variance with those of Manier et al. [10], who reported that the major part of pulmonary blood flow is distributed in a mode near to, or slightly above, a $\dot{V}A/\dot{Q}$ ratio of 1. Findings similar to those of Manier et al. have also been reported by Huet et al. [8]. On the other hand, our results appear similar to those reported by Dantzker et al. after acute pulmonary thromboembolization in dogs [4]. These authors observed a few minutes after experimental embolization an increase in blood flow and ventilation to units with $\dot{V}A/\dot{Q}$ ratios less than 1 in all dogs and development of lung units with $\dot{V}A/\dot{Q}$ ratios between 10 and 100 in two-thirds of the dogs. In time, namely over the ensuing 2 hours, the $\dot{V}A/\dot{Q}$ distribution and the arterial PO_2, depending on the type of embolization, either went back to preembolization values or showed a tendency to return toward preembolization measurements. These observations indicate the important effect of the time elapsed after embolization on the parameters of gas exchange and on the shape of the $\mathring{V}A/\mathring{Q}$ distributions.

As to the size of the shunt, as assessed in our patients by the inert gas technic, it was usually small. It averaged 2.7 % and only in one instance amounted to 11 %. Our results are consistent with most of the data reported in the literature which indicate that an arteriovenous shunt or an intracardial shunt through a patent faramen ovale are only occasionally findings of functional significance in patients with acute pulmonary embolism [2, 7]. Shunts of limited size seem to develop in time [8] and may be ascribed to reperfusion of atelectasic embolized lung regions.

As to the size of the dead space, as assessed again in our patients by the inert gas technic, it amounted to 31.0 ± 14.4 % and resulted in somewhat lower values than the physiologic dead space (48.2 ± 12.7 %) measured simultaneously with the Bohr formula modified by Enghoff. Most of our patients with acute pulmonary embolism developed, as we have seen, lung regions with high ventilation-perfusion ratios, thus, explaining the increase in Bohr-Enghoff physiological dead space (CO_2 dead space) and the discrepancy between this and ventilation to unperfused lung or, to be precise, to regions with $\mathring{V}A/\mathring{Q}$ > 100, that is, the definition of the dead space by the inert gas technic. As suggested by Dantzker et al. [4], it is then possible by using the inert gas approach to identify the components of the physiological dead space quantitatively and thereby clarify the change produced by pulmonary embolization. In our case, some 17 % of VDphy/VT should be ascribed to development of areas with high ventilation-perfusion ratios ($\mathring{V}A/\mathring{Q}$ between 5 and 100, approximately).

Regional lung function and inert gas elimination

Perfusion lung scintigraphy demonstrated more extensive perfusion defects in the 7 patients who developed low and high $\mathring{V}A/\mathring{Q}$ units (Fig. 2). In them, the number of unperfused lung segments averaged 74 %. If we look closely at these perfusion scans, we observe numerous lung areas with reduced perfusion, sometimes very much reduced, and one or two areas, usually small, with increased perfusion (Fig. 3B). The small areas with increased perfusion likely represent the lung regions where the flow has been diverted from the embolized regions. At the ventilation lung scintigrams it appears that ventilation is also

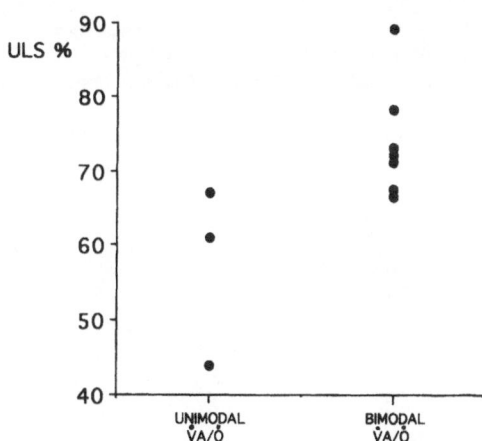

Fig. 2. Patients with acute pulmonary embolism and unimodal aspect of $\mathring{V}A/\mathring{Q}$ distributions exhibit a smaller number of unperfused lung segments (ULS) with respect to those with bimodal $\mathring{V}A/\mathring{Q}$ distributions (n = 10).

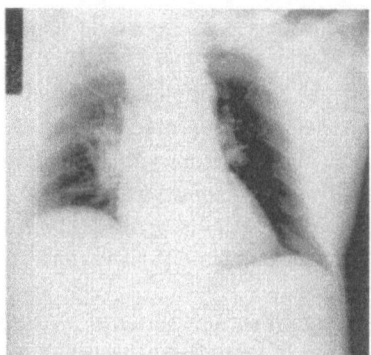

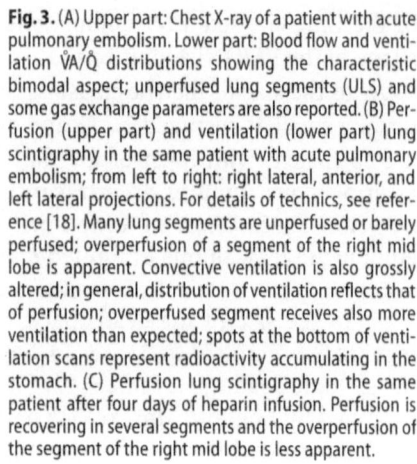

Fig. 3. (A) Upper part: Chest X-ray of a patient with acute pulmonary embolism. Lower part: Blood flow and ventilation V̇A/Q̇ distributions showing the characteristic bimodal aspect; unperfused lung segments (ULS) and some gas exchange parameters are also reported. (B) Perfusion (upper part) and ventilation (lower part) lung scintigraphy in the same patient with acute pulmonary embolism; from left to right: right lateral, anterior, and left lateral projections. For details of technics, see reference [18]. Many lung segments are unperfused or barely perfused; overperfusion of a segment of the right mid lobe is apparent. Convective ventilation is also grossly altered; in general, distribution of ventilation reflects that of perfusion; overperfused segment receives also more ventilation than expected; spots at the bottom of ventilation scans represent radioactivity accumulating in the stomach. (C) Perfusion lung scintigraphy in the same patient after four days of heparin infusion. Perfusion is recovering in several segments and the overperfusion of the segment of the right mid lobe is less apparent.

AP
Before heparin

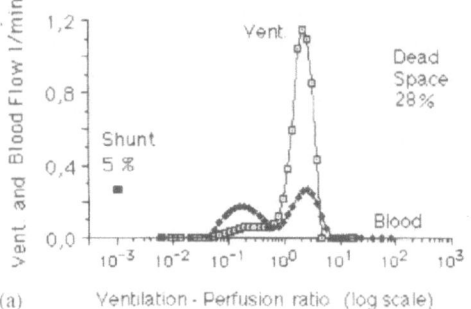

(a)   Ventilation - Perfusion ratio (log scale)

ULS	= 78	%
PHa	= 7,430	u
PaCO2	= 32	mmHg
PaO2	= 54	mmHg
PaO2st	= 41	mmHg
VDphy/Vt	= 49	%

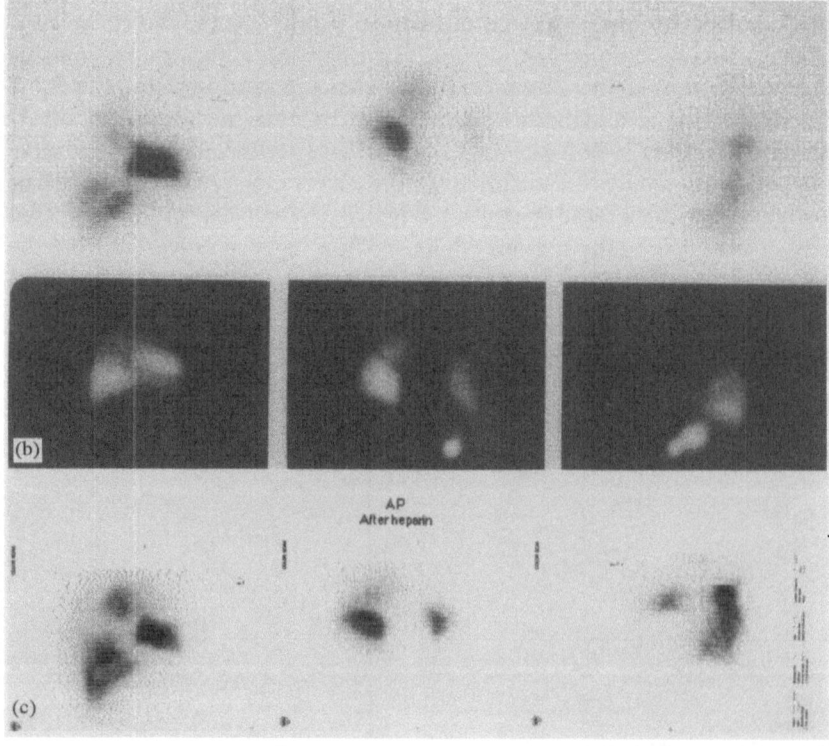

AP
After heparin

diverted to the same regions but to a smaller extent (Fig. 3B). Thus, lung units with a low $\mathring{V}A/\mathring{Q}$ ratio may develop. The conclusions are in agreement with the observation, by the inert gas elimination method, of an increase in blood flow to lung units with $\mathring{V}A/\mathring{Q}$ ratios less than 1 (Fig. 3A).

In the ventilation lung scan, areas with reduced perfusion appear to receive a fair amount of ventilation (Fig. 3B). Thus, lung units with high $\mathring{V}A/\mathring{Q}$ ratios are likely to develop (Fig. 3A). It should be remarked that, according to the perfusion lung scan, rarely pulmonary embolization causes complete abolition of segmental blood flow (Fig. 3B). These observations are in keeping with the results of the inert gas technic which shows that lung units with high $\mathring{V}A/\mathring{Q}$ ratios usually develop in acute pulmonary embolism whereas ventilation to unperfused lung, i.e., dead space by inert gas technic, appears only moderately increased (Fig. 3A).

Following treatment, small lung areas of increased perfusion tend to disappear soon at lung perfusion scan (Fig. 3C). This may explain why distributions with low $\mathring{V}A/\mathring{Q}$ units have not usually been reported in pulmonary embolism. Regions of overperfusion may easily disappear by natural evolution of the condition or following the administration of heparin.

Mechanisms of gas exchange disturbances

Based on the $\mathring{V}A/\mathring{Q}$ distributions obtained by inert gas elimination and on the regional perfusion and ventilation observed at lung scintigraphy, we may attempt to explain the gas exchange data found in our patients with acute pulmonary embolism. First of all, the changes in CO_2 dead space. The physiologic dead space/VT amounted to 48.2 % in the 10 patients who were studied by the inert gas technic and 45 % in all the 33 patients. It was somewhat larger than the inert gas dead space, which amounted to 31 % and we have already examined the reason of this, but its increase with respect to the expected control value was far less than the amount of unperfused lung as estimated from the unperfused lung segments (68.9 and 63 % in the 10 and 33 patients, respectively). Even the alveolar dead space (34 and 32 %, respectively) was less than expected. If the distribution of ventilation had remained unchanged, alveolar dead space should have increased by a fraction equal to the original alveolar ventilation of the occluded lung regions. However, since the ventilation of the occluded lung regions was partially diverted, as already seen, to the perfused lung regions, this may explain why the increase of the alveolar dead space was less than expected. Furthermore, since the occlusion of the embolized lung vessels was rarely complete, this may explain in part the discrepancy between the different measures of the dead space and the estimated amount of unperfused lung.

As to the hypoxemia encountered in acute pulmonary embolism, the mechanism mainly responsible for it appears from the inert gas and the regional perfusion studies to be the redistribution of pulmonary blood flow with the development of low $\mathring{V}A/\mathring{Q}$ units (shift of perfusion from large embolized to small nonembolized regions with development of overperfusion on the latter). The small difference (5.0 mmHg) between measured PaO_2 and that predicted by inert gas elimination may be ascribed to diffusion impairment. Right-to-left shunting only occasionally appears as a mechanism of hypoxemia following acute massive pulmonary embolism. Furthermore, a reduction in cardiac output and O_2 transport in acute pulmonary embolism with the resultant fall in mixed venous oxygen tension ($P\bar{v}O_2 = 30.9 \pm 3.9$ mmHg in the 10 patients) may contribute to the development of hypoxemia even though the degree of its influence will depend on the presence of lung units with $\mathring{V}A/\mathring{Q}$ inequalities and, therefore, on the development of such units. Under these conditions, a lowered oxygen hemoglobin affinity, due to a raised red blood cell level of 2,3-DPG, may also play a role.

Hemodynamic alterations

The cardiac output, measured applying the Fick principle to arteriovenous O_2 difference, was on the average reduced (4.7 ± 1.7 L/min) in the 10 patients with acute pulmonary embolism studied with the inert gas technic [18]. The mean pulmonary artery pressure was considerably increased (38.3 ± 17.3 mmHg). After 1 week heparin infusion, cardiac output increased slightly, whereas mean pulmonary artery pressure dropped by some 20 mmHg on average.

Chronic pulmonary embolism

One patient was studied in a chronic condition, affected by pulmonary hypertension due to recurrent pulmonary embolism [12, 13]. The mechanisms of hypoxemia are the same observed in the acute phase, namely alterations of the $\mathring{V}A/\mathring{Q}$ distributions and decrease of $P\bar{v}O_2$. This observation and others reported in the literature [3, 9, 16] suggest that in patients with chronic pulmonary embolism low or very low $\mathring{V}A/\mathring{Q}$ units tend to persist. Their persistence may be explained by a lasting combination of relative overperfusion and underventilation. When $\mathring{V}A/\mathring{Q}$ inequality occurs in presence of an abnormally low $P\bar{v}O_2$, clinically significant hypoxemia develops.

Clinical implications

From the practical point of view, it has been suggested to make use of the CO_2 dead space in the diagnosis of acute pulmonary embolism [1]. If we plot the physiologic dead space as a fraction of tidal volume against the arterialalveolar gradient of CO_2, we observe that the limit of 40 % for VDphy/VT would not suggest the diagnosis of pulmonary embolism in 13 of our 33 patients with the diagnosis of acute pulmonary embolism. Similar results are obtained with alveolar dead space calculated from arterialalveolar CO_2 gradient, as proposed by some authors [5, 19]. We take these observations to signify that the sensitivity of VDphy/VT (20/13 + 20 = 0.16) is too low. In other words, the diagnostic value of CO_2 dead space in pulmonary embolism is limited only to patients with major pulmonary embolization. On the other hand, a marked increase of CO_2 dead space when accompanied by hypoxemia and hypocapnia appears a specific feature of pulmonary embolism as shown when on the diagram VDphy/VT vs aADCO$_2$ we report the range of the values of the same variables observed in adult respiratory distress syndrome (ARDS) at comparable levels of hypoxemia. Patients with ARDS, who also have hypocapnia and hypoxemia, do not exhibit the very high values of VDphy/VT and aADCO$_2$ observed in some patients with pulmonary embolism. This observation may have some useful clinical application in the differential diagnosis between pulmonary embolism and ARDS. When, in a patient with hypoxemia and hypocapnia, VDphy/VT is larger than 50 % or aADCO$_2$ is greater than 10 mmHg, the diagnosis of pulmonary embolism is highly probable.

As to the evolution with time of the gas exchange disturbances in pulmonary embolism, we observe that, whereas some recovery may take place in the course of few hours or days, normalization even after appropriate treatment may not be complete several months later (Fig. 1) [11].

Conclusions

Thus, we may conclude that in pulmonary embolism in man:

- The increase in physiologic and alveolar dead space underestimates the percent of unperfused alveoli as assessed by lung perfusion scintigraphy.
- The decrease of PaO_2 is rather marked. Due to the accompanying decrease of $PaCO_2$, PaO_2 standardized to a $PaCO_2$ of 40 mmHg is even lower.
- There is a remarkable increase of $AaDO_2$.
- There is redistribution of pulmonary blood flow with development of high and low $\mathring{V}A/\mathring{Q}$ units.
- Redistribution of ventilation is also present but shift of ventilation from embolized to nonembolized regions is much less than that of perfusion.
- The ventilation shift and incomplete obstruction of embolized vessels explain the limited increase of both CO_2 dead space and inert gas dead space.
- Perfusion shift with development of overperfused lung regions may explain the major part of PaO_2 decrease.
- Right-to-left shunts, decrease of $P\bar{v}O_2$ and of oxygenhemoglobin affinity may contribute to the arterial hypoxemia.
- Whereas some gas exchange disturbances regress soon, especially under appropriate treatment, others are not completely normalized after several months.
- The combined persistence of low or very low $\mathring{V}A/\mathring{Q}$ units and of abnormally low $P\bar{v}O_2$ is responsible for clinically significant hypoxemia in patients with chronic pulmonary embolism.

Acknowledgement Supported in part with funds from the CNR Cardiorespiratory Group and the Italian Ministry of the University and of Scientific and Technologic Research.

References

1. Burki NK (1986) The dead space to tidal volume ratio in the diagnosis of pulmonary embolism. Am Rev Respir Dis 133: 679–685
2. D'Alonzo GE, Bower JS, DeHart P, Dantzker DR (1983) Case Reports. The mechanisms of abnormal gas exchange in acute massive pulmonary embolism. Am Rev Respir Dis 128: 170–172
3. Dantzker DR, Bower JS (1979) Mechanisms of gas exchange abnormality in patients with chronic obliterative pulmonary vascular disease. J Clin Invest 64: 1050–1055
4. Dantzker DR, Wagner PD, Tornabene VW, Alazraki NP, West JB (1978) Gas exchange after pulmonary thromboembolization in dogs. Circulation Res 42: 92–103
5. Eriksson L, Wollmer P, Olsson C-G, Albrechtsson U, Larusdottir H, Nilsson R, Sjögren A, Jonson B (1989) Diagnosis of pulmonary embolism based upon alveolar dead space analysis. Chest 96: 357–362
6. Giannella Neto A, Fornai E, Paoletti P, Prediletto R, Fazzi P, Di Ricco G, Marini C, Perissinotto A, Giuntini C (1982) Ventilation and gas exchange in massive pulmonary embolism. Bull europ Physiopath resp 18 (suppl. 4): 127–138
7. Herve PH, Petitpretz P, Simonneau G, Salmeron S, Laine JF, Duroux P (1983) Correspondence. The mechanisms of abnormal gas exchange in acute massive pulmonary embolism. Letter to the Editor & Reply from the Authors. Am Rev Respir Dis 128: 1101–1102
8. Huet Y, Lemaire F, Brun-Buisson C, Knaus WA, Teisseire B, Payen D, Mathieu D (1985) Hypoxemia in acute pulmonary embolism. Chest 88: 829–836
9. Kapitan KS, Buchbinder M, Wagner PD, Moser KM (1989) Mechanisms of hypoxemia in chronic thrombo-embolic pulmonary hypertension. Am Rev Respir Dis 139: 1149–1154
10. Manier G, Castaing Y, Guenard H (1985) Determinants of hypoxemia during the acute phase of pulmonary embolism in humans. Am Rev Respir Dis 132: 332–338
11. Marini C, Di Ricco G, Rossi G, Rindi M, Palla R, Giuntini C (1988) Fibrinolytic effects of urokinase and heparin in acute pulmonary embolism: A randomized clinical trial. Respiration 54: 162–173
12. Moser KM, Auger WR, Fedullo PF, Jamieson SW (1992) Chronic thromboembolic pulmonary hypertension: Clinical picture and surgical treatment. Eur Respir J 5: 334–342

13. Palla A, Formichi B, Santolicandro A, Di Ricco G, Giuntini C (1993) From not detected pulmonary embolism to diagnosis of chronic thromboembolic pulmonary hypertension: A retrospective study. Respiration 60: 9–14
14. Perret C, Enrico JF, Troillet F (1971) The arterial-alveolar carbon dioxide tension gradient in acute pulmonary embolism. In: Giuntini C (ed) Central Hemodynamics and Gas Exchange. Minerva Medica, Turin, pp 421–435
15. Prediletto R, Paoletti P, Fornai E, Perissinotto A, Petruzzelli S, Formichi B, Ruschi S, Palla A, Giannella-Neto A, Giuntini C (1990) Natural course of treated pulmonary embolism: Evaluation by perfusion lung scintigraphy, gas exchange, and chest roentgenogram. Chest 97: 554–561
16. Riedel M, Stanek V, Widlimsky J, Prerovsky I (1982) Longterm follow-up of patients with pulmonary thromboembolism: Late prognosis and evolution of hemodynamic and respiratory data. Chest 81: 151–158
17. Robin ED, Forkner CE Jr, Bromberg PA, Croteau JR, Travis DM (1960) Alveolar gas exchange in clinical pulmonary embolism. New Engl J Med 262: 283–287
18. Santolicandro A, Prediletto R, Fornai E, Formichi B, Begliomini E, Giannella-Neto A, Giuntini C (1995) Mechanisms of hypoxemia and hypocapnia in pulmonary embolism. Am J Respir Crit Care Med 152: 336–347
19. Wollmer P (1988) Diagnosis of pulmonary embolism. Appl Cardiopulm Pathophysiol 2: 13–22

C. Giuntini · A. Santolicandro · R. Prediletto · P. Paoletti · B. Formichi
E. Fornai · E. Begliomini · R. Puntoni · A. Perissinotto · A. Giannella Neto
Prof. Dr. C. Giuntini (✉)
Clinica Medica II
Universita deglistudi di Pisa
Via Paradisa
I-56124 Cisanello Pisa

Clinical course and prognosis of acute pulmonary embolism

S. Konstantinides, A. Geibel, W. Kasper

Summary Effective treatment of acute pulmonary embolism (PE) requires prompt identification of patients at high risk of death or severe cardiovascular complications during the hospital stay. Determination of prognostic parameters in this heterogeneous patient population is far more important than calculation of a crude mortality rate due to PE. The multicenter Management Strategy and Prognosis in Pulmonary Embolism Registry examined the in-hospital clinical course of 1001 consecutive patients with acute PE. Overall mortality was 22 %, with 91 % of deaths directly related to PE. Clinical signs of acute right heart failure due to major PE (arterial hypotension, shock, circulatory collapse) were clearly associated with an adverse outcome. Mortality ranged from 8 to 65 % depending on the severity of clinical instability at presentation. Importantly, a significantly increased death rate was also observed in patients with echocardiographically detected right ventricular dilation (84 vs. 16 %), a reliable noninvasive index of impending right heart failure. The independent prognostic effect of this finding was confirmed by multivariate analysis (Odds Ratio, 2.44; $P = 0.004$). Thus, the combination of clinical and echocardiographic findings permits accurate risk stratification of patients with acute PE. Evidence is also accumulating that these prognostic factors can be used to identify candidates for early thombolytic treatment.

Key words Pulmonary embolism – echocardiography – prognosis – mortality – thrombolysis

Despite major advances in cardiovascular diagnosis and treatment, acute pulmonary embolism (PE) is still one of the leading causes of death among hospitalized patients. It is particularly disappointing in this regard that mortality associated with PE has remained virtually unchanged during the past 30 years [15, 16]. These facts underline the necessity of a more effective therapeutic approach to patients with clinically suspected PE. Development of treatment strategies, however, requires adequate knowledge of the natural course of venous thromboembolism and, in particular, prompt identification of patients at high risk of death or major complications during the hospital stay. Yet a review of the literature reveals that many issues regarding the prognosis of acute PE remain poorly understood. Thus, one-year mortality was reported to be as low as 1 % in a multicenter study performed by the British Thoracic Society to find out the optimal duration of anticoagulation for venous thromboembolism [19]. On the other hand, 18 % of patients with massive PE died in the series of Hall et al. [8] and death rates approached [7] or exceeded 30 % [1] in patients presenting with cardiogenic shock due to right heart failure. In another major study, the Prospective Investigation of Pulmonary Embolism Diagnosis (PIOPED), in-hospital mortality was 9.5 % but death was directly related to the thromboembolic event in only 10 patients (2.5 % of the study population). Twenty years earlier, the Urokinase in Pulmonary Embolism Trial (UPET) had come to similar conclusions [21, 22]. The authors of the PIOPED further reported that age and underlying disease were important prognostic indicators in their patients and argued that "pulmonary embolism is an unusual cause of death" (3). However, the strict scintigraphic and angiographic criteria required to confirm PE in PIOPED and UPET virtually precluded the study of severely compromised, high-risk patients.

The conflicting and apparently confusing results of the aforementioned reports simply reflect the fact that patients with acute PE comprise a heterogeneous population whose prognosis and clinical course should be stratified rather than "globally" determined. Furthermore, they raise the important question whether studies primarily designed to set accurate diagnostic or therapeutic standards can also "tell the whole story" regarding the clinical course of PE.

Three major factors determine the pathophysiology of acute PE: (1) the extent of pulmonary arterial embolic obstruction; (2) the severity of pre-existing cardiopulmonary dysfunction; and (3) the peripheral venous clot burden which determines the risk of recurrent thromboembolic events [10, 13]. The interactions of these factors result in the development of pulmonary artery hypertension and right ventricular pressure overload. The abrupt or progressive increase in afterload leads, in turn, to enlargement and dysfunction (hypokinesis) of the right ventricle. It was recently demonstrated that the presence of right ventricular dilatation, which can be rapidly and reliably diagnosed by bedside echocardiography, is associated with increased in-hospital mortality in patients presenting with clinically suspected PE [13]. These findings are in accordance with current theories which emphasize that death due to acute PE is death resulting from right heart failure [17]. To confirm this thesis, however, it was important to show in large numbers of patients that clinical, echocardiographic or hemodynamic findings indicating overt *or impending* right heart failure are the most relevant predictors of outcome in the setting of acute PE [2].

Resolving controversial issues on the clinical course of acute pulmonary embolism: Results of a multicenter registry

The Management Strategy and Prognosis of Pulmonary Embolism Registry (MAPPET) was conducted between September 1993 and December 1994. The registry focused on current management strategies as well as on the clinical outcome of 1001 consecutive patients with acute *major* pulmonary embolism recruited by a total of 204 centers throughout Germany. The aim of the study was to test the following hypotheses: 1) the extent of diagnostic work-up and, in particular, the frequency of nuclear imaging or pulmonary angiographic studies for definite confirmation of pulmonary embolism decreases as the severity of hemodynamic instability at presentation increases; 2) patients who are most unstable, i.e., in cardiogenic shock or in need of cardiopulmonary resuscitation at the time of diagnosis are those who most frequently receive aggressive treatment, especially early thrombolysis; and 3) the degree of clinical and hemodynamic instability due to acute right heart failure is the most important determinant of inhospital mortality.

The inclusion criteria of the registry consisted of the following clinical, echocardiographic and cardiac catheterization findings signifying acute right heart failure and/or pulmonary hypertension due to pulmonary embolism: (1) *arterial hypotension*, defined as systolic blood pressure below 90 mmHg or a pressure drop of at least 40 mmHg for a time period exceeding 15 minutes; (2) *cardiogenic shock*, in which the presence of arterial hypotension as defined above was accompanied by clinical signs of organ hypoperfusion and hypoxia (altered level of consciousness, urine output below 30 mL/h, cold and clammy extremities); (3) *circulatory collapse* necessitating cardiopulmonary resuscitation; (4) at least two of the following two-dimensional and Doppler *echocardiographic findings* indicating acute right ventricular pressure overload and/or pulmonary hypertension *in the absence of* left ventricular or mitral valve disease [11, 12]: (i) right ventricular dilatation (i.e., right ventricle appearing larger than the left ventricle from the apical or subcostal view), (ii) paradoxical septal wall motion, (iii) loss of inspiratory collapse of the inferior vena cava, (iv) tricuspid regurgitation jet velocity over 2.8 m/s or over 2.5 m/s in the absence of inspiratory collapse of the inferior vena cava, and, finally, (5) diagnosis of *precapillary pulmonary hypertension* (mean pulmonary artery pressure > 20 mmHg in the presence of normal pulmonary artery occlusion pressures) by right heart catheterization.

Patients with clinically suspected pulmonary embolism were included in the Registry if they met at least one of the above criteria at presentation together with: (1) a diagnostic pulmonary angiogram, or, (2) a lung scan indicating high probability of pulmonary embolism, or, (3) at least three of the following findings: (i) syncope, (ii) tachycardia (heart rate > 100 bpm), (iii) dyspnoea and/or tachypnoea (breathing rate > 24 per minute or need for mechanical ventilation), (iv) arterial hypoxemia (partial arterial pressure of oxygen < 70 mmHg while breathing room air or < 80 mmHg under supplemental oxygen of at least 2 liters per minute) in the absence of pulmonary infiltrates on chest X-ray, and (v) ECG signs of right heart strain (at least one of the following: complete or incomplete right bundle branch block, S waves in lead I combined with Q waves in lead III, or T wave inversion in the precordial leads V_1 to V_3).

Four patient groups were prospectively defined based on the severity of clinical and hemodynamic instability at presentation: *Group* 1, patients with evidence of right ventricular pressure overload and/or pulmonary hypertension on the echocardiogram, or with confirmation of precapillary pulmonary hypertension on right heart catheterization, in the absence of arterial hypotension at presentation; *Group* 2, patients presenting with arterial hypotension as defined above but without clinical signs of cardiogenic shock or the need for catecholamine support of blood pressure; *Group* 3, patients with arterial hypotension accompanied by cardiogenic shock or judged by the attending physicians to require the administration of catecholamines; and *Group* 4, patients with circulatory collapse who underwent cardiopulmonary resuscitation at presentation.

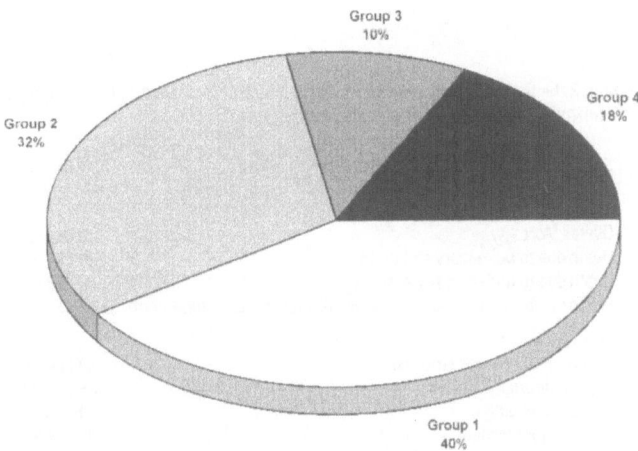

Fig. 1. Distribution of patients included in the Management Strategy and Prognosis of Pulmonary Embolism Registry according to the severity of hemodynamic compromise at presentation (4 prospectively defined groups).

Table 1. Predisposing conditions for acute pulmonary embolism in the Management and Prognosis in Pulmonary Embolism Registry (n = 1001 patients)

Underlying disease/predisposing factor	n (% of the patient population)
Recent major surgery (within 10 days)	274 (27 %)
Recent major trauma or fracture (within 10 days)	106 (11 %)
Gestation/recent delivery	14 (1.4 %)
History of previous venous thrombosis	289 (29 %)
History of previous pulmonary embolism	117 (12 %)
Chronic pulmonary disease	105 (11 %)
History of congestive heart failure	316 (32 %)
Cancer	122 (12 %)
Stroke	22 (2.2 %)

The mean age of the patients at diagnosis was 63 ± 15 years. The distribution of the study population according to the severity of clinical instability (Groups 1 through 4) is shown in Fig. 1. *Group* 1 comprised 407 patients, *Group* 2 316, *Group* 3 102, and *Group* 4 176 patients. Overall, most of the patients (70 %) had an acute onset of symptoms (less than 48 hours) and 784 patients (78 %) had at least one known risk factor for venous thromboembolism in their history (Table 1).

The majority of the registry patients (74 %) underwent two-dimensional and Doppler echocardiographic studies. The presence of right heart pressure overload and/or pulmonary hypertension was thus established in 303 patients of Group 1 (74 %), 221 patients of Group 2 (70 %), 69 patients of Group 3 (68 %), and 115 patients of Group 4 (65 %). On the other hand, 227 patients of the study population (23 %) had invasive confirmation of pulmonary hypertension by right heart catheterization.

Thromboembolic pulmonary vessel occlusion was confirmed by angiography in 174 patients (17 %), by a high probability lung scan in 549 patients (55 %), and by at least one of these imaging studies in 68 % of the patients.

In-hospital course and mortality

Overall in-hospital mortality was 22 %. There was a substantial increase in death rate from 8.1 % in patients who were hemodynamically stable at presentation (Group 1) to 65 % in

Table 2. Clinical course of acute pulmonary embolism (* defined as bleeding requiring red cell transfusion or discontinuation of therapeutic anticoagulation or thrombolytic treatment)

Events	Group 1 n = 407	Group 2 n = 316	Group 3 n = 102	Group 4 n = 176
Overall Mortality	33 (8.1 %)	48 (15 %)	25 (25 %)	114 (65 %)
Death due to pulmonary embolism	29 (7.1 %)	43 (14 %)	23 (23 %)	106 (60 %)
Death due to underlying disease	3 (0.7 %)	3 (1.0 %)	1 (1.0 %)	2 (1.1 %)
Death due to complications of diagnostic procedures or treatment	1 (0.3 %)	2 (0.6 %)	1 (1.0%)	6 (3.4 %)
Non-fatal events				
Recurrent pulmonary embolism	57 (14 %)	61 (19 %)	22 (22 %)	32 (18 %)
Arterial thromboembolism	5 (1.2 %)	4 (1.3 %)	0	5 (2.8 %)
Cerebral bleeding	1 (0.3 %)	3 (1.0 %)	0	1 (0.6 %)
Other major bleeding *	30 (7.4 %)	24 (7.6 %)	12 (12 %)	21 (12 %)

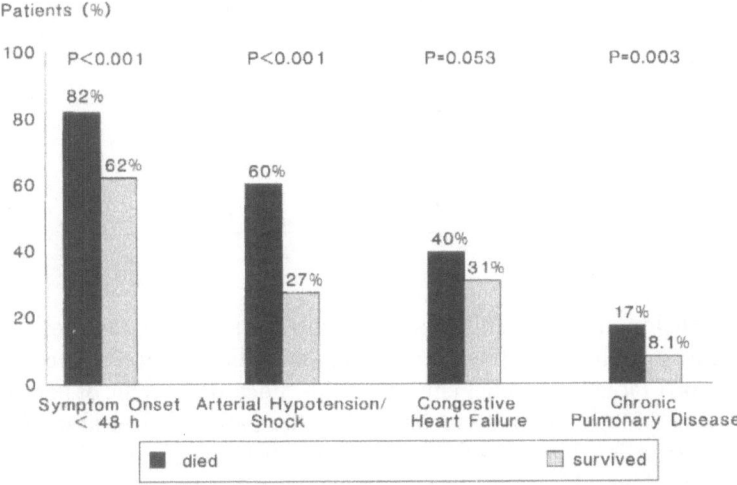

Fig. 2. Association between clinical findings at diagnosis and 30-day mortality using Fisher's exact test.

clinically unstable patients necessitating cardiopulmonary resuscitation (Group 4: P < 0.001 vs. Group 1). In most of the cases (91 %), death occurring during the inhospital phase was directly related to the thromboembolic event (Table 2). Only a few patients died from their underlying disease or due to complications of diagnostic or therapeutic procedures (0.9 and 1.0 %, respectively).

Figures 2 and 3 demonstrate the effect of baseline characteristics on the clinical outcome of the registry patients as assessed by univariate analysis (Fisher's exact test). Multiple logistic regression analysis showed the following findings at diagnosis to be significant predictors of outcome: (1) acute symptom onset; (2) clinical instability (indi-

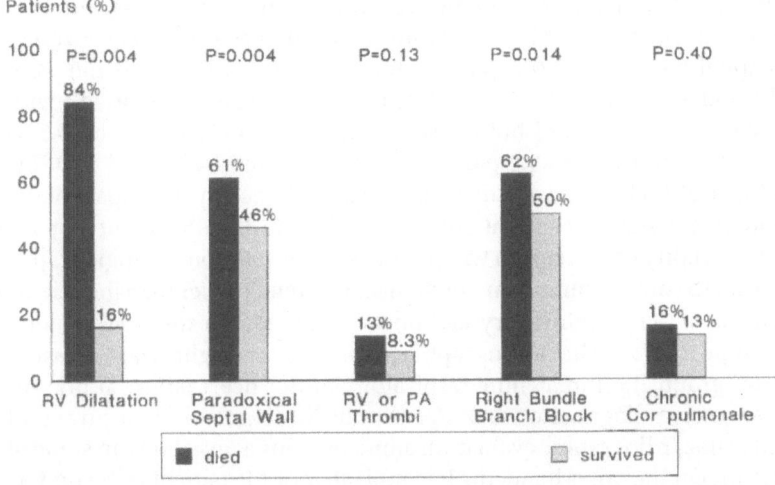

Fig. 3. Association between echocardiographic and ECG findings at diagnosis and 30-day mortality using Fisher's exact test. Chronic cor pulmonale was diagnosed if systolic pulmonary pressure was found to be > 70 and/or mean pressure > 40 mmHg.

Table 3. Predictors of outcome in patients with acute major pulmonary embolism (CI denotes confidence interval, RV right ventricular)

Characterstic	Odds ratio (95 % CI)	P value
Acute symptom onset	1.89 (1.08–3.29)	0.026
Arterial hypotension	1.69 (1.00–2.84)	0.050
Chronic pulmonary disease	2.42 (1.23–4.77)	0.011
Endotracheal intubation	3.76 (1.43–9.90)	0.007
Cardiopulmonary resuscitation	3.68 (1.35–10.05)	0.011
RV dilatation (Echo)	2.44 (1.34–4.47)	0.004

cated by arterial hypotension, need for endotracheal intubation or cardiopulmonary resuscitation); (3) preexisting pulmonary disease; and (4) echocardiographically detected right ventricular dilatation (Table 3). No other clinical, ECG, echocardiographic or hemodynamic parameters were independently associated with the patients' clinical course during the in-hospital period. Finally, it was found that patients with definite confirmation of PE by pulmonary angiography or lung scan had a much lower death rate compared with those patients in whom the diagnosis was based on clinical, ECG, and echocardiographic findings alone (11 vs. 45 %; $P < 0.001$).

Clinically apparent recurrence of pulmonary embolism was diagnosed in 172 of the study patients (17 %). The recurrence rates were similar among the four patient groups. Arterial thromboembolic events as well as cerebral hemorrhage were observed in very few patients within each group. Finally, the occurrence of other major bleeding episodes requiring red cell transfusions or discontinuation of treatment ranged from 7.4 to 12 % (Table 2).

Comparison with previous studies

The patients included in the present registry had major pulmonary embolism according to prospectively defined clinical and hemodynamic criteria. Overall, 93 % of our patients had confirmation of pulmonary artery hypertension by right heart catheterization or evidence of acute right heart strain provided by ECG or echocardiographic findings. Furthermore, 28 % of the patients were hemodynamically unstable at presentation requiring catecholamine support of blood pressure or even cardiopulmonary resuscitation. The in-hospital mortality of this patient population was 22 %. This rate is in accordance with the high mortality rates reported by other investigators in patients with massive pulmonary embolism [1, 7, 8] but considerably higher than the 8 and 9.5 % mortality of the hemodynamically stable patients included in the UPET and PIOPED trials, respectively [3, 21, 22]. This apparent discrepancy is explained by the impact of the patients' clinical and hemodynamic status at presentation on the diagnostic work-up for PE. In MAPPET, the mortality of patients in whom lung scan or pulmonary angiography was performed in order to confirm pulmonary embolism was much lower than in patients in whom the diagnosis of acute pulmonary embolism was made on the basis of high clinical suspicion supported by echocardiographic signs of acute right heart pressure overload. In the latter group, life-threatening respiratory and/or heart failure at presentation prohibited extensive diagnostic work-up. Certainly, diagnostic inaccuracy of bedside clinical and echocardiographic evaluation alone remains a possibility in some of these unstable patients. On the other hand, the low mortality of the patients who underwent nuclear imaging or angiographic studies in our registry (11 %) closely approaches the mortality of the patients in the UPET and PIOPED trials (8–9.5 %) and thus indicates that diagnostic strategies seeking definite confirmation of pulmonary embolism may lead to "selection" of a patient population with a relatively benign clinical outcome.

Therapeutic implications of the registry findings:
Identification of candidates for thrombolytic treatment

During the past 3 decades, several studies compared the efficacy of streptokinase [9, 18] or alteplase (recombinant tissue plasminogen activator) [4–6] with conventional intravenous heparin anticoagulation in patients with acute PE. These trials consistently demonstrated the superiority of thrombolysis in restoring patency of the occluded pulmonary vessels. It could further be shown that rapid clot lysis was accompanied by resolution of pulmonary hypertension [4] and echocardiographically detected right ventricular pressure overload [6]. However, the impact of the hemodynamic benefits of thrombolysis on the clinical outcome of the patients had not been systematically investigated and, thus, the indications for thrombolytic treatment in the setting of acute PE remained the subject of debate [20, 23]. In the Management Strategy and Prognosis of Pulmonary Embolism Registry, the clinical course of patients treated with thrombolytic agents within 24 hours of diagnosis was compared to that of patients who initially received heparin alone. All patients included in the registry had major PE according to the aforementioned criteria. However, statistical analysis focused on these patients who were clinically stable at presentation. The end points of the study were 30-day mortality, clinically apparent recurrence of pulmonary embolism, and the occurrence of major bleeding complications during the hospital stay. Early thrombolysis was shown to be independently associated with a significant reduction in overall mortality [odds ratio, 0.46; 95 % confidence interval, 0.21–1.00; $P = 0.051$). The death rate of patients in the thrombolysis treatment group was 4.7 % compared with 11.1 % in patients of the heparin group [14]. Recurrence of PE was also significantly reduced after thrombolytic treatment (7.7 vs. 18.7 %; $P < 0.001$). Cerebral hemorrhage occurred in 2 patients in each group. These intriguing results which provide a first link between the hemodynamic effects of thrombolysis and the clinical outcome of patients with major PE have to be confirmed by a prospective, randomized trial in order to provide undisputable indications for thrombolysis in venous thromboembolism.

Conclusions

Based on the results of the large multicenter registry presented above, it can now be stated that the presence of right ventricular failure is the most important prognostic factor in patients with acute PE. Clinical signs of overt right heart failure such as cardiogenic shock or circulatory collapse necessitating cardiopulmonary resuscitation are obviously associated with a particularly poor outcome during the hospital stay. However, the most important message for the physician in the emergency room or intensive care unit is the fact that detection of right ventricular dilatation with echocardiography rapidly and reliably identifies patients with impending hemodynamic compromise. The findings of MAPPET further suggest that these high-risk patients may benefit from early thrombolytic treatment even if their critical condition is initially masked by an apparently "stable" or "compensated" cardiovascular status.

References

1. Alpert JS, Smith R, Carlson J, Ockene IS, Dexter L, Dalen JE (1976) Mortality in patients treated for pulmonary embolism. JAMA 236: 1477–1480
2. Cannon CP, Goldhaber SZ (1996) Cardiovascular risk stratification of pulmonary embolism. Am J Cardiol 78: 1149–1151
3. Carson JL, Kelley MA, Duff A, Weg JG, Fulkerson WJ, Palevsky HI, Schwartz S, Thompson BT, Popovich J, Hobbins TE, Spera MA, Alavi A, Terrin ML (1992) The clinical course of pulmonary embolism. N Engl J Med 326: 1240–1245
4. Dalla-Volta S, Palla A, Santolicandro A, Giuntini C, Pengo V, Visioli O, Zonzin P, Zanuttini D, Barbaresi F, Agnelli G, Morpurgo M, Marini MG, Visani L (1992) PAIMS 2: Alteplase combined with heparin versus heparin in the treatment of acute pulmonary embolism. Plasminogen Activator Italian Multicenter Study 2. J Am Coll Cardiol 20: 520–526
5. Goldhaber SZ, Vaughan DE, Markis JE, Selwyn AP, Meyerovitz MF, Loscalzo J, Soo Kim D, Kessler CM, Dawley DL, Sharma GVRK, Sasahara A, Grossbard EB, Braunwald E (1986) Acute pulmonary embolism treated with tissue plasminogen activator. Lancet 2: 886–889
6. Goldhaber SZ, Haire WD, Feldstein ML, Miller M, Toltzis R, Smith JL, Taveira da Silva AM, Come PC, Lee RT, Parker JA, Mogtader A, McDonough TJ, Braunwald E (1993) Alteplase versus heparin in acute pulmonary embolism: Randomised trial assessing right-ventricular function and pulmonary perfusion. Lancet 341: 507–511
7. Gulba DC, Schmid C, Borst HG, Lichtlen P, Dietz R, Luft FC (1994) Medical compared with surgical treatment for massive pulmonary embolism. Lancet 343: 576–577
8. Hall RJC, Sutton GC, Kerr IH (1977) Long-term prognosis of treated acute massive pulmonary embolism. Br Heart J 39: 1128–1134
9. Hirsh J, Gale GS, McDonald IG, McCarthy RA, Pitt A (1968) Streptokinase therapy in acute major pulmonary embolism: Effectiveness and problems. Br Med J 4: 729–734
10. Hull RD, Raskob GE, Coates G, Panju AA, Gill GJ (1989) A new noninvasive management strategy for patients with suspected pulmonary embolism. Arch Intern Med 149: 2549–2555
11. Kasper W, Meinertz T, Henkel B, Eissner D, Hahn K, Hofmann T, Zeiher A, Just H (1986) Echocardiographic findings in patients with proven pulmonary embolism. Am Heart J 112: 1284–1290
12. Kasper W, Geibel A, Tiede N, Bassenge D, Kauder E, Konstantinides S, Meinertz T, Just H (1993) Distinguishing between acute and subacute massive pulmonary embolism by conventional and Doppler echocardiography. Br Heart J 70: 352–356
13. Kasper W, Konstantinides S, Geibel A, Tiede N, Krause T, Just H (1997) Prognostic significance of right ventricular afterload stress detected by echocardiography in patients with clinically suspected pulmonary embolism. Heart 77: 346–349
14. Konstantinides S, Geibel A, Olschewski M, Heinrich F, Grosser KD, Rauber K, Iversen S, Redecker M, Kienast J, Just H, Kasper W (1997) Association between thrombolytic treatment and the prognosis of hemodynamically stable patients with major pulmonary embolism: Results of a multicenter registry. Circulation 96: 882–888
15. Lilienfeld DE, Chan E, Ehland J, Godbold JH, Landrigan PJ, Marsh G (1990) Mortality from pulmonary embolism in the United States: 1962 to 1984. Chest 98: 1067–1072
16. Lindblad B, Sternby NH, Bergquist D (1991) Incidence of venous thromboembolism verified by necropsy over 30 years. Br Med J 302: 709–711
17. Lualdi JC, Goldhaber SZ (1995) Right ventricular dysfunction after acute pulmonary embolism: Pathophysiologic factors, detection, and therapeutic implications. Am Heart J 130: 1276–1282
18. Miller AH, Sutton GC, Kerr IH, Gibson RV, Honey M (1971) Comparison of streptokinase and heparin in treatment of isolated acute massive pulmonary embolism. Br Med J 2: 681–684
19. Research Committee of the British Thoracic Society (1992) Optimum duration of anticoagulation for deep-vein thrombosis and pulmonary embolism. Lancet 340: 873–876
20. Stein PD, Hull RD, Raskob G (1994) Risks for major bleeding from thrombolytic therapy in patients with acute pulmonary embolism. Ann Intern Med 121: 313–317
21. Urokinase in Pulmonary Embolism Trial: phase 1 results: a cooperative study (1970) JAMA 214: 2163–2172
22. Urokinase in Pulmonary Embolism Trial: phase 2 results: a cooperative study (1974) JAMA 229: 1606–1613
23. Verstraete M (1995) Thrombolytic treatment. Br Med J 311: 582–583

S. Konstantinides, M.D. (✉) · A. Geibel
Klinikum der Georg-August-Universität, Zentrum Innere Medizin
Abteilung Kardiologie und Pneumologie
Robert-Koch-Str. 40
D-37075 Göttingen, Germany

W. Kasper
St. Josefs-Hospital Wiesbaden, Medizinische Klinik
Solmsstraße 15
65189 Wiesbaden, Germany

Clinical implications of a patent foramen ovale in patients with massive pulmonary embolism

A. Geibel, S. Konstantinides, W. Kasper

Summary   The aim of our investigations was to prospectively evaluate the clinical relevance of a patent foramen ovale in patients with acute massive pulmonary embolism with regard to mortality, the occurrence of cardiovascular complications and the extent of arterial hypoxemia.

In 85 patients and in a second study in 139 patients with acute massive pulmonary embolism a right-to-left shunt was diagnosed by contrast echocardiography. A patent foramen ovale was found in 39 % of the patients in the first and in 35 % in the second study.

With regard to the extent of arterial hypoexemia the oxygen tension was significantly lower in patients with a patent foramen ovale (55 ± 14 mm Hg vs 62 ± 16 mm Hg). Furthermore in the second study, clinical symptoms presumptive of paradoxical embolism occurred in 13 patients (27 %) with a patent foramen ovale and in 2 patients (2.2 %) without a patent foramen ovale. During the inhospital stay, patients with a patent foramen ovale had a death rate of 33 % as opposed to 14 % in patients without a patent foramen ovale. Logistic regression analysis demonstrated that after adjustment for the clinical characteristics the only independent predictors of inhospital mortality were arterial hypotension at presentation ($p < 0.01$) and a patent foramen ovale ($p < 0.001$). Patients with a patent foramen ovale also had a significantly higher incidence of cardiovascular complications. Overall, the risk of a complicated in-hospital course was 5.2 times higher in the patient group with a patent foramen ovale.

These investigations underlines the prognostic impact of a patent foramen ovale in high-risk patients with acute massive pulmonary embolism.

Key words   Pulmonary embolism – patent foramen ovale – paradoxical embolism – contrast echocardiography – prognosis

Introduction

The clinical relevance of a patent foramen ovale, an embryological remnant, has remained obscure for many decades [3, 9, 27]. However, recent developments of adequate imaging techniques have allowed the visualization of a patent foramen ovale during life and furthermore facilitate detailed evaluation of the interatrial septum with regard to the assessment of its functional anatomy and hemodynamics [7, 10, 11, 18, 28, 29]. However, apart from isolated reports of paradoxical embolism in patients with a patent foramen ovale no systematic evaluation has been made to explore the clinical relevance of a right-to-left shunt at atrial level in patients with pulmonary embolism and elevated right heart pressures [22, 24, 25, 30, 31]. Therefore, the aim of our investigations was to prospectively evaluate the hypothesis that a patent foramen ovale is an important prognostic determinant in patients with acute massive pulmonary embolism with regard to mortality, the occurrence of cardiovascular complications and the extent of arterial hypoxemia.

Incidence and pathological consequences of a patent foramen ovale

The prevalence of a patent foramen ovale in adults varied in necropsy series from 25 to 35 % whereas that in healthy volunteers ranged between 5 and 31 % [9, 23, 26, 35, 36]. In a series of 965 autopsy specimens from the Mayo Clinic, the size of the foramen ovale in normal hearts varied between 1 and 19 mm with a mean of 4.9 mm [9]. Neither the incidence nor the size varied significantly between sexes but did correlate with age. The overall incidence was 27.3 %, declining from 34.3% in the first three decades to 25.4 % in the fourth to the eighth decades. In patients older than 80 years, the incidence decreased to 20.2 %. The reason for these differences remains speculative and includes age-dependent closure of the patent foramen ovale or it could be simply a selection bias, if adults with a patent foramen ovale would be more likely to die earlier.

The anatomic configuration establishes the characteristic of a foramen ovale as a potential one-way passage for blood from the right to the left atrial cavity. The extent of the shunt is determined by the size of the patent foramen ovale and the pressure differences between the right and left atrium. A right-to-left shunt through a patent foramen ovale may occur under specific physiological conditions, such as coughing and the Valsalva maneuver and under different heart and lung diseases in which right atrial pressure exceeds left [7, 8, 20, 26, 32]. The potential pathological consequences of a patent foramen ovale are those encountered with a right-to-left shunt and include hypoxemia in the presence of a hemodynamically significant shunt and the risk of paradoxical embolism.

Methods of detection of a patent foramen ovale during life

Patent foramen ovale presents no abnormalities by history, physical examination, electrocardiogram, and X-ray. Both noninvasive and invasive methods have been used in the detection of the intracardiac shunt. Routine right and left cardiac catheterizations do not usally allow the definite diagnosis of a patent foramen ovale. Transthoracic and transesophageal echocardiography are the preferred methods for detection and visualization of a patent foramen ovale [10, 23, 26]. Beside color flow Doppler, the establishment of contrast echocardiography as a simple, accurate, and safe procedure for diagnosis of right-to-left shunt at the atrial level has enhanced the sensitivity to detect a patent foramen ovale [Fig. 1; 7, 11, 18, 26]. As an alternative technique, the transcranial Doppler ultrasound is established in clinical routine providing direct evidence of paradoxical cerebral echo contrast embolization [33].

Clinical relevance of a patent foramen ovale in patients with acute pulmonary embolism

Hypoxemia

The pathophysiology of arterial hypoxemia in patients with acute pulmonary embolism is not well understood [5, 12, 37]. In addition to hypoxemia caused by the pathophysiological consequences of the pulmonary embolism itself, an intracardiac right-to-left shunt may further decrease arterial oxygenation [8, 22]. In a first study published in 1992,

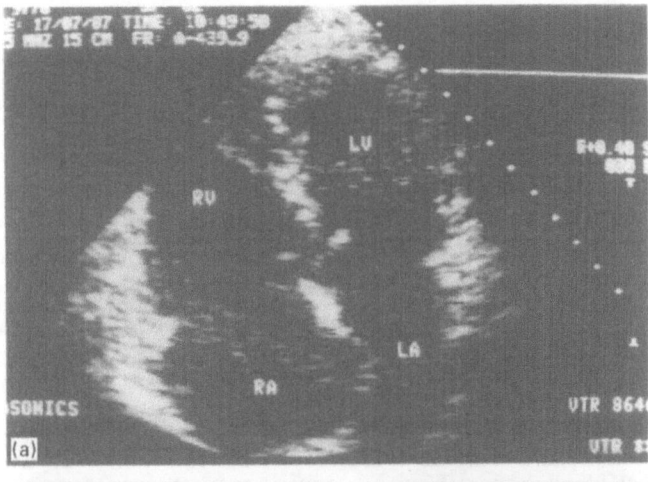
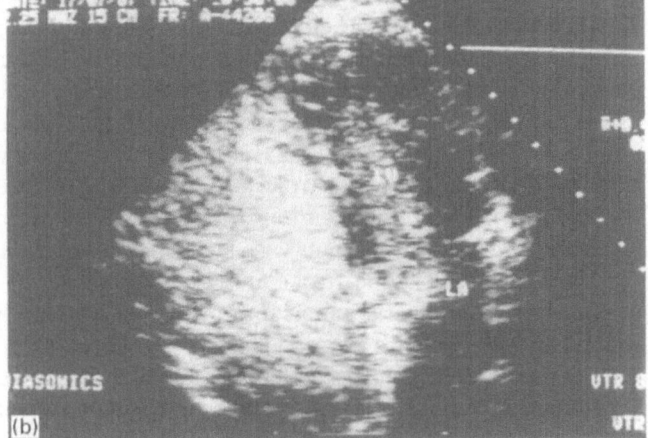

Fig. 1. The transthoracic echocardiogram demonstrates a patient suffered an acute pulmonary embolism with dilatation of the right ventricle (1a). After echo contrast injection (Gelifundol 5 %) from the left cubital vein, echo contrast appears in the left atrium and left ventricle (1b) indicating the presence of a patent foramen ovale. LA: left atrium; LV: left ventricle; RA: right atrium; RV: right ventricle.

we prospectively investigated the clinical relevance of right-to-left shunt in the presence of a patent foramen ovale in 85 patients with acute massive pulmonary embolism [18]. Significant differences were observed in the arterial oxygen tension depending on the presence or absence of a patent foramen ovale. Under room air, patients with a patent foramen ovale had an oxygen tension of 55 ± 14 mm Hg, which was significantly lower (p = 0.038) compared to patients without a patent foramen ovale in whom oxygen tension was 62 ± 16 mm Hg. When arterial oxygen tension was adjusted by pulmonary vascular resistance, the difference in arterial oxygenation between patients with and without a patent foramen ovale was significant (Fig. 2). Our results are in accordance with several incidental findings suggesting that an intracardiac right-to-left shunt through a patent foramen ovale may contribute to arterial hypoxemia [8, 22].

Paradoxical embolism

Paradoxical embolism first described by Cohnheim 1877 is commonly diagnosed at necropsy and can only be detected during life when a right atrial thrombus crossing the

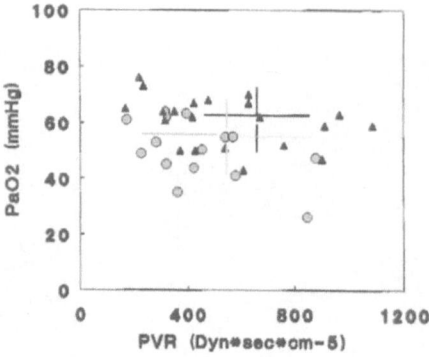

Fig. 2. Arterial oxygen tension (PaO₂) on breathing room air in relation to total pulmonary vascular resistance. PaO₂ is influenced by the presence of a patent foramen ovale (○ = Patent foramen ovale present; ▲ = Patent foramen absent).

foramen ovale can be identified (4; Fig. 3). However, direct observation of the thrombus is rare and remains confined to isolated reports [25, 29–31]. In clinical practice, the diagnosis of paradoxical embolism has to be established by the following indirect criteria: (1) evidence of systemic embolization, (2) detection of an abnormal communication between the right and left circulation, and (3) the presence of venous thrombosis or pulmonary embolism [13, 28]. In initial studies, especially in young patients with stroke, association between a patent foramen ovale and the clinical signs of paradoxical arterial embolism was suggested [6, 10, 23, 36]. However, other investigators could not confirm these results in patients with stroke [14]. The clinical relevance of a patent foramen ovale in patients with pulmonary embolism is not known. Therefore, in a second prospective study we examined 139 patients with acute massive pulmonary embolism with regard to the incidence of ischemic stroke and peripheral arterial embolism depending on the presence or absence of a patent foramen ovale. The study population consisted of 69 women and 70 men with a mean age of 59 ± 17 years. Their clinical characteristics at the time of diagnosis are shown in Table 1. All patients had echocardiographic evidence of pulmonary hypertension and/or right ventricular pressure overload according to the previously published criteria [17, 18, 19]. In addition, confirmation of pulmonary embolism was provided by nuclear imaging and/or pulmonary angiographic examination or by autoptic findings in 110 patients (79 %).

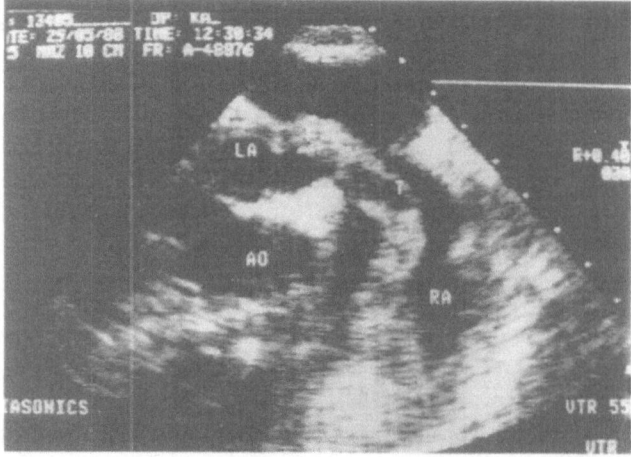

Fig. 3. The transesophageal echocardiogram visualizes an impending paradoxical embolism. A large mobile thrombus protrudes from the right into the left atrium through a patent foramen ovale. AO: ascending aorta; LA: left atrium; RA: right atrium; T: thrombus.

Table 1. Clinical characteristics at diagnosis (n = 139 patients; * Clinical and laboratory findings signifying renal, intestinal, or limb ischemia)

Characteristics	n (% of the patient population)
Acute symptom onset (within 4 days)	97 (70)
Syncope	35 (25)
Focal neurological deficits	7 (5.0)
Peripheral arterial occlusion*	7 (5.0)
Cardiogenic shock	21 (15)
Cardiac arrest	8 (5.7)
Recent major surgery (within 14 days)	28 (20)
Recent major trauma or fracture (within 14 days)	8 (5.8)
History of venous thrombosis	45 (32)
History of pulmonary embolism	7 (5.0)
Congestive heart failure	21 (15)
Chronic pulmonary disease	7 (5.0)
Cancer	16 (12)
Gestation	2 (1.4)
Stroke	3 (2.1)

Right-to-left shunt through a patent foramen ovale was diagnosed by contrast echocardiography in 48 patients (35 %). There was no difference in systolic pulmonary pressure between patients with and without a patent foramen ovale (58 ± 17 vs 57 ± 19 mm Hg; p = 0.6).

Clinical symptoms presumptive of paradoxical embolism occurred in 13 patients (27 %) with a patent foramen ovale and in 2 patients (2.2 %) without a patent foramen ovale. Ischemic stroke was diagnosed in 6 patients (13 %) with a patent foramen ovale compared to 2 patients (2.2 %) without a patent foramen ovale (p = 0.02). Seven patients (15 %) with a patent foramen ovale suffered a peripheral arterial thromboembolic event (p < 0.001).

Prognostic impact of a patent foramen ovale in patients with acute massive pulmonary embolism

In-hospital mortality

Based on the experience of the increased risk of paradoxical embolism and severe arterial hypoxemia, we investigated the clinical outcome in the aforementioned study population depending on the presence or absence of a patent foramen ovale. During the hospital stay, 29 patients (21 %) died. Death was directly related to the pulmonary embolic event in 26 patients (90 %). One patient died of septic shock on the fourth postoperative day following emergency pulmonary embolectomy, a second patient with Salmonella osteomyelitis and sepsis, and a third patient with malignant tumor died due to the underlying disease.

With regard to in-hospital mortality, patients with a patent foramen ovale had a death rate of 33 % as opposed to 14 % in patients without a patent foramen ovale (p = 0.015). Logistic regression analysis demonstrated that, after adjustment for the clinical characteristics listed in Table 1 as well as for the echocardiographic detection of right heart thrombi, the only independent predictors of in-hospital death were arterial hypotension at presentation (p < 0.001) and a patent foramen ovale (p < 0.001; Table 2).

Table 2. Determinants of outcome in patients with acute massive pulmonary embolism (* Complicated in-hospital course was defined as the occurrence of one of the following events: death, ischemic stroke, peripheral arterial embolism, major bleeding, or the need for endotracheal intubation or cardiopulmonary resuscitation. OR denotes odds ratio, CI confidence interval, BP blood pressure, and PA pulmonary artery)

Patient characteristics	Overall in-hospital mortality	Complicated in-hospital course*
Patent foramen ovale	11.35 (2.89–44.52) p < 0.001	5.21 (2.32–11.71) p < 0.001
Age over 60 years	1.28 (0.45–3.66) p = 0.64	1.46 (0.67–3.19) p = 0.34
Acute symptoms onset (within 4 days)	3.72 (0.88–15.72) p = 0.07	0.91 (0.40–2.09) p = 0.82
Arterial hypotension (systolic BP < 90 mm Hg)	26.29 (5.76–120) p < 0.001	7.57 (2.10–27.26) p < 0.002
Cardiac arrest	3.05 (0.46–19.83) p = 0.24	6.09 (0.62–59.6) p = 0.12
Malignant tumor	2.31 (0.53–10.17) p = 0.27	1.52 (0.46–5.05) p = 0.50
Right heart or proximal PA- thrombi (echocardiography)	1.70 (0.49–5.95) p = 0.41	1.06 (0.36–3.05) p = 0.93

Clinical events

Clinical events were defined as death, ischemic stroke, peripheral arterial embolism, major bleeding, or the need for endotracheal intubation or cardiopulmonary resuscitation. Beside ischemic stroke and peripheral arterial thromboembolic events as mentioned before major bleeding occurred in 30 patients (22 %). Cerebral bleeding events were documented in 3 patients (2.1 %). Major bleeding events were observed in 32 % of patients who received thrombolytic treatment as opposed to 15 % in the patient group who underwent conventional heparin anticoagulation.

Endotracheal intubation was performed in 17 patients (35 %) with a patent foramen ovale compared to 15 patients (16 %) without an intraatrial communication. Cardiopulmonary reanimation were found slightly increased when patients with and without a patent foramen ovale were compared (19 % vs 11 %; p = 0.3). According to multiple logistic regression analysis, patent foramen ovale had a highly significant independent effect on the occurrence of major in-hospital complications (odds ratio 10.8 : 1; p < 0.001). Arterial hypotension at presentation was also shown to be an independent predictor of a complicated in-hospital course (Table 2).

In patients with acute massive pulmonary embolism, the independent prognostic determinants with regard to mortality and a complicated clinical course were the presence of a patent foramen ovale and arterial hypotension. The overall mortality in the present study was 21 % with a significant difference between patients with and without a patent foramen ovale. Previous series have reported in-hospital death rates between 8 and 9.5 % in patients with acute pulmonary embolism [2, 15, 34]. A mortality rate of between 18 and 32 % has been reported in clinically unstable high risk patients [1, 15, 16]. Our results are in accordance with these observations. Moreover, beside clinical instability the presence of a patent foramen ovale is additionally a major independent predictor for clinical outcome. Multiple logistic regression analysis demonstrated that, after adjustment for all clinical and echocardiographic findings by multivariate analysis in patients with a patent foramen ovale, the risk of death was more than 10 times higher and the risk of a complicated in-hospital course was more than 5 times higher compared to patients without this atrial communication. A patent foramen ovale was found to be associated with a higher occurrence of ischemic stroke, peripheral arterial embolism, major bleeding, and with the need for endotracheal intubation or cardiopulmonary resuscitation. This prospective study underlines the prognostic impact of a patent foramen ovale in high-risk patients with acute massive pulmonary embolism. The recognition of the prognostic determinants with regard to the clinical outcome in these patients should influence the diagnostic and therapeutic management strategies in these high-risk patients [15, 21].

References

1. Alpert JS, Smith R, Carlson J, Ockene IS, Dexter L, Dalen JE (1976) Mortality in patients treated for pulmonary embolism. JAMA 236: 1477–80
2. Carson JL, Kelly MA, Duff A, Weg JG, Fulkerson WJ, Palevsky HI, Schwartz JS, Thompson BT, Popovich J, Hobbins TE (1992) The clinical course of pulmonary embolism. N Engl J Med 326: 1240–45
3. Cheng TO (1976) Paradoxical embolism. A diagnostic challenge and its detection during life. Circulation 53: 565–68
4. Cohnheim J (1877) Thrombose und Embolie. Vorlesung über allgemeine Pathologie. Vol 1. Berlin: Hirschwald, p 134
5. D'Alonzo G, Bower JS, DeHart P, Dantzker DR (1983) The mechanisms of abnormal gas exchange in acute massive pulmonary embolism. Am Rev Respir Dis 128: 170–72
6. Di Tullio M, Sacco RL, Gopal A, Mohr JP, Homma S (1992) Patent foramen ovale as a risk factor for crytogenic stroke. Ann Intern Med 117: 461–65
7. Dubourg O, Bourdarias JP, Farcot JC, Gueret P, Terdjam M, Ferrier A, Rigaud M, Bardet JC (1984) Contrast echocardiographic visualization of cough-induced right to left shunt through a patent foramen ovale. J Am Coll Cardiol 4: 587–94
8. Hale GS, Clarebrough JK, Fox P, Blair N, McDonald IG, Chestermann C (1979) Severe pulmonary embolism complicated by right-to-left shunting: Diagnosis and implications in management. Aust NZ J Med 9: 953
9. Hagen PT, Scholz DG, Edwards WD (1984) Incidence and size of patent foramen ovale during the first 10 decades of life; An autopsy study of 965 normal hearts. Mayo Clin Proc 59: 17–20
10. Hausmann D, Mügge A, Becht I, Daniel WG (1992) Diagnosis of a patent foramen ovale by transesophageal echocardiography and association with cerebral and peripheral embolic events. Am J Cardiol 70: 668–72
11. Higgins JR, Strunk BL, Schiller NB (1984) Diagnosis of paradoxical embolism with contrast echocardiography. Am Heart J 107: 375–77
12. Jardin F, Gurdjian F, Desfonds P, Fouil-ladieu JL, Margairaz A (1979) Hemodynamic factors influencing arterial hypoxemia in massive pulmonary embolism with circulatory failure. Circulation 59: 909–12
13. Johnson BJ (1951) Paradoxical embolism. J Clin Pathol 4: 316–32
14. Jones EF, Calafiore P, Donnan GA, Tonkin AM (1994) Evidence that patent foramen ovale is not a risk factor for cerebral ischemia in the elderly. Am J Cardiol 74: 596–99
15. Kasper W, Konstantinides S, Geibel A, Olschewski M, Heinrich F, Grosser KD, Rauber K, Iversen S, Redecker M, Kienast J (1997) Management strategies and determinants of outcome in acute major pulmonary embolism: Results of a multicenter registry. J Am Coll Cardiol 30: 1165–71
16. Kasper W, Konstantinides S, Geibel A, Tiede N, Krause T, Just H (1997) Prognostic significance of right ventricular afterload stress detected by echocardiography in patients with clinically suspected pulmonary embolism. Heart 77: 346–49
17. Kasper W, Geibel A, Tiede N, Bassenge D, Kauder E, Konstantinides S, Meinertz T, Just J (1993) Distinguishing between acute and subacute massive pulmonary embolism by conventional and Doppler echocardiography. Br Heart J 70: 352–56
18. Kasper W, Geibel A, Tiede N, Just H (1992) Patent foramen ovale in patients with hemodynamically significant pulmonary embolism. Lancet 340: 561–64
19. Kasper W, Geibel A, Tiede N, Hofmann T, Meinertz T, Just H (1989) Echocardiographic diagnosis of pulmonary embolism. Herz 14: 82–101
20. Keidar S, Grenadier E, Binenboim C, Palant A (1984) Transient right to left atrial shunt detected by contrast echocardiography in the acute stage of pulmonary embolism. J Clin Ultrasound 12: 417–19
21. Konstantinides S, Geibel A, Olschewski M, Heinrich F, Grosser K, Rauber K, Iversen S, Redecker M, Kienast J, Just H, Kasper W (1997) Association between thrombolytic treatment and the prognosis of hemodynamically stable patients with major pulmonary embolism. Circulation 96: 882–888
22. Lang I, Steurer G, Weissel M, Burghuber OC (1988) Recurrent paradoxical embolism complicating severe thromboembolic pulmonary hypertension. Eur Heart J 9: 678–81
23. Lechat P, Mas JL, Lascault G, Loron P, Theard M, Klimczag M, Drobinski G, Thomas D, Grosgogeat Y (1988) Prevalence of patent foramen ovale in patients with stroke. N Engl J Med 318: 1148–52

24. Leonard RCF, Neville E, Hall RJC (1982) Paradoxical embolism: A review of cases diagnosed during life. Eur Heart J 3: 362–70
25. Loscalzo J (1986) Paradoxical embolism: Clinical presentation, diagnostic strategies, and therapeutic options. Am Heart J 112: 141–45
26. Lynch JJ, Schuchard GH, Gross CM, Wann LS (1984) Prevalence of right-to-left shunting in the healthy population: Detection by Valsalva maneuver contrast echocardiography. Am J Cardiol 53: 1478–80
27. Meister SG, Grossmann W, Dexter L, Dalen JE (1972) Paradoxical embolism. Diagnosis during life. Am J Med 53: 292–98
28. Movsowitz C, Podolsky LA, Meyerowitz CB, Jacobs LE, Kotler MN (1992) Patent foramen ovale: A non-functional embryologic remnant or a potential cause of significant pathology. J Am Soc Echocardiogr 5: 259–70
29. Nagelhout DA, Pearson AC, Labovitz AJ. Diagnosis of paradoxic embolism by transesophageal echocardiography. Am Heart J 121: 1552–54
30. Nellessen U, Daniel WG, Matheis G, Oelert H, Depping K, Lichtlen PR (1985) Impending paradoxical embolism from atrial thrombus: Correct diagnosis by transesophageal echocardiography and prevention by surgery. J Am Coll Cardiol 5: 1002–04
31. Nelson CW, Snow FR, Barnett M, McRoy L, Wechsler AS, Nixon JV (1991) Impending paradoxical embolism: Echocardiographic diagnosis of an intra cardiac thrombus crossing a patent foramen ovale. Am Heart J 122: 859–62
32. Rodgers DM, Singh S, Meister SG (1984) Contrast echocardiographic documentation of paradoxical embolism. Am Heart J 107: 1270–71
33. Teague SM, Sharma MK (1991) Detection of paradoxical cerebral echo contrast embolization by trans-cranial Doppler ultrasound. Stroke 22: 740–45
34. The Urokinase Pulmonary Embolism Trial. A national cooperative study (1973) Circulation 47 (II): 1–108
35. Thompson T, Evans W (1930) Paradoxical embolism. Q J Med 23: 135–50
36. Webster MW, Chancellor AM, Smith HJ, Swift DL, Sharpe DN, Bass NM, Glasgow GL (1988) Patent foramen ovale in young stroke patients. Lancet ii: 11–12
37. Wilson JE, Pierce AK, Johnson (1971) Hypoxemia in pulmonary embolism, a clinical study. J Clin Invest 50: 481–91

A. Geibel (✉) · S. Konstantinides
Universitätsklinik Freiburg,
Innere Medizin III – Kardiologie und Angiologie
Hugstetterstr. 55
79 106 Freiburg, Germany

W. Kasper
St. Josefs-Hospital Wiesbaden
Medizinische Klinik I
Solmsstraße 15
65189 Wiesbaden

The value of echocardiography in the diagnostic work-up of patients with suspected acute pulmonary embolism

W. Kasper, S. Konstantinides, A. Geibel

Summary Echocardiography can be used as a differential diagnostic procedure in the diagnostic workup of patients with clinically suspected pulmonary embolism. If RV pressure overload is ruled out in those patients, mortality from thrombembolism seems to be low irrespective of whether pulmonary embolism is present or absent. If, on the other hand, RV pressure overload is present, the prognosis is worse and is dependent on the presence of arterial hypotension at presentation and a patent foramen ovale. Clinicians no longer insist on definite confirmation of pulmonary embolism by nuclear imaging studies or pulmonary angiography especially if the patient is clinically unstable at presentation. It is, thus, evident that echocardiography has gained an important diagnostic position for the management of patients with suspected pulmonary embolism.

Introduction

Echocardiography has increased our understanding of the pathophysiological consequences of acute pulmonary thromboembolism. Right ventricular (RV) pressure overload as a result of major pulmonary obstruction can be easily detected by using echocardiography. This finding can be particularly useful in the differential diagnosis of acute dyspnea and/or hemodynamic instability (7). It has also been shown recently that echocardiography is capable of identifying patients at high risk of death or serious complications due to acute pulmonary embolism [6, 10, 12].

The course of acute pulmonary embolism is related to the degree of pulmonary embolic obstruction, the severity of pre-existing cardiopulmonary dysfunction, and the presence of peripheral venous thrombosis as a potential threat for recurrent thromboembolic events [11]. The interaction of these factors may lead to RV pressure overload which can be readily detected by two-dimensional and Doppler echocardiographic imaging. In particular, the following findings have been shown to be diagnostic of acute *major* pulmonary embolism [4, 7] : 1) RV dilation; 2) asynergic RV free wall motion; 3) thickening (i.e., hypertrophy) of the RV free wall; 4) an abnormal motion pattern of the interventricular septum; 5) tricuspid regurgitation jet velocity > 2.82 m/s; and 6) dilation of the inferior vena cava and right pulmonary artery.

It should be noted that some of the echocardiographic findings listed above can also be encountered in patients with significant left ventricular or mitral valve dysfunction, chronic pulmonary disease, congenital heart disease, right ventricular infarction and, perhaps, heart sarcoidosis (6). In most cases, however, these disorders can be readily excluded at the bedside based on the clinical examination, the ECG, as well as the radiologic and echocardiographic findings.

Diagnostic sensitivity and specificity of echocardiography

During a six year period we studied by echocardiography a total of 698 consecutive patients with clinically suspected pulmonary embolism. Of these, 547 patients (79 %) had further diagnostic work-up in order to confirm or exclude acute pulmonary embolism by pulmonary angiography or ventilation/perfusion lung scan and an interpretable echocardiogram. Pulmonary embolism was confirmed in a total of 288 patients (53 %) and excluded in 259 patients (47 %). RV pressure overload was initially present in 185 patients (34 %).

Echocardiographic imaging had a sensitivity of 52 %, a specificity of 86 %, a positive predictive value of 81 %, and a negative predictive value of 62 % for diagnosis of acute pulmonary embolism. If only those patients with echocardiographically detected RV afterload stress were considered in the statistical analysis, sensitivity was slightly lower (45 %) and specificity higher (97 %). Importantly, the positive predictive value of echocardiography was as high as 93 % in this patient population.

Thus, echocardiography has a high positive predictive value and is, in our experience, a valuable substitute for other diagnostic procedures, especially in situations where it is difficult to perform pulmonary angiograms or ventilation/perfusion lung scans such as in clinically unstable patients. On the other hand, the low negative predictive value of cardiac ultrasound indicates that a normal echocardiogram does not exclude minor pulmonary embolism.

RV pressure overload and prognosis

The prognostic impact of RV pressure overload diagnosed by the echocardiographic findings listed above was studied in a subgroup of 317 patients with clinically suspected pulmonary embolism [6]. Objective confirmation of pulmonary embolism and diagnosis of deep vein thrombosis were both more common in patients with RV pressure overload than in those without it (83 vs. 40 % and 46 vs. 22 %, respectively, $p < 0.001$ for both comparisons). This was also true for the detection of thrombi in the right heart and major pulmonary arteries (12 vs. 1 patient; $p < 0.01$; Table 1). Aggressive therapeutic interventions such as thrombolysis or surgical embolectomy, as well as the implantation of vena cava filters, catecholamine administration for blood pressure support or cardiopulmonary resuscitation where also required more often in the former patient group (Table 2).

In-hospital mortality from venous thrombembolism amounted to 13 % in the presence of RV pressure overload vs. 0.9 % in the remaining patients ($p < 0.001$). Patients with *acute* RV pressure overload did even worse: twelve patients died in this subgroup (24 %) com-

Table 1. RV-afterload stress and prognosis: diagnostic work-up. Data presented are % of patients; RVAS = Right ventricular afterload stress; PE = pulmonary embolism; DVT = deep venous thrombosis

RVAS	Present (n = 87)	Absent (n = 230)	p-Value
PE confirmed	83	40	< 0.001
DVT confirmed	46	22	< 0.001
PE excluded	2.3	44	< 0.001
DVT excluded	24	20	n.s.
Right side thrombi	14.9	0.4	< 0.001

Table 2. RV-afterload and prognosis: therapeutic strategy. Data presented are % of patients; RVAS = right ventricular afterload stress; CPR = cardio pulmonary resuscitation

RVAS	Present (n = 87)	Absent (n = 230)	p-Value
Thrombolysis	42.5	5.2	< 0.001
Surgical embolectomy	5.8	0	< 0.001
Caval filter implantation	8.1	2.2	< 0.02
Catecholamin support	19.5	2.6	< 0.001
CPR	18.4	2.1	< 0.001

Table 3. RV-afterload and prognosis: clinical outcome. Data presented are % of patients; RVAS = right ventricular afterload stress; PE = pulmonary embolism

RVAS	Present (n = 87)	Absent (n = 230)	p-Value
Total mortality	18.4	5.7	< 0.001
Due to PE	12.6	0.9	< 0.001
Acute RVAS	23.5		
Chronic RVAS	11.0		
Right side thrombi	46.0		
1-year mortality	12.6	1.3	< 0.001

pared with 4 of 36 patients with *chronic* RV pressure overload (11 %). Patients with right-heart or pulmonary artery thrombi also had an unfavorable in-hospital course with death in 6/13 patients (46 %). During one year of follow-up after hospital discharge, only one patient of the study population died from consequences of venous thrombembolism; this patient had a negative ultrasound examination at diagnosis. The total one-year mortality of patients without RV pressure overload, thus, rose to 1.3 % but still remained much lower than the 13 % mortality of patients who initially had echocardiographic evidence of major pulmonary embolism (Table 3).

In conclusion, patients without RV pressure overload on the initial echocardiogram had a favorable in-hospital and long-term clinical course irrespective of whether pulmonary embolism was confirmed or excluded by further diagnostic work up. These results suggest that the mortality from venous thrombembolism is mainly determined by the *acute* hemodynamic consequences of pulmonary embolism.

Patent foramen ovale and pulmonary embolism

In the setting of increased right atrial pressure due to right heart failure, a patent foramen ovale may give rise to significant right-to-left shunt. This shunt can contribute to arterial hypoxemia and may result in paradoxic embolic events [5]. In a prospective study, we examined 139 consecutive patients with massive pulmonary embolism for the presence or absence of a patent foramen ovale by contrast echocardiography. A patent foramen ovale was found in 48 patients (35 %; Table 4). Patients with a patent foramen ovale had an in-hospital death rate of 33 % as opposed to 14 % in patients without atrial communication (p < 0.001). Likewise, the incidence of stroke and peripheral arterial embolism and the need for endotracheal intubation was higher in these patients compared to those without a patent foramen ovale. Logistic regression analysis revealed that the only independent predictors of inhospital mortality were a patent foramen ovale and arterial

Table 4. Patent foramen ovale and prognosis: clinical outcome. Data presented are % of patients. PFO = patent foramen ovale, CPR = cardio pulmonary resuscitation

PFO	Present (n = 48)	Absent (n = 91)	p-Value
In-hospital mortality	33	14	< 0.015
Ischemic stroke	13	2.2	0.02
Cerebral bleeding	4.2	1.1	n.s.
Peripheral arterial embolism	15	0	< 0.001
Endotracheal intubation	35	16	0.02
CPR	19	11	n.s.

hypotension at presentation in this group of patients, all of whom demonstrated a RV pressure overload pattern echocardiographically [9].

Right-side thrombi and pulmonary embolism

Echocardiography can diagnose the presence of right-side thrombi in up to 17 % of patients with acute pulmonary embolism [8]. In a European survey concerning the clinical implications of echocardiographically detected right-side thrombi, Kronik and co-workers demonstrated that most thrombi were found in the right atrium and half of these had a mobile structure resembling a worm or a snake [1]. Such thrombi had been shown to originate in the peripheral venous system and were partly entrapped within the right-side chambers during their passage towards the pulmonary circulation. Almost every patient with such a thrombotic structure suffered a pulmonary embolism in this survey, and the in-hospital mortality was extremely high (44 %). These findings are in accordance with our prospective evaluation [6].

Management strategies in acute pulmonary embolism

At present there is no doubt that echocardiography is a useful, noninvasive, bedside diagnostic tool for evaluating patients with clinically suspected or proven pulmonary embolism. The question, thus, arises whether the echocardiographic findings can affect the *management* of patients with suspected acute major pulmonary embolism. This question was addressed in a prospective multicenter registry investigating management strategies and determinants of outcome in acute major pulmonary embolism, the so called MAPPET trial [3]. Patients were included in the registry from 204 participating centers all over Germany. The inclusion criteria of the registry were based on clinical, echocardiographic, and cardiac catheterization findings indicating acute right heart failure and/or pulmonary hypertension due to pulmonary embolism. Four patient groups with increasing clinical and hemodynamic instability were prospectively defined, signifying increasing severity of acute right ventricular failure:

Group 1:   patients with RV pressure overload in the absence of arterial hypotension (n = 407).

Group 2:   patients with transient arterial hypotension, not needing catecholamine support of blood pressure (n = 316).

Group 3:   patients with cardiogenic shock, or those requiring the administration of catecholamines (n = 102).

Table 5. Diagnostic work-up

Method (%)	Group 1 (n = 407)	Group 2 (n = 316)	Group 3 (n = 102)	Group 4 (n = 176)
ECG	99.5	99	100	92
Echo	80	73	68	66
Lung scan	68	60	57	24
Right heart catheter	29	23	26	24
Pulmonary angiography	23	15	14	14

Group 4:   patients with circulatory collapse requiring cardiopulmonary resuscitation at presentation (n = 176).

The relative frequencies with which non-invasive and invasive methods were used in each of these groups are given in Table 5. Besides an electrocardiogram, echocardiography was the most frequently performed diagnostic procedure (74 %). Lung scan or pulmonary angiography was more often performed in clinically stable patients (79 %) but much less frequently in those with circulatory collapse (32 %; Fig. 1). The diagnosis of major pulmonary embolism based on clinical findings and echocardiography "alone" was independently associated with older age (> 65 years), pregnancy, and signs of clinical instability such as arterial hypotension, tachycardia, and the need for endotracheal intubation or cardiopulmonary resuscitation. There was also a substantial increase in

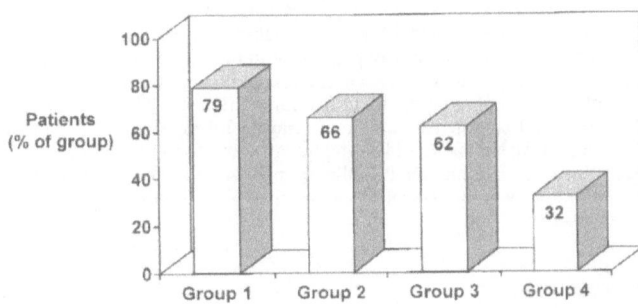

Fig. 1

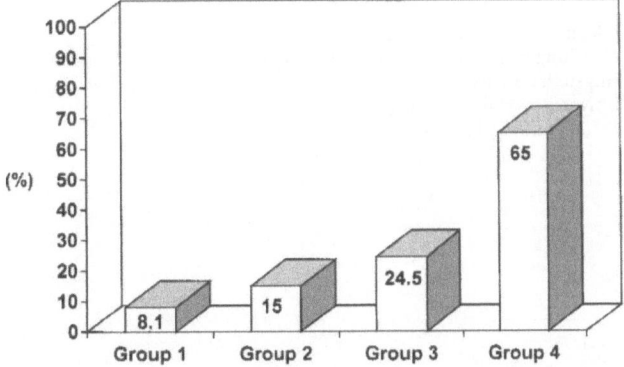

Fig. 2

mortality with increasing clinical instability, ranging from 8.1 % in group 1 to 65 % in group 4 (Fig. 2).

The fact that the majority of the registry patients underwent echocardiography at presentation signifies an important trend in the diagnostic approach to patients with clinically suspected pulmonary embolism. Thus, current management strategies for acute major pulmonary embolism differ greatly from standard management policies which have been recommended up to now [2]. Prospective trials on the outcome of patients with acute pulmonary embolism should take these widely used diagnostic and treatment modalities into account to accurately address clinical needs.

References

1. The European cooperative study on the clinical significance of right heart thrombi (1989) Eur Heart J 10: 1046–1059
2. Ginberg JS (1996) Management of venous thromboembolism. N Engl J Med 335: 1816–1828
3. Kasper W, Konstantinides S, Geibel A, Olschewski M, Heinrich F, Grosser KD, Rauber K, Iversen S, Redecker M, Kienast J (1997) Management strategies and determinants of outcome in acute major pulmonary embolism: Results of a multicenter registry. J Am Coll Cardiol 30: 1165–1171
4. Kasper W, Geibel A, Tiede N, Bassenge D, Kauder E, Konstantinides S, Meinertz T, Just H (1993) Distinguishing between acute and subacute massive pulmonary embolism by conventional and Doppler echocardiography. Br Heart J 70: 352–356
5. Kasper W, Geibel A, Tiede N, Just H (1992) Patent foramen ovale in patients with hemodynamically significant pulmonary embolism. Lancet 340: 561–564
6. Kasper W, Konstantinides S, Geibel A, Tiede N, Krause T, Just H (1997) Prognostic significance of right ventricular afterload stress detected by echocardiography in patients with clinically suspected pulmonary embolism. Heart 77: 346–349
7. Kasper W, Meinertz T, Henkel T, Eissner D, Hahn K, Hofmann T, Zeiher A, Just H (1986) Echocardiographic findings in patients with proved pulmonary embolism. Am Heart J 112: 1284–1290
8. Konstantinides S, Geibel A, Kasper W (1996) Role of cardiac ultrasound in the detection of pulmonary embolism. Semin Respir Crit Care Med 17: 39–49
9. Konstantinides S, Geibel A, Kasper W, Olschewski M, Blümel L, Just H (1998) Patent foramen ovale is a major determinant of outcome in patients with massive pulmonary embolism. Circulation: in press
10. Konstantinides S, Geibel A, Olschewski M, Kasper W, Just H (1997) Acute pulmonary embolism: The value of echocardiography for identification of high risk patients. Circulation 96: I-25 (Abstract)
11. Mark A, Kelley, Jeffrey L, Carson, Harold I, Palevsky J, Sanford Schwartz (1991) Diagnosing pulmonary embolism: New facts and strategies. Ann Int Med 114: 300–306
12. Ribeiro A, Lindmarker P, Juhlin-Damfelt A, Johnsson H, Jorfeldt L (1997) Echocardiography Doppler in pulmonary embolism: Right ventricular dysfunction as a predictor of mortality rate. Am Heart J 134: 479–487

W. Kasper (✉)
St. Josefs-Hospital
Medizinische Klinik
Solmsstraße 15
65189 Wiesbaden, Germany

S. Konstantinides · A. Geibel
Abteilung Innere Medizin III, Kardiologie
Hugstetter Str. 55
Universitätsklinik Freiburg
79106 Freiburg, Germany

Scintigraphy-ventilation/perfusion scanning and imaging of the embolus

P. D. Stein

Summary *Purpose:* This is a review of data on ventilation/perfusion (V/Q) imaging obtained in the collaborative study, Prospective Investigation of Pulmonary Embolism Diagnosis (PIOPED). Special emphasis is given to data obtained subsequent to the main PIOPED publication. New criteria for the interpretation of V/Q scans are based on data obtained by retrospective evaluation of the data from PIOPED.

Background: PIOPED was a prospective randomized double blind investigation of the validity of V/Q scans, based on an angiographic diagnosis of acute pulmonary embolism (PE) in 251 patients and an angiographic exclusion of PE in 480 patients and based on follow-up of patients with normal V/Q scans who did not undergo angiography.

Results: The original PIOPED criteria for interpretation of V/Q scans are reviewed. The positive predictive value of V/Q scans based on these criteria is shown. Clinical assessment in combination with objective readings of V/Q scans is evaluated. The positive predictive value of V/Q scans is assessed according to the complexity of associated disease. The validity of the perfusion scan alone is evaluated. Revised criteria for the interpretation of V/Q scans are described. Criteria for a very low probability interpretation are proposed. The importance of small perfusion defects is described. The diagnostic value of matched ventilation, perfusion and chest radiographic abnormalities is described. The concept of segmental equivalent perfusion defects is assessed. The concept of a mismatched vascular defect, whether moderate or large size, is described. An interpretation of V/Q scans based on the presence of a mismatched perfusion defect in patients stratified according to prior cardiopulmonary disease is described.

Conclusion: Retrospective analysis of the data from PIOPED has permitted an extensive assessment of the diagnostic validity of V/Q scans since the original PIOPED publication. New criteria for interpretation of V/Q scans have been proposed.

Key words Pulmonary embolism – thromboembolism – thromboembolic disease – scintigraphy – ventilation lung scan – perfusion lung scan – pulmonary angiography

Observations from PIOPED

The Prospective Investigation of Pulmonary Embolism Diagnosis (PIOPED) was a national collaborative study designed to determine the sensitivities and specificities of V/Q lung scans in patients with suspected acute PE [2]. The criteria for the interpretation of V/Q scans developed for PIOPED have become widely used [2]. The PIOPED criteria were developed on the basis of 2 or more mismatched segmental equivalent defects being indicative of a high probability of PE. A mismatched segmental equivalent defect is 1 large mismatched segmental defect or 2 moderate size segmental defects. A large segmental defect is > 75 % of a segment. A moderate size segmental defect is ≥ 25 % of a segment but ≤ 75 % of a segment. These criteria assume that a mismatched moderate size segmental equivalent defect is of less diagnostic value than a mismatched large segmental defect [11]. One of the diffculties with this system of grading is the interpretation of the size of the mismatched defect. The distinguishability of large vs moderate size segmental defects requires skill and judgement. Experienced readers of radionuclide lung scans often underestimate the size of segmental defects [10].

The PIOPED criteria for interpretation of V/Q lung scans defined a "very low probability" V/Q scan, but the results of PIOPED reported "nearly normal/normal" interpretations. The latter interpretation includes nearly normal V/Q lung scans and entirely normal V/Q lung scans. A nearly normal V/Q lung scan category included readings of very low probability by one central scan reader and low probability by the other, very low probability by both, very low probability by one and normal by the other. An entirely normal V/Q lung scan was one that was agreed upon by both central scan readers as being normal.

Among the general population of patients suspected of PE, a high probability V/Q scan using original PIOPED criteria was indicative of PE in 87 % [2]. Among patients in whom the V/Q scan probability interpretation was intermediate, PE was present in 30 %. Therefore, the intermediate or indeterminate interpretation was nondiagnostic.

Among patients – whom a low probability interpretation of the V/Q lung scan was made, PE was present in 14 %. Some physicians believe that this percentage of patients with PE who have a low probability V/Q scan is too high to adequately exclude PE [7]. Therefore, patients with low probability V/Q scans require further diagnostic studies [7, 21, 22].

A nearly normal or normal V/Q lung scan by original PIOPED criteria showed PE in only 4 % of patients. Conversely, such an interpretation excluded PE in 96 % of patients.

A normal V/Q scan entirely excluded PE in the experience of PIOPED and others [2, 6, 8, 13]. There were 21 patients in PIOPED who had V/Q scans read as normal by both central readers. Three underwent angiography and none showed thromboemboli. None of the remaining 18 patients received anticoagulants and none had clinically evident PE on follow-up. Sporadic case reports suggest that PE may occur in the presence of a normal perfusion lung scan. If these reports are correct, such cases are extremely rare. The major theoretical reasons for PE associated with a normal perfusion scan are central, non-obstructing, nonlateralized PE or minimal defects on the perfusion scan that are not appreciated [16]. Patients with a single, small, or partially occluding embolus may not show a perfusion defect because of limitations of perfusion scanning.

In PIOPED, only 13 % of patients had high probability V/Q scans. Intermediate V/Q scan readings occurred in 39 % of patients. Low probability V/Q scans occurred in 34 % and nearly normal V/Q scans in 14 %.

Clinical assessment in combination with lung scans

Clinical assessment used in combination with the findings of V/Q lung scans strengthened the diagnostic value of the V/Q scan [2]. In PIOPED, if both the independent clinical assessment and findings by V/Q lung scans were high probability for PE, the diagnosis was correct in 96 % of patients [2] (Table 1). If both the independent clinical assessment and findings by V/Q lung scanning were low probability PE was present in only 4 % of patients. Unfortunately, these concordant diagnostic combinations were uncommon, occurring in only 28 % of patients with clinically suspected PE. Either clinical uncertainty or uncertainty regarding the V/Q lung scan findings (i.e., intermediate V/Q scan pattern)

Table 1. Clinical assessment and ventilation/perfusion lung scan probability in PIOPED

V/Q scan	Clinical Assessment					
	Highly likely PE/Pts	%	Uncertain PE/Pts	%	Unlikely PE/Pts	%
High probability	28/29	96	70/80	88	5/9	56
Intermediate prob	27/41	66	66/236	28	11/68	16
Low probability	6/15	40	30/191	16	4/90	4
Near normal/normal	0/5	0	4/62	6	1/61	2
Total	61/90	68	170/569	30	21/228	9

Highly likely = 80–100 % likelihood of PE based on clinical assessment; Uncertain = 20–79 % likelihood of PE based on clinical assessment; Unlikely = 0–19 % likelihood of PE based on clinical assessment; PE = pulmonary embolism; V/Q = ventilation/perfusion scan; Pulmonary embolism was diagnosed by pulmonary angiography in 248 patients and by autopsy in 4 patients. Pulmonary embolism was excluded by pulmonary angiography in 465 patients. Pulmonary embolism was excluded by outcome assessment (the absence of adverse events during 1 year follow-up while not receiving anticoagulants) in 170 patients. Table modified from (PIOPED) [2].

was present in 72 % of patients. The probability of PE with various V/Q scan probabilities combined with various concordant and discordant clinical suspicions is shown in Table 1.

Complexity of disease

As the complexity of associated cardiopulmonary disease increased, the likelihood that the V/Q lung scan interpretation would be intermediate probability (indeterminate) also increased [9, 14, 15]. Using the original PIOPED criteria, an intermediate probability interpretation of the V/Q lung scan was made in 13 % of patients with a normal chest radiograph, 33 % of patients with no prior cardiopulmonary disease, and 43 % of patients with any prior cardiopulmonary disease. With even more complex disease (chronic obstructive pulmonary disease) (COPD), 60 % of patients had intermediate probability interpretations of the V/Q lung scans. Among each of these categories of patients, the positive predictive value of high, low, and nearly normal V/Q lung scans was similar [9, 14, 15].

Perfusion scan alone

A high probability perfusion scan read with the chest radiograph had no less positive predictive value for acute PE than did a high probability combination V/Q scan [24]. Similarly, a low probability or near normal/normal perfusion scan excluded PE with no less validity than did a low probability or near normal/normal V/Q scan [24]. Somewhat more patients who had only perfusion scans had intermediate (indeterminate) probability interpretations than did those with V/Q scans, but this difference was not statistically significant. Useful information can be obtained if the interpretation of the perfusion is high or low probability, or near normal/normal. If the perfusion scan is interpreted as intermediate probability for PE, a subsequent ventilation scan may change the interpretation to a more definitive probability. A promptly obtained perfusion scan may spare patients an unnecessary hospitalization or unnecessary anticoagulant therapy while awaiting further diagnostic tests [25].

Good results have been shown with obtaining perfusion lung scans before ventilation scans when the ventilation scans were obtained with 99mTc-diethylenetriamine penta-acetate (DPTA) [3]. Performing the perfusion scan prior to the ventilation scan permitted the ventilation study to be tailored for optimal positioning to determine if mismatched defects were present. Direct overlay of the ventilation image on the perfusion image allowed detection of some previously unrecognized perfusion defects.

Investigators in the PISA-PED study used only perfusion lung scans; they did not use ventilation lung scans [12]. Combining clinical assessment with the perfusion scan showed good results when clinical assessment and the perfusion scan reading were concordant. Only the minority of patients (21 %) had discordant clinical and perfusion scan assessments, and these patients required pulmonary angiography. These results at first glance appear better than the results of PIOPED. In the PISA-PED study, however, 24 % of patients had normal perfusion scans, whereas in PIOPED, only 2 % had normal scintiscans. The two study populations, therefore, were dissimilar.

Revised PIOPED criteria

After PIOPED was concluded the nuclear physicians in PIOPED determined that most of the original criteria appropriately categorized V/Q scans [5]. However, it was recommended that three criteria should be reconsidered:

- Two large segmental mismatches may not be the optimum threshold for high probability, and in some cases should be considered for intermediate probability. However, due to the small number of cases with this finding, no definite, statistically founded recommendation could be made.
- A single moderate mismatched perfusion defect is appropriately categorized as intermediate, rather than as low probability.
- Extensive matched V/Q abnormalities are appropriate for low probability, provided that the chest radiograph is clear. Single-matched defects may be better categorized as intermediate probability. Due to the small number of cases with this finding, no definite, statistically founded recommendation could be made.

Criteria for very low/probability interpretation of ventilation perfusion lung scans

The modifications of the PIOPED criteria for low probability were made on the assumption that patients with low probability interpretations of V/Q scans should have a positive predictive value of PE < 20 % [5]. A "very low probability" interpretation with a positive predictive value less than 10 % would be more useful than a "low probability" interpretation [7]. In view of this, we evaluated the individual characteristics and combinations of characteristics of the low probability V/Q lung scan in order to identify criteria that can be used for a "very low probability" interpretation (< 10 % positive predictive value) [23]. The data were limited, and statistically significant differences were not shown between positive predictive values of V/Q criteria that we categorize as "very low probability" and criteria that we categorize as "low probability". We believe, nevertheless, that the trends suggested by the data can be applied in a useful fashion.

Nonsegmental perfusion abnormalities (enlargement of the heart, mediastinum or hila or elevated diaphragm) perfusion defects smaller than opacities on the chest radiograph, and matched V/Q abnormalities in 2 or 3 zones of a single lung showed a positive predictive value < 10 %. A matched V/Q defect in only 1 zone of the lung showed a positive predictive value for PE higher than 10 % and should not be considered a criterion for very low probability, but can be considered a criterion for low probability. Perfusion defects associated with small pleural effusions (obliteration of the costophrenic angle) showed a positive predictive value of 29 % and should be considered a criterion for intermediate probability [23].

PE in patients with small perfusion defects

Perfusion lung scans with 1 to 3 small subsegmental defects satisfy the criterion for a very low probability (< 10 % positive predictive value) for PE and perfusion lung scans with > 3 small subsegmental defects satisfy the criterion for a low probability (< 20 % positive predictive value) for PE) [20]. A small subsegmental perfusion defect was defined as less than 25 % of a segment in the presence of a regionally normal chest radiograph [2]. Evaluation of small perfusion defects was independent of findings on the ventilation scan; a regionally normal chest radiograph was required.

Matched defects of ventilation, perfusion and the chest radiograph: the triple matched defect

The finding of a matched V/Q defect with associated matching chest radiographic opacity (the triple match) has been reported to be an intermediate (nondiagnostic) finding, with a positive predictive value for acute PE of 26 % [26]. This was similar to the positive predictive value for PE of a perfusion defect which matched the chest radiograph, 27 % [1]. The triple match can be caused by PE creating a pulmonary "infarction" (usually pulmonary hemorrhage) but other etiologies are more common [26]. Worsley and associates showed that matching V/Q defects and chest radiographic opacities isolated to the upper and middle zones represent a low probability of PE (less than 20 % positive predictive value), whereas triple matched defects in the lower zone represent an intermediate probability for PE (20 % to 79 % positive predictive value) [26].

Refinement of the PIOPED data for evaluation of triple matched defects were made by elimination of nonrandomized patients, elimination of lungs with mismatched perfusion defects, and elimination of lungs with a pleural effusion [4]. These refined data indicated that the positive predictive value of triple matched defects with PE (radiographic pulmonary infarcts) in the upper lung zone or middle lung zone was low. The positive predictive value of combined upper and middle zones was only 4 %. In the lower lung zone, however, the positive predictive value of a triple matched defect was 23 %. When a triple matched defect with PE occurred, it was most likely to be 1 to 2 segments in size (25–50 % of a zone).

Table 2. Positive predictive value of cumulative number of mismatched segmental equivalent perfusion defects among patients with no prior cardiopulmonary disease and patients with prior cardiopulmonary disease

Segmental equivalents	Patients with no prior cardiopulmonary disease (n = 421) # PE/# PTS (%)	Patients with prior cardiopulmonary disease (n = 629) # PE/# PTS (%)	All patients (n = 1050) # PE/# PTS (%)
≥ 0.0	173/421 (41)	205/629 (33)*	378/1050 (36)
≥ 0.5	123/154 (80)	130/192 (68)**	253/346 (73)
≥ 1.0	102/118 (86)	113/155 (73)*	215/273 (79)
≥ 1.5	91/102 (89)	99/128 (77)**	190/230 (83)
≥ 2.0	79/87 (91)	91/114 (80)***	170/201 (85)
≥ 2.5	72/80 (90)	87/105 (83)	159/185 (86)
≥ 3.0	65/73 (89)	81/97 (84)	146/170 (86)
≥ 3.5	60/67 (90)	77/88 (88)	137/155 (88)
≥ 4.0	57/63 (90)	74/84 (88)	131/147 (89)
≥ 4.5	50/53 (94)	70/78 (90)	120/131 (92)
≥ 5.0	49/52 (94)	65/72 (90)	114/124 (92)
≥ 5.5	47/50 (94)	61/66 (92)	108/116 (93)
≥ 6.0	42/44 (95)	59/64 (92)	101/108 (94)
≥ 6.5	40/42 (95)	56/61 (92)	96/103 (93)
≥ 7.0	38/40 (95)	51/56 (91)	89/96 (93)
≥ 7.5	34/36 (94)	43/47 (91)	77/83 (93)

* P < 0.01, ** P < 0.02, *** P < 0.05: No prior cardiopulmonary disease vs Prior cardiopulmonary disease. These probabilities were calculated with chi square and are higher than reported in Stein and associates (17) because Yates' correction, which was unnecessarily conservative, was used in the previous analysis.

Probability assessment of V/Q scans based on the number of mismatched segmental equivalent perfusion defects in all patients and patients stratified according to the presence or absence of prior cardiopulmonary disease

Table 2 can be utilized by readers of V/Q lung scans to assign to their patients an individualized percentage probability of PE and specificity based on the observed number of mismatched segmental equivalent defects [17]. This strengthens the diagnostic value of V/Q lung scans and gives more useful information than categorical diagnoses of "high," "intermediate," and "low" probability. Stratification of patients by prior disease status enhances the ability of V/Q scan readers to assign an accurate positive predictive value to both clinical categories of patients [17]. Among patients with no prior cardiopulmonary disease, a high positive predictive value of PE is shown with fewer mismatched segmental equivalent defects than were required in PIOPED.

Probability assessment based on the number of mismatched vascular defects and stratification according to prior cardiopulmonary disease

The diagnosis of PE on the basis of the number of mismatched segmental equivalents assumes that a mismatched moderate size segmental perfusion defect is of less diagnostic value than a mismatched large size segmental perfusion defect [11]. This assumption has not been fully tested. There is considerable skill and judgement required in distinguishing a moderate size mismatched segmental perfusion defect (25 % to 75 % of a segment) from a large size mismatched segmental perfusion defect (> 75 % of a segment). We showed that V/Q lung scans can be assessed without the necessity of distinguishing

Table 3. Positive predictive value of pulmonary embolism in relation to the cumulative number of mismatched vascular perfusion defects (large and/or moderate size segmental perfusion defects)

Cumulative number of defects	All patients (n = 1064)	(%)	No prior CPD (n = 421)	(%)	Any prior CPD (n = 629)	(%)
≥ 0	383/1064	(36)	173/421	(41)	205/629	(33)*
≥ 1	255/350	(73)	123/154	(80)	130/190	(68)**
≥ 2	200/244	(82)	94/106	(89)	105/136	(77)***
≥ 3	170/201	(85)	79/87	(91)	90/112	(80)***
≥ 4	149/172	(87)	67/75	(89)	81/96	(84)
≥ 5	130/144	(90)	55/60	(92)	75/84	(89)
≥ 6	116/124	(94)	49/52	(94)	67/72	(93)
≥ 7	103/110	(94)	43/45	(96)	60/65	(92)
≥ 8	93/100	(93)	41/43	(95)	52/57	(91)

CPD = Cardiopulmonary disease * P < 0.01, ** P < 0.02, *** P, 0.05: Prior cardiopulmonary disease vs No prior cardiopulmonary disease. These probabilities are higher than reported by Stein and associates [18] because the chi square probabilities previously calculated used the unnecessarily conservative Yates correction.

large mismatched segmental defects from moderate size mismatched segmental defects [18]. This makes the interpretation of V/Q lung scans easier and more objective. The size of the mismatched defect, providing it was ≥ 25 percent of a segment, was of no consequence. The positive predictive value of the cumulative number of mismatched vascular defects (mismatched large and/or moderate size segments) is shown in Table 3.

Stratification of patients according to the presence or absence of prior cardiopulmonary disease enhanced the positive predictive value of the number of mismatched vascular defects in each category (Table 3). Among patients with no prior cardiopulmonary disease, ≥ 1 vascular defect indicated a positive predictive value for PE of 80 % and ≥ 2 mismatched vascular defects indicated a positive predictive value of 89 %. Among patients with prior cardiopulmonary disease ≥ 1 mismatched vascular perfusion defect indicated a positive predictive value of 68 % and ≥ 2 mismatched vascular perfusion defects indicated a positive predictive value of 77 %. Tables can be used to assess a positive predictive value and specificity for individual patients stratified according to prior cardiopulmonary disease and according to the number of mismatched vascular perfusion defects.

The addition of clinical assessment to stratification according to prior cardiopulmonary disease further optimizes the interpretation of V/Q lung scans

By combining prior clinical assessment with stratification of patients according to the presence or absence of prior cardiopulmonary disease, a family of curves was derived which allowed an accurate assessment of the positive predictive value of PE based upon the number of mismatched segmental equivalent defects or upon the number of mismatched vascular defects [19]. Among patients with no prior cardiopulmonary disease, a high likelihood clinical assessment in combination with ≥ 1 mismatched vascular perfusion defects resulted in a positive predictive value for PE of 100 % (Table 4) [19].

Among patients with no prior cardiopulmonary disease and an intermediate likelihood clinical assessment, a positive predictive value for PE ≥ 80 % was shown with ≥ 2 mismatched vascular perfusion defects. To achieve ≥ 90 % positive predictive value for PE, ≥ 5 mismatched vascular perfusion defects were required.

Table 4. Positive predictive value of pulmonary embolism in relation to the cumulative number of mismatched vascular defects and clinical assessment among patients with no prior cardiopulmonary disease (n = 324)

Mismatched vascular defects	High clinical likelihood # PE/# PTS (%)	Intermed clin likelihood # PE/# PTS (%)	Low clinical likelihood # PE/# PT
≥ 0	27/31 (87)*	107/251 (43)	16/42 (38)+
≥ 1	19/19 (100)**	79/101 (78)	9/15 (60)++
≥ 2	16/16 (100)	60/70 (86)	7/8 (88)
≥ 3	16/16 (100)	50/56 (89)	4/5 (80)
≥ 4	15/15 (100)	42/48 (88)	2/3 (67)
≥ 5	11/11 (100)	36/39 (92)	1/2 (50)
≥ 6	10/10 (100)	31/32 (97)	1/2 (50)
≥ 7	8/8 (100)	28/29 (97)	1/2 (50)
≥ 8	8/8 (100)	26/27 (96)	1/1 (100)

PE = Pulmonary embolism; PTS = patients; *$P < 0.001$, **$P < 0.05$: high vs intermediate; + $P < 0.001$, ++ $P < 0.01$: high vs low. Probabilites are higher than reported by Stein and associates [19] because chi square probabilities previously were calculated using Yates' correction, which was unnecessarily conservative.

Table 5. Positive predictive value of pulmonary embolism in relation to the cumulative number of mismatched vascular perfusion defects and clinical assessment among patients with prior cardiopulmonary disease (n = 569)

Mismatched vascular defects	High clinical likelihood # PE/# PTS (%)	Intermed clin likelihood # PE/# PTS (%)	Low clinical likelihood # PE/# PT
≥ 0	24/30 (80)*	144/396 (36)+	13/143 (9)#
≥ 1	17/19 (89)	99/139 (71)+	3/15 (20)#
≥ 2	16/18 (89)	81/103 (79)++	2/7 (29)##
≥ 3	13/14 (93)	71/86 (83)	1/6 (29)
≥ 4	13/14 (93)	63/72 (88)	1/5 (20)
≥ 5	12/13 (92)	59/64 (92)	1/4 (25)
≥ 6	11/11 (100)	52/55 (95)	1/3 (33)
≥ 7	10/10 (100)	46/49 (94)	1/3 (33)
≥ 8	7/7 (100)	42/45 (93)	0/2 (0)

PE = pulmonary embolism; PTS = patients; INTERMED = intermediate; CLIN = clinical; *$P < 0.001$ high vs intermediate; #$P < 0.001$, ##$P < 0.01$ high vs low; +$P < 0.001$, ++$P < 0.01$ intermediate vs low; probabilites are higher than reported by Stein and associates (19) because chi square probabilities previously were calculated using Yates' correction, which was unnecessarily conservative.

Among patients with prior cardiopulmonary disease who had a high probability clinical assessment and prior cardiopulmonary disease, ≥ 1 mismatched vascular perfusion defect resulted in a positive predictive value for PE ≥ 89 % (Table 5) [19].

Among patients with an intermediate probability clinical assessment, ≥ 3 mismatched vascular defects indicated a positive predictive value ≥ 80 %. To achieve ≥ 90 % positive predictive value for PE, ≥ 5 mismatched vascular defects were required (Table 5) [19].

Presentation of the data as continuous numbers of mismatched defects provided a positive predictive value for PE based upon the V/Q scan characteristics of any particular patient. This flexibility was not possible with the criteria used for V/Q scan interpretation data as presented in PIOPED, which employed fixed numbers of defects for various probabilities of PE [19].

References

1. Biello DR, Mattar AG, McKnight RC, Siegel BA (1979) Ventilation/perfusion studies in suspected pulmonary embolism. Amer J Radiol 133: 1033–1037
2. A Collaborative Study by the PIOPED Investigators (1990) Value of the ventilation/perfusion scan in acute PE: Results of the Prospective Investigation of Pulmonary Embolism Diagnosis (PIOPED). J Am Med Assoc 263: 2753–2759

3. Freitas JE, Sarosi MG, Nagle CC, Yeomans ME, Freitas AE, Juni JE (1995) Modified PIOPED criteria used in clinical practice. J Nucl Med 36: 1573–1578
4. Gottschalk A, Stein PD, Henry JW, Relyea B (1996) Matched ventilation/perfusion defects and chest radiographic abnormalities: Re-evaluation of the triple matched defect in the assessment of acute pulmonary embolism. J Nucl Med 37: 1636–1638
5. Gottschalk A, Sostman HD, Coleman RE, Juni JE, Thrall J, McKusick KA, Froelich JW, Alavi A (1993) Ventilation-perfusion scintigraphy in the PIOPED study. Part II. Evaluation of the scintigraphic criteria and interpretations. J Nucl Med 34: 1119–1126
6. Hull RD, Raskob GE, Coates G, Panju A (1990) Clinical validity of a normal perfusion lung scan in patients with suspected pulmonary embolism. Chest 97: 23–26
7. Hull RD, Raskob GE (1991) Low-probability lung scan findings: A need for change. Ann Internal Med 114: 142–143
8. Kipper MS, Moser KM, Kortman KE, Ashburn WL (1982) Longterm follow-up of patients with suspected pulmonary embolism and a normal lung scan. Chest 82: 411–415
9. Lesser BA, Leeper KV, Stein PD, Saltzman HA, Chen J, Thompson BT, Hales CA, Popovich J Jr, Greenspan RH, Weg JG (1992) The diagnosis of pulmonary embolism in patients with chronic obstructive pulmonary disease. Chest 102: 17–22
10. Morrell NW, Nijran KS, Jones BE, Biggs T, Seed WA (1993) The underestimation of segmental defect size in radionuclide lung scanning. J Nucl Med 34: 370–374
11. Neumann RD, Sostman HD, Gottschalk A (1980) Current status of ventilation-perfusion imaging. Semin Nucl Med 10: 198–217
12. PISA-PED Investigators. (1995) Invasive and noninvasive diagnosis of pulmonary embolism. Chest 107: 33S–38S
13. Stein PD (1982) Low-dose heparin for prevention of pulmonary embolism and significance of normal lung scan. ACCP Bulletin 21: 12–14
14. Stein PD, Alavi A, Gottschalk A, Hales CA, Saltzman HA, Vreim CE, Weg JG (1991) Usefulness of non-invasive diagnostic tools for diagnosis of acute pulmonary embolism in patients with a normal chest radiograph. Am J Cardiol 67: 1117–1120
15. Stein PD, Coleman RE, Gottschalk A, Saltzman HA, Terrin ML, Weg JG (1991) Diagnostic utility of ventilation/perfusion lung scans in acute pulmonary embolism is not diminished by pre-existing cardiac or pulmonary disease. Chest 100: 604–606
16. Stein PD, Gottschalk A (1994) Critical review of ventilation/perfusion lung scans in acute pulmonary embolism. Prog Cardiovasc Dis 37: 13–24
17. Stein PD, Gottschalk A, Henry JW, Shivkumar K (1993) Stratification of patients according to prior cardiopulmonary disease and probability assessment based upon the number of mismatched segmental equivalent perfusion defects: Approaches to strengthen the diagnostic value of ventilation/perfusion lung scans in acute pulmonary embolism. Chest 104: 1461–1467
18. Stein PD, Henry JW, Gottschalk A (1993) Mismatched vascular defects: An easy alternative to mismatched segmental equivalent defects for the interpretation of ventilation/perfusion lung scans in pulmonary embolism. Chest 104: 1468–1472
19. Stein PD, Henry JW, Gottschalk A (1993) The addition of clinical assessment to stratification according to prior cardiopulmonary disease further optimizes the interpretation of ventilation/perfusion lung scans in pulmonary embolism. Chest 104: 1472–1476
20. Stein PD, Henry JW, Gottschalk A (1996) Small segmental perfusion defects in suspected pulmonary embolism. J Nucl Med 37: 1313–1316
21. Stein PD, Hull RD, Saltzman HA, Pineo G (1993) Strategy for diagnosis of patients with suspected acute pulmonary embolism. Chest 103: 1553–1559
22. Stein PD, Hull RD, Pineo G (1995) Strategy that includes serial and noninvasive leg tests for diagnosis of thromboembolic disease in patients with suspected acute pulmonary embolism: Estimated percentage of patients, based on data from PIOPED, in whom a noninvasive diagnosis or exclusion of thromboembolic disease might be safely made. Arch Intern Med 155: 2101–2104
23. Stein PD, Relyea B, Gottschalk A (1996) Evaluation of the positive predictive value of specific criteria used for the assessment of low probability ventilation/perfusion lung scans. J Nucl Med 37: 577–581
24. Stein PD, Terrin ML, Gottschalk A, Alavi A, Henry JW (1992) Value of ventilation/perfusion scans compared to perfusion scans alone in acute pulmonary embolism. Am J Cardiol 69: 1239–1241
25. van Beek EJR, Kuyer PMM, Schenk BE, Brandjes DPM, tenCate JW, Buller HR (1995) A normal perfusion lung scan in patients with clinically suspected pulmonary embolism. Chest 108: 170–173
26. Worsley DF, Kim CK, Alavi A, Palevsky HI (1993) Detailed analysis of patients with matched ventilation/perfusion defects and chest radiographic opacities. J Nucl Med 34: 1851–1853

P. D. Stein (✉)
Henry Ford Heart and Vascular Institute
Cardiac Wellness Center
6525 Second Avenue
Detroit, MI 48282-3006, USA

MR-angiography in the diagnosis of pulmonary embolism

P. Steiner, T. H. Hany, G. McKinnon, F. Follath, J. F. Debatin

Summary The purpose of this article is to describe the role of 3 dimensional (3D), breath-hold, contrast enhanced magnetic resonance angiography (MRA) in the diagnosis of acute pulmonary embolism. In a volunteer study, two MRA techniques were adopted. One of which enabled acquisition of the pulmonary vasculature in 18 s. The other technique was coupled with a higher spatial resolution, leading to a scan time of 23 s. Additionally, the impact of breathing motion on vessel delineation was assessed. The breathheld 23 second scans revealed excellent image quality and near complete visualization of central and segmental, as well as 81 % of subsegmental, pulmonary arteries. Imaging time can be shortened to 18 seconds with only marginal loss in visualization performance (p < 0.05). Respiratory motion was found to cause significant worsening of image quality and vessel detectability. To maintain relevance in a clinical setting, imaging time can be minimized at the cost of a reduction in spatial resolution. According to data available from patient studies, the sensitivity, specificity, positive and negative predictive values of 3D MRA in comparison to conventional angiography amounts to 100, 95, 87, and 100 %, respectively.

However, breathhold duration and spatial resolution need further optimization if 3D MRA should replace conventional angiography as the gold standard in the future.

Conclusion: The preliminary experience suggest that gadoliniumenhanced, three dimensional, breathhold, magnetic resonance angiography shows promise as a safe, rapid, accurate and cost-effective imaging technique for the diagnosis of pulmonary embolism. In combination with its ability to perform deep venous studies and the potential aspect of MR-perfusion studies of the lung parenchyma, pulmonary MRA might in the future turn out to be the "one stop shop" for diagnosing pulmonary embolism.

Key words Pulmonary magnetic resonance imaging – 3 dimensional magnetic resonance angiography – pulmonary embolism – contrast enhanced magnetic resonance imaging

Introduction

Effective therapy is available for venous thromboembolism, but the therapy itself can produce significant morbidity. Thus, an accurate diagnosis is mandatory. The clinical presentation and laboratory findings in pulmonary embolism (PE) are non-specific; therefore, additional evaluation with imaging studies is essential.

Due to its exquisite resolution, invasive pulmonary angiography remains the gold standard in the evaluation of patients with suspected acute PE. Associated major and minor complications of up to 5 % [23] have motivated the exploration of other less invasive imaging techniques, including nuclear scintigraphy [21], echocardiography [1], and most recently spiral CT and electron-beam CT [20, 26]. Despite initial enthusiasm, none of these has been able to provide sufficient diagnostic sensitivity and specificity to obviate the need for invasive pulmonary angiography [6, 16].

In comparison to CT, magnetic resonance imaging (MRI) is an imaging modality which is associated with a lack of radiation exposure, an unsurpassed soft tissue contrast, multiplanar reconstruction capabilities, and the ability to visualize vessels without administration of intravenous contrast material. This article focuses on the potential value of MRI in diagnosing pulmonary embolism.

Magnetic resonance angiography

As part of the ongoing search for a non-invasive and accurate means for diagnosing acute pulmonary embolism, MR angiography (MRA) has been evaluated [7, 22]. Until recently, these MR techniques exploited the phenomenon that flowing blood within vessels induces MR signal intensities different to surrounding stational tissue. However, visualization of pulmonary artery vessels remained problematic. This was mostly due to the long MR acquisition times and the associated patient movement. Other reasons for suboptimal image quality were the presence of respiratory and cardiac motion, air-tissue interface susceptibility variations, arterial-venous overlap, and the low contrast between slow flowing blood and intravascular clots. Finally, the spatial resolution turned out to be insufficient for delineation of segmental and sub-segmental pulmonary rami [5, 10].

Ultrafast, breathhold, contrast enhanced 3-D magnetic resonance angiography

Breathholding during data acquisition [4] and the intravenous application of para-magnetic contrast [17] have been shown to be beneficial for vascular imaging in MR. Intravenous administration of paramagnetic contrast induces a shortening of the T1 relaxation time of blood [19]. The resulting vascular enhancement is no longer flow dependent, but instead solely reflects T1-shortening. Furthermore it has become apparent that 3D data collection strategies are superior to 2D acquisitions, as they provide more vascular detail with fewer artifacts and enable acquisition of thinner slices resulting in higher spatial resolution [28]. Eventually, the availability of faster magnetic resonance hardware, namely gradient systems, reduced the time needed for 3D MR acquisition of whole body systems like the thorax from several minutes to about 20 s. The combination of dynamic intravenous gadolinium injection and this fast 3-D MR technique made it possible to perform high resolution angiography during a single suspended breath. This technique has already proved successful in detecting abnormalities in the thoracic and abdominal aorta and visceral arteries [13, 18]. Exploiting the availability of such previously mentioned ultrafast gradients, we were able to perform contrast-enhanced 3D MR-angiographies capable of acquiring 48 MR-sections within a comfortable breathhold. Fueled by this prerequisite, we started studying the value of MR for pulmonary artery visualization in volunteers [24] and patients.

MR-technique

Imaging was performed on a 1.5-T MR scanner (Signa Horizon Echospeed, General Electric Medical Systems, Milwaukee, WI) equipped with an ultrafast, three-axis gradient system. A phased-array surface coil was employed for signal reception. Subjects and patients were imaged in the supine position with the arms placed above the head. The MR acquisition volume consisted of 48 contiguous coronal sections. The section thickness was adapted to assure coverage of the entire arterial pulmonary vasculature and ranged between 2.0 and 3.0 mm. The high-perfomance gradient system permitted repetition (TR) and echo times (TE) of 3.8 and 1.7 ms, respectively. A flip angle of 40° was used. A 32 cm field of view (FOV) coupled with either a 160×160 or 192×192 matrix rendered an in plane resolution of 2×2 mm or 1.7×1.7 mm, respectively. Imaging times for the 3D volume amounted to 18 (160×160 matrix) or 23 s (192×192 matrix).

In MR imaging the central part of the k-space is responsible for the contrast within the picture. This part of k-space is acquired in the midportion of the MR acquisition. In order to achieve optimal vessel opacification during that part of the MR acquisition, a test bolus technique was adopted. 5 ml gadolinium-DTPA (Magnevist, Schering AG, Berlin, Germany) followed by a saline flush was injected. A region of interest was used to measure signal intensities within the pulmonary outflow tract. The time to half peak enhancement was defined as the start delay between start of contrast injection and start of MRA. During pulmonary MRA the contrast material was injected at a dose of 0.3 mmol/kg (= 0.6 ml/kg body weight) followed by a 20 ml saline flush. The contrast was administered as a bolus via a 20 gauge intravenous catheter placed into an antecubital vein, using an automated injector (Spectris, Medrad, Pittsburgh, U.S.A.) at a rate of 3 ml/s.

Volunteer study

In a volunteer study [24], we investigated the impact of two different spatial resolution techniques on image quality. Furthermore, we were interested to which degree breathing affects pulmonary vessel delineation. Ten healthy volunteers (5 men, 5 women, mean age 24 years) were enrolled in the study. Each volunteer was imaged twice within a period of no longer than eight days. The first time the subjects were instructed to hold their breath (endinspiration) during data acquisition. The second time the data were acquired during shallow breathing. Half the subjects were imaged using a 160×160 matrix, and the other half with a 192×192 matrix. The performance of the technique was determined by evaluating the degree of pulmonary arterial depiction. Analysis was based on maximum intensity projections (MIP) reconstructions as well as 3 mm thick 3D multiplanar reformations in the axial and coronal planes. Additionally, interactive viewing of the 3D data was possible on a work station in cine display.

The pulmonary outflow tract (main pulmonary artery and both central pulmonary arteries), the lobar arteries (right side: interlobar trunk, upper, middle, and lower lobe artery; left side: upper and lower lobe), and the associated 19 segmental arteries were assessed with regard to their visibility. Grading was performed on a 'per segment' basis using a four point scale: 1 = not seen; 2 = seen, cannot exclude thrombus; 3 = seen, can exclude thrombus; 4 = well seen, can exclude thrombus. Additionally, for each subsegmental artery, the number of depicted first order bifurcations into subsegmental rami was determined.

Fig. 1 summarizes the mean visibility scores with associated standard deviations for the pulmonary outflow tract as well as lobar and segmental arteries for all four evaluated acquisitions. Respiratory motion had a dominant impact upon the ability to visualize pulmonary arteries. Lobar and particularly the more peripheral segmental pulmonary arteries were not seen as well on the non-breathheld sequences compared to either of the two breathheld image sets (p < 0.001). The differences in segmental arterial visibility were more pronounced in the middle and lower lobes than in the upper lobes (p < 0.001). No

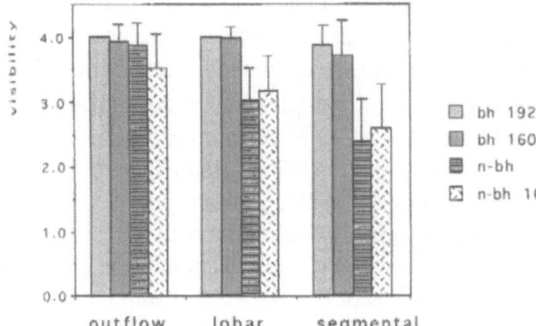

Fig. 1. Visibility of pulmonary outflow tract, lobar, and segmental pulmonary arteries. Notations: bh 192 = breathheld sequence, matrix 192 × 192; bh 160 = breathheld sequence, matrix 160 × 160; n-bh 192 = non-breathheld sequence, matrix 192 × 192: n-bh 160 = non-breathheld sequence, matrix 160 × 160. Outflow = pulmonary outflow tract; lobar = lobar pulmonary arteries; segmental = segmental pulmonary arteries

such difference between upper and lower lobe segmental artery visibility was observed on the breathheld image sets.

Comparison of the two breathheld techniques demonstrated no difference with regard to visualization of the outflow tracts and lobar pulmonary arteries. Segmental artery visibility scores revealed a marginally significant difference favoring the 192 × 192 matrix acquisition ($p < 0.05$). When the data were collected in apnoea, image quality was sufficient to exclude the presence of thrombi (visibility score 3 or 4) in 100 % of outflow and lobar pulmonary arteries (Fig. 2). Furthermore, thrombi could be excluded in 98.9 %

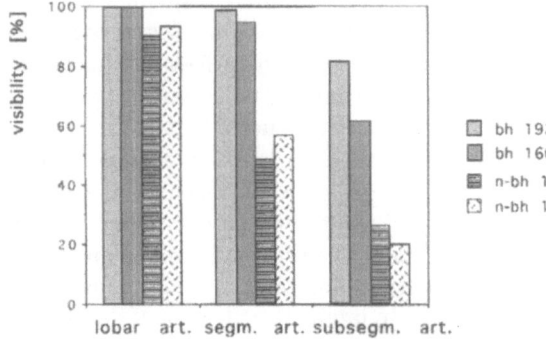

Fig. 2. Procentual visibility of lobar, segmental, and sub-segmental pulmonary arteries. Notations: bh 192 = breathheld sequence, matrix 192 × 192; bh 160 = breathheld sequence, matrix 160 × 160; n-bh 192 = non-breathheld sequence, matrix 192 × 192; n-bh 160 = non-breathheld sequence, matrix 160 × 160. lobar art. = lobar pulmonary arteries; segm. art. = segmental pulmonary arteries; subsegm. art. = subsegmental pulmonary arteries

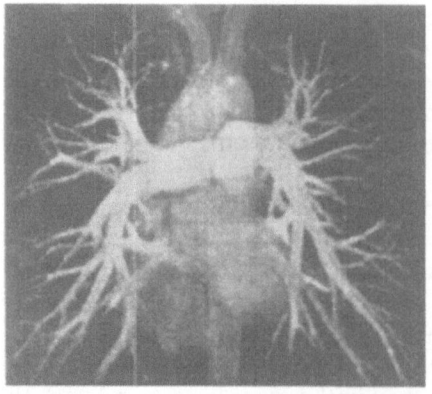

Fig. 3. Maximum intensity projection of a contrast enhanced 3D pulmonary MRA with 192 × 192 matrix (23 second scan, breathhold). In this anterior-posterior projection, subsegmental and even subsubsegmental pulmonary arteries are visualized

and 94.7 % of segmental arteries, depending on whether the data were collected with a 192 × 192 or 160 × 160 matrix, respectively. Non-breathheld data sets performed significantly poorer (p < 0.001).

Even fifth order branches, the subsegmental pulmonary arteries, were visualized to a significant degree. On average, 81 % and 61 % were seen when analysis was based upon breathheld 192 × 192 and 160 × 160 acquisitions, respectively (Fig. 3). Only 26 % and 20 % on the other hand were adequately seen on the non-breathheld 192 × 192, and 160 × 160 data sets, respectively (Fig. 4). As evidenced by these numbers, the presence of respiratory motion had a far greater effect on the ability to visualize sub-segmental arteries than a

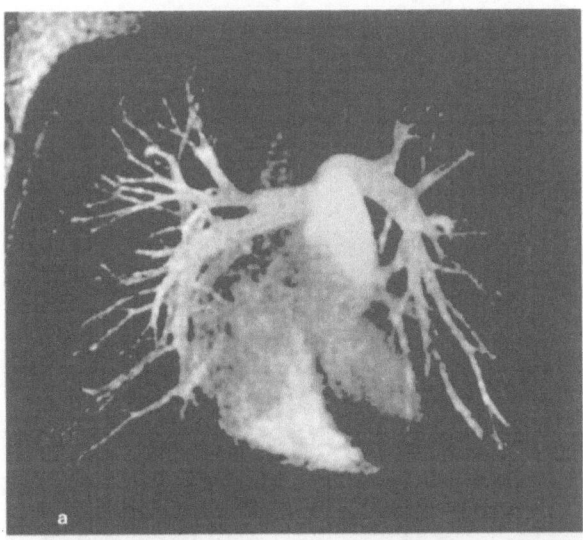

Fig. 4a

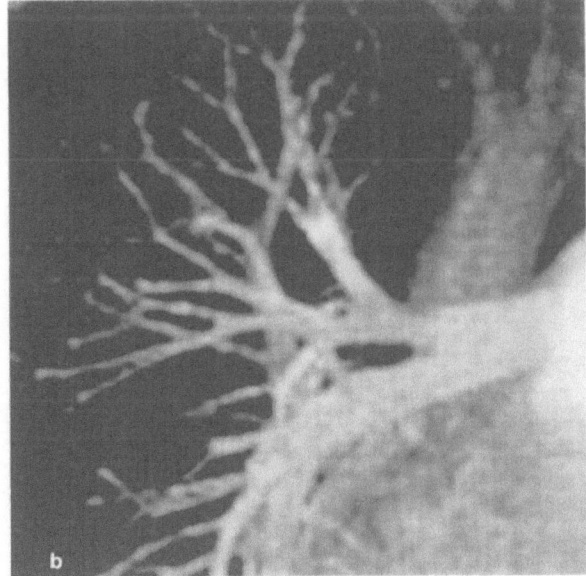

Fig. 4b

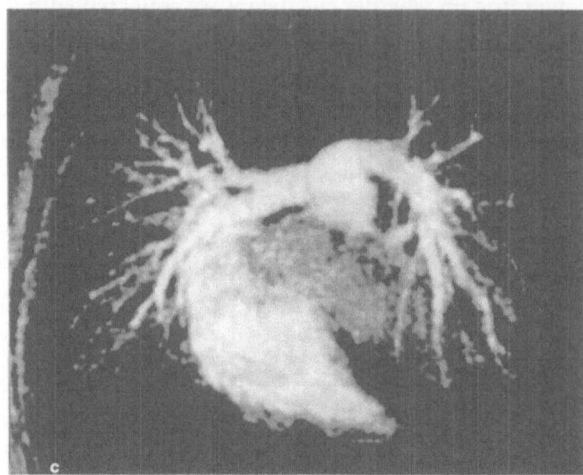

Fig. 4. MRA using a 192 × 192 matrix demonstrating central and peripheral pulmonary vessels (a) as well as some overlap by pulmonary veins in the magnified view of the right upper lobe. (b) Comparison with the non-breathheld scan (c) of the same subject demonstrates loss of anatomical information. Visualization of segmental and subsegmental vessels within the middle and lower lobes is affected by breathing motion

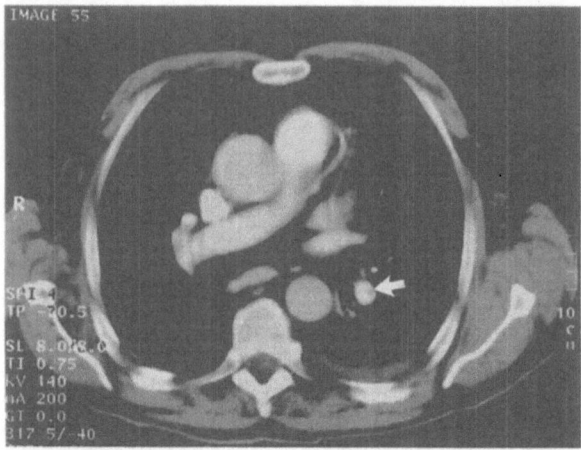

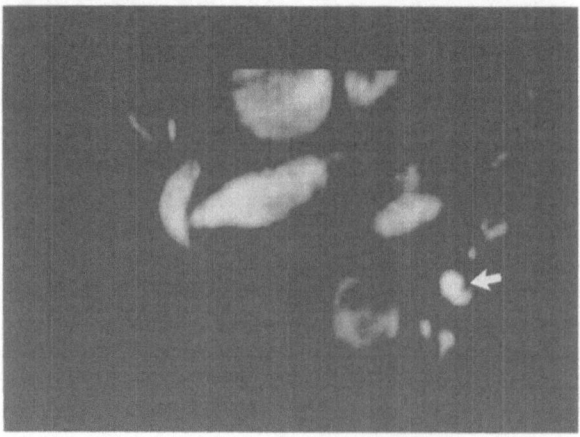

Fig. 5. Spiral CT (a) and MRA (b) of a patient with acute PE. Note the small thrombus in the left lower lobe pulmonary artery (arrow)

reduction in spatial resolution. Both differences, however, were found to be statistically significant ($p < 0.05$).

Patient studies

Subsequently, breathhold, contrast enhanced 3D pulmonary MRA were performed in 15 patients (aged 45–82 years) with clinical suspicion of acute pulmonary embolism. All patients had clinical signs of PE according to the Greenfield classification grade II–III [25]. In 9 patients 23 s scans and in the remaining 18 s scans were performed. Conventional angiography (n = 7), spiral CT (n = 4), and ventilation/perfusion scintigraphy (n = 10) were conducted within 24 hours of MRA. The people interpreting the MRA were blinded to the results of the complementary imaging modalities. Intravascular filling defects and complete vessel cut offs were defined as positive signs of PE. Nonvisualization of a vessel alone was considered insufficient evidence for the diagnosis. Vessels down to the level of segmental pulmonary arteries were assessed.

Three patients were not able to hold the breath for the required time period. However, all MRA were considered interpretable. Seven patients were found to have positive evidence for PE on the basis of all complementary imaging modalities. In 8 patients PE was excluded. In all patients with PE, MRA revealed positive signs of intravascular thrombi (Fig. 5). In the remaining 7 patients MRA was correctly negative. Spiral CT (n = 1) and ventilation-perfusion scintigraphy (n = 2) produced three false positive results. PE was excluded by conventional angiography in these patients. MRA was correctly negative in all these patients.

Discussion

The presented ultrafast contrast-enhanced 3D MRA strategy provides near complete visualization of central and segmental, as well as 81 % of subsegmental, pulmonary arteries, as long as the data are acquired in apnoea. The use of ultrafast gradient systems has reduced the acquisition time for a 3D volume, covering the entire pulmonary arterial tree in 44 thin contiguous sections with high inplane spatial resolution, to 23 seconds. By reducing spatial in-plane resolution, imaging times can be shortened to 18 seconds with only marginal loss in visualization performance. The presence of respiratory motion during data acquisition, on the other hand, causes a dramatic worsening of image quality. Reflecting the effect of breathing on lung motion the segmental arteries were affected more than central vessels. As a result of the volunteer study it seems conceivable that limited spatial resolution acquired in apnoea is clearly preferable to high spatial resolution corrupted by respiratory motion. Therefore, preventing respiratory motion in severely ill patients might indeed warrant further reductions in spatial resolution.

The data of our preliminary patient study underline the value of the pulmonary MRA. If the software and hardware prerequisites are met, contrast enhanced pulmonary MRA may play a interesting role in the diagnosis of acute PE. A study published recently [15] supports our results. In this study 30 patients underwent both MRA and conventional angiography. Due to hardware restrictions of the MR scanner in use, the breathhold period was even longer than in our series and amounted to 27 s. Nevertheless, breathing motion was observed in only 3 patients and corroborated the depiction of some segmental pulmonary arteries. Eight of the 30 patients had PE. All 5 lobar emboli and 16 of

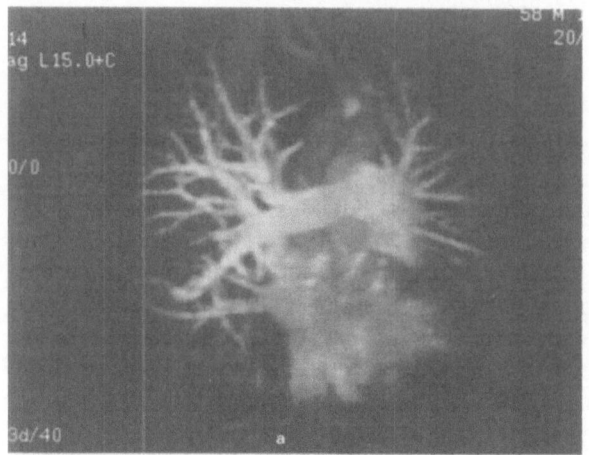

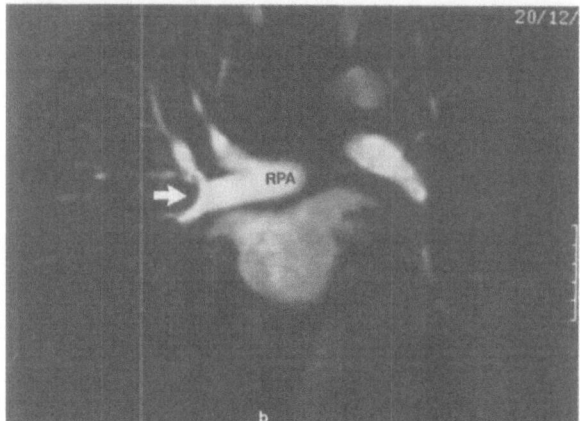

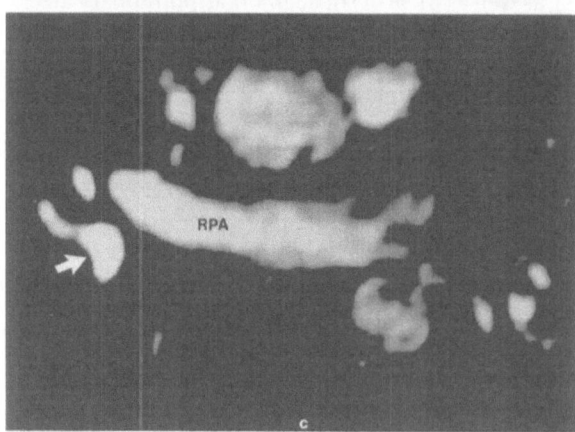

Fig. 6. 30° right anterior oblique MIP (a), coronal reformatted image (b), and axial reformatted image (c) of a patient with partially occluding thrombi in the proximal part of the right lower lobe pulmonary artery. Due to venous overlap, the clot was not seen on the MIP. The coronal reformat clearly demonstrates the thrombus (arrow). Note that differentiation between thrombus and lung parenchyma is not possible. The partially occluding character of the clot is also revealed by the axial image (arrow). RPA = right main pulmonary artery

17 segmental emboli identified on standard angiograms were also identified on MR images. The single segmental thrombi missed was in a patient with breathing motion artifacts. As compared with standard pulmonary angiography gadolinium enhanced MRA had a sensitivity, specificity, positive and negative predictive value of 100, 95, 87, and 100 %. These accuracies are well within the range of reported results from spiral and electron beam CT.

Although some patients seem to be able to hold their breath for as long as 27 s, it is obvious that shortening of imaging times is of paramount importance to any breathheld pulmonary MRA strategy in order to attain relevance in a clinical setting with dyspnoeic patients. Although higher spatial resolutions did indeed allow visualization of significantly more sub-segmental pulmonary arteries, data sets acquired with lower spatial resolution still permitted complete assessment of the diagnostically relevent central and segmental pulmonary arteries. The associated reduction of the imaging time to 18 seconds will vastly enhance the ability of many patients, particularly those with cardiopulmonary diseases, to hold their breath during the data acquisition. In patients not able to hold their breath at all, it is conceivable that the use of navigator sequences, tracking the motion of the diaphragm, would be beneficial. These techniques have been shown to enhance the visualization of coronary arteries [27]. The presence of atelectasis and pleural effusions in the affected lung might make tracking the diaphragm difficult however. Other vessel tracking techniques have been proposed [3, 14]. In the setting of pulmonary embolism, their impact needs yet to be evaluated.

Adequate intravascular signal does require sufficient T1-shortening of the arterial blood. Based on previously published work, this is accomplished by administering gadolinium-DTPA. Even at a dose of 0.3 mmol/kg, the administered MR contrast volume is still less than half of the iodinated contrast volume that is required for conventional or CT angiography. In the meantime, new data have shown that similar results can be achieved with a dose of 0.2 mmol/kg [9]. Contrast volume reduction could be of particular benefit in hemodynamically unstable patients suspected of suffering from pulmonary embolisms.

In the current study protocol an individual scan delay pattern was maintained for volunteers and patients. To maximize the diagnostic utility of the paramagnetic contrast agent, its administration should be timed to solely opacify the pulmonary arteries. The use of automated injectors in combination with a test bolus [8], automative bolus onset detection or time resolved 3D data acquisition techniques [12] promise to further enhance the performance of this technique.

Even with optimal contrast bolus timing, some degree of pulmonary venous opacification is unavoidable. Utilization of multiple standard MIP views (60° left anterior oblique to 60° right anterior oblique) might reduce that problem to some extent. The required post-processing effort is limited, since only vessels containing paramagnetic contrast are rendered bright in this 3D MRA technique. In contrast to CT angiography, calcified structures, including ribs and spine, as well as calcified hilar lymph nodes remain dark and, thus, do not obscure visualization of the pulmonary arteries. Venous overlap can be further reduced by incorporating source images, multiplanar reformations, as well as interactive cine-mode viewing of the data on a work station. For definitive identification of clot, especially partially occluding thrombi, these reformatted images are definitely of greater value than MIPs and are the basis of pulmonary MRA interpretation (Fig. 6).

In conclusion, short single-breathheld contrast enhanced MRA provides high quality images of central and peripheral pulmonary arteries in healthy subjects. Preliminary data concerning patient applications are promising. However, larger clinical trials will have to determine the ultimate efficacy of this technique.

Further MRI-developments

MRA is known to be an accurate non-invasive method for diagnosing deep venous thrombosis. Sensitivities and specificities were found to be between 90 and 100 % for visualizing thrombi in the calf, thigh or pelvis [2]. While that application has been established for some time, first experiences with regard to MR ventilation studies of the lungs utilizing Helium gas have recently been reported. This technique might potentially enable visualization of lung parenchyma similar to scintigraphic ventilation studies [11].

The group in Rotterdam has further developed their MRA technique, which now enables them to acquire as much as 20 coronal slices of the lung in 1 s (29). The MRA experiment can be repeated several times so that in conjunction with intravenous gadolinium injection, MR perfusion studies can be obtained. As shown by these few examples, MR can potentially be used as multifunctional method. It might have the potential of replacing some of the common and currently widely used diagnostic methods.

Potential role of MRA in the diagnostic workup of pulmonary embolism

For a new test to replace ventilation-perfusion scanning or conventional pulmonary angiography for the definitive diagnosis of pulmonary embolism, it must be accurate, readily available, cost effective, and acceptable to both the physician and the patient. According to the most recently published studies, MRA met most of these criteria. In terms of charges to the patient, MRA is more expensive than ventilation-perfusion scanning but cheaper than conventional angiography. When one takes into account the high number of indeterminate findings on ventilation-perfusion scans, however, the effective cost of magnetic resonance angiography per diagnosis is considerably lower than the cost of ventilation-perfusion scanning. However, certain limitations must also be addressed:

As the MR hardware prerequisites are not yet widely met, only preliminary data from a limited number of research groups are available. Therefore, conclusions with regard to the role of MR pulmonary angiography have to be drawn with caution. In order to gain widespread use the spatial and temporal resolution of breathhold, MRA has to be improved. With rapid improvements being made in MR, it is likely that the resolution of magnetic resonance angiograms will soon rival that of conventional pulmonary angiograms. Until now, only vessels down to the level of segmental pulmonary arteries can be accurately visualized in clinical settings. However, the need to visualize more peripheral vessels remains controversial. Furthermore, the clinical significance of small emboli in subsegmental vessels remains uncertain. Non-invasive imaging with MR, as well as with CT, may thus be acceptable despite the possibility of missing small emboli. In comparison to spiral CT, which offers additional information about the lung structure itself, the differentiation between vessel wall and thrombus is difficult in MRA. This might potentially obscure the delineation of smaller wall adherent thrombi.

There are several options with regard to the optimal diagnostic algorithm for the workup of patients with suspected acute pulmonary embolism. Eventually, the question which diagnostic method to choose will always depend on the clinical status of the patient, the technology available, personnel experience, and last but not least on regional prevailing trends.

In conclusion, the preliminary experience suggest that gadolinium-enhanced, three dimensional, breathhold, magnetic resonance angiography shows promise as a safe, rapid, accurate, and cost-effective imaging technique for the diagnosis of pulmonary embolism. In combination with its ability to perform deep venous studies and the potential aspect of MR perfusion studies of the lung parenchyma, pulmonary MRA might in the future turn out to be the "one stop shop" for diagnosing pulmonary embolism.

References

1. Come PC (1992) Echocardiographic evaluation of pulmonary embolism and its response to therapeutic interventions. Chest 101: 151S–162S
2. Evans AJ, Sostman HD, Knelson MH, Spritzer CE, Newman GE, Paine SS, BeamCA (1993) Detection of deep venous thrombosis: prospective comparison of MR imaging with contrast venography. Amer J Roentgenol 161: 131–140
3. Franck A, Selby K, van Tyen R, Nordell B, Saloner D (1995) Cardiac-gated MR angiography of pulsatile flow: k-space strategies. J Magn Reson Imag 5: 297–307
4. Foo KF, MacFall JR, Sostman HD, Hayes CE (1993) Single-breath-hold venous or arterial flow-suppressed pulmonary vascular MR imaging with phased-array coils. J Magn Reson Imag 3: 611–616
5. Gefter WB, Hatabu H (1993) Evaluation of pulmonary vascular anatomy and blood flow by magnetic resonance. J Thorac Imaging 7: 208–225
6. Goodman LR, Curtin JJ, Mewissen MW, Foley WD, Lipchik RJ, Crain MR, Sagar KB, Collies BD (1995) Detection of pulmonary embolism in patients with unresolved clinical and scintigraphic diagnosis: helical CT versus angiography. Amer J Roentgenol 164: 1369–1374
7. Grist TM, Sostman HD, MacFall JR, Foo TKF, Spritzer OE, Witty L, Newman GE, Debatin JF, Tapson V, Saltzman HA (1993) Pulmonary angiography with MR imaging: Preliminary clinical experience. Radiology 189: 523–530
8. Grist TM, Sproat IA, Kennel TW, Korosec FR, Swan JS (1996) MR angiography of the renal arteries during a breath-hold using gadolinium-enhanced 3D TOF with k-space zero-filling and a contrast timing scan (abstr.). In: Book of abstracts: Society of Magnetic Resonance in Medicine 1996. New York, NY: Society of Magnetic Resonance in Medicine, pp 163
9. Hany TF, Schmidt M, Steiner P, Debatin JF (in press) Optimization of contrast dosage for gadolinium-enhanced 3D MRA of the pulmonary and renal arteries. Magnetic Resonance Imaging
10. Hatabu H, Gefter WB, Axel L, Palevsky HI, Cope C, Reichek N, Dougherty L, Listernd J, Kressel HY (1994) MR imaging with spatial modulation of magnetization in the evaluation of chronic central pulmonary thromemboli. Radiology 190: 791–796
11. Kauzcor HU, Hofmann D, Kreitner KF, Nilgens H, Surkau R, Thelen M (1996) MR imaging assessment of pulmonary ventilation with inhalation of hyperpolarized He-3 gas: Work in progress. Radiology 201 (P): 201
12. Korosec FR, Grist TM, Frayne R, Polacin JA, Mistretta CA (1996) Timeresolved contrast-enhanced 3D MR angiography (abstr.) In: Book of abstracts: Society of Magnetic Resonance in Medicine 1996. New York, NY: Society of Magnetic Resonance in Medicine, pp. 238
13. Leung DA, McKinnon GE, Davis CP, Pfammatter T, Krestin GP, Debatin JF (1996) Breath-hold, contrast enhanced, three dimensional MR angiography. Radiology 201: 569–571
14. Lin W, Haacke EM, Masaryk TJ, Smith AS (1992) Automated local maximumintensity projection with three-dimensional vessel tracking. J Magn Reson Imag 2: 519–526
15. Meaney JFM, Weg JG, Chenevert TL, Stafford-Jonson D, Hamilton BH, Prince MR (1997) Diagnosis of pulmonary embolism with magnetic resonance angiography N Engl J Med 336: 1422–1427
16. PIOPED investigators: Value of ventilation/perfusion scan in acute pulmonary embolism. J Amer Med Assoc 1990; 263: 2753–2759
17. Prince MR (1994) Gadolinium-enhanced MR aortography. Radiology 191: 155–164
18. Prince MR, Narasimham DL, Stanley JC, Chenevert TL, Williams DM, Marx MV, Cho KJ (1995) Breath-hold gadolinium enhanced MR arteriography of the abdominal aorta and its major branches. Radiology 197: 785–792
19. Prince MR, Yucel EK, Kaufmann JA, Harrison DC, Geller SC (1993) Dynamic gadolinium-enhanced three dimensional abdominal MR arteriography. JMRI 3: 877–881
20. Remy-Jardin M, Remy J, Wattinne L, Giraud F (1992) Central pulmonary thromboembolism: diagnosis with spiral volumetric CT with the single breathhold technique – comparison with pulmonary angiography. Radiology 185: 381–387
21. Royal HD (1989) Radionuclide imaging of the lung. Curr Opin Radiol 1: 446–459
22. Sostman HD, Debatin JF, Spritzer CE, Coleman RE, Grist TM, MacFall JR (1993) MRI in venous thrombo-embolic disease. Eur Radiol 3: 53–61

23. Stein PD, Athanasoulis C, Alavi A et al. (1992) Complications and validity of pulmonary angiography in acute pulmonary embolism. Circulation 85: 462–468
24. Steiner P, McKinnon GC, Romanowski B, Goehde SC, Hany T, Debatin JF (1997) Contrast-enhanced, ultra-fast 3D pulmonary MR angiography in a single breath-hold: Initial assessment of imaging perfomance. JMRI 7: 177–182
25. Stewart JR, Greenfield LJ (1982) Transvenous vena caval filtration and pulmonary embolectomy. Surg Clin North Am 62: 411–430
26. Teigen CL, Maus TP, Sheedy PF, Stanson AW, Johnson CM, Breen JF, Mc Kusick MA (1995) Pulmonary embolism: Diagnosis with contrastenhanced electron-beam CT and comparison with pulmonary angiography. Radiology 194: 313–319
27. Wang Y, Rossman PJ, Grimm RC, Riederer SJ, Ehman RL (1996) Navigator-echo-based real-time respiratory gating and triggering for reduction of respiration effects in three-dimensional coronary MR angiography. Radiology 198: 55–60
28. Wielopolski PA, Haacke EM, Adler LP (1992) Three dimensional MR pulmonary vascular imaging: preliminary experience. Radiology 183: 465–472
29. Wielopolski PA, Oudkerk M, De Bruin HG (1996) Three dimensional MR pulmonary perfusion imaging with Gadopentate Dimeglumine. Radiology 201 (P): 230

T. H. Hany · G. McKinnon · J. F. Debatin
MR-Center
Department of Diagnostic Radiology
University Hospital Zurich
Rämistr. 100
CH-8091 Zurich, Switzerland

F. Follath
Department of Internal Medicine
University Hospital Zurich
Rämistr. 100
CH-8091 Zurich, Switzerland

P. Steiner (✉)
Department of Diagnostic Radiology
University Hospital Hamburg
Martinistr. 52
D-20246 Hamburg, Germany

Mechanism of blood coagulation. Newer aspects of anticoagulant and antithrombotic therapy

W. Jeske, D. A. Hoppensteadt, R. Pifarre, J. M. Walenga, J. Fareed

Mechanisms of blood coagulation

Introduction

Hemostasis as defined by Virchow in the last century is a fine balance between blood flow, humoral factors, and cellular elements of the vascular system. Today, biotechnology has advanced our understanding of the thrombotic process and its regulation. Whereas in the past, heparin and warfarin have been the sole antithrombotic agents available, specific sites in the thrombotic network at both plasmatic and cellular sites can now be targeted. Antibodies against specific platelet receptors as well as specific antithrombin and anti-Xa agents are being developed. Mutations of endogenous inhibitors have been identified as causes of congenital thrombophilias. The use of heparin has also advanced. Heparin is no longer solely a surgical anticoagulant, but is used to treat a variety of conditions including venous thrombosis, unstable angina, and myocardial infarction and is used in procedures such as angioplasty and stent implantation. The mechanism of heparin's action has become more complex with the discovery of tissue factor pathway inhibitor, selectins, and other cellular targets where the drug is able to produce its effects.

Blood is normally maintained in the fluid state so that nutrients can be delivered to the various tissues of the body. When the integrity of the vascular system has been compromised, it becomes necessary for the blood to clot. The initial response to a break in the continuity of the vasculature is the formation of the platelet plug. Platelets in the flowing blood rapidly adhere to the exposed subendothelial vessel wall matrix and become activated. During this activation process, components of the platelet α and β granules (ATP, ADP, factor V, 5-HT) are released causing further platelet aggregation. Also during these morphologic changes, activated platelets express protein and cell receptors and procoagulant phospholipids are expressed upon their surface.

The negatively charged phospholipid phosphatidylserine is asymmetrically distributed in mammalian cell membranes, primarily on the inner leaflet. Upon exposure to collagen or thrombin, the distribution of phospholipids changes with increasing phosphatidylserine in the external membrane leaf [12]. The increased expression of phosphatidylserine on the outer leaflet of the membrane creates a procoagulant surface on which several steps of the coagulation cascade take place.

The platelet plug initially arrests the loss of blood. This, however, is not a permanent blockade. The formation of a fibrin based clot acts to stabilize the initial platelet plug. The coagulation system is a complex network of zymogens which must be activated to ultimately form the fibrin strands of the blood clot. Upon activation, most of these coagulation proteins are converted into active serine proteases which are similar to trypsin and chymotrypsin. Traditionally, coagulation has been viewed as having two distinct branches [28, 80], the intrinsic and the extrinsic pathways. Today it has been established that the two pathways are linked prior to the generation of factor Xa [103].

Intrinsic pathway of coagulation

In the intrinsic pathway, factor XII becomes activated in the contact phase of coagulation. This occurs when factor XII, factor XI, prekallikrein, and high molecular weight kininogen come together on a negatively charged surface. While this reaction can take place in the laboratory on a negatively charged surface such as glass or kaolin, the physiologic surface is unknown. It has been proposed that this could be a tissue rich in collagen or sulphatides [119]. By binding to the negatively charged surface, factor XII is converted to its active form through an unknown mechanism. The formation of factor XIIa is amplified by a positive feedback loop. Factor XIIa is capable of converting prekallikrein to kallikrein. Likewise, kallikrein converts factor XII to its active form. Factor XIIa also converts factor XI to factor XIa which in turn activates factor IX. Factor IX along with its cofactor factor VIII, calcium ions, and phospholipid membranes form the "tenase" complex which converts factor X to factor Xa thereby initiating the common pathway of coagulation. The phospholipid membrane in these complexes serves to lower the Km of the reaction. The phospholipid allows the enzyme to become saturated more easily and serves to localize the coagulation response to where it is most needed. The cofactor, factor V, increases the catalytic efficiency of the enzyme [52]. Factor Xa joins with its cofactor factor V, calcium ions and phospholipid membranes to form the prothrombinase complex. The prothrombinase complex then acts to convert prothrombin into the active enzyme thrombin. Factors V and VII are activated through proteolytic cleavage by factor Xa or thrombin. They are not, however, active proteases. Factor V is believed to have two rate enhancing effects on the prothrombinase complex. In the prothrombinase complex, factor Xa and factor V are present in stoichiometric amounts resulting in an unknown alteration in the active site of factor Xa which increases its catalytic efficiency [81]. Factor V also binds to prothrombin thus sequestering it at the site of assembly of the prothrombinase complex. Overall, these two actions of factor V result in a 300,000-fold increase in the rate of prothrombin conversion.

Thrombin serves many functions in coagulation. First, thrombin cleaves the soluble protein fibrinogen to generate the insoluble fibrin monomer. Fibrinogen circulates as a disulfide-linked dimer containing two A-α chains, two B-β chains and two gamma chains. Cleavage of fibrinogen by thrombin results in the release of fibrinopeptides A and B and the exposure of charged domains at opposite ends of the molecule. Exposure of these charged domains leads to polymerization of the monomers. The release of fibrinopeptides A and B occur at different rates with fibrinopeptide A preferentially removed in mammalian systems [14, 121]. Removal of fibrinopeptide A leads to end-to-end fibrin polymerization whereas loss of fibrinopeptide B allows side-to-side polymerization of the end-to-end linked monomers. It is these monomers which are cross-linked by the transaminase factor XIIIa to form the meshwork of the thrombus. Thrombin also acts to augment its own generation by being a part of several positive feedback loops in the coagulation cascade. In these loops, thrombin activates factors XII, XI, VIII, and V. By activating the precursors to its own generation, thrombin greatly amplifies its own generation. Thrombin also activates platelets, activates the inhibitor Protein C through binding with thrombomodulin [35], and stimulates activated endothelial cells to release tissue plasminogen activator.

Extrinsic pathway of coagulation

The extrinsic pathway of coagulation is activated when circulating factor VII encounters tissue factor. Tissue factor is a transmembrane glycoprotein which is normally expressed by subendothelial fibroblast-like cells which surround the blood vessel. An intact endothelium normally shields the circulating blood from exposure to tissue factor. The tissue factor molecule consists of a 219 amino acid hydrophilic extracellular domain, a 23 amino acid hydrophobic region which spans the membrane, and a 21 amino acid cytoplasmic tail which anchors the molecule to the cell membrane [5, 93]. Other sites of tissue factor expression include activated monocytes, activated endothelial cells, and atherosclerotic plaques.

Factor VII exhibits a weak procoagulant activity on its own, typically accounting for about 1–2 % of the total factor VII/VIIa activity [97]. Upon binding to tissue factor, a 10,000,000-fold increase in factor VIIa enzymatic activity is observed [31]. Both factor VII and factor VIIa bind to tissue factor with equal affinity [100]. How factor VII is initially activated is not known, though it is hypothesized that factor Xa can activate factor VII in a back activation reaction. The factor VIIa – tissue factor complex can then activate factor X leading to the generation of thrombin and ultimately to the formation of fibrin strands.

It was shown in 1977 and more recently appreciated that the tissue factor – factor VIIa complex also activates factor IX to factor IXa, thus, interacting with "intrinsic" pathway enzymes [103]. This is believed to be important for maintaining the clotting process. Direct activation of factor X by factor VIIa – tissue factor can rapidly initiate coagulation, but both of these enzymes are quickly inhibited by the endogenous inhibitor tissue factor pathway inhibitor. By activating factor IX, the tissue factor – VIIa complex initiates two pathways for thrombin generation. The small amounts of factor Xa generated prior to TFPI inhibition are sufficient to cleave prothrombin and generate a small amount of thrombin. This thrombin is then capable of back-activating factors V, VIII and possibly XI, thereby sustaining clot formation through generation of thrombin via the intrinsic pathway. It has been observed that the activation of factor X by the factor IXa-VIII complex in the presence of calcium and phospholipids is 50 times greater than by the tissue factors-VIIa complex [82]. Factor XI activation has been shown to occur in the presence of thrombin and a polyanion cofactor [43, 98]. Activation with the cofactor has been observed to be poor. A physiologic cofactor has not been elucidated. It has been reasoned that if the direct activation of factor X by VIIa-tissue factor is the sole source of thrombin generation, there would be no manifestation of hemophilia, genetic deficiency of either factor IX or factor VIII.

Role of platelets

Platelets are disc-shaped, anuclear cells which circulate in a non-adhesive state in the undamaged circulation [105]. These cells contain a contractile system and a number of storage granules. The α storage granules contain platelet factor 4 (PF4), β-thrombo-globulin, platelet derived growth factor (PDGF), fibrinogen, factor V, and von Willebrand factor [69]. The dense or β-granules contain ATP, ADP, and serotonin [50, 57].

The first step toward platelet aggregation is platelet adhesion. Normally, platelets do not adhere to the vessel walls due to the non-thrombogenic properties of the endo-thelium. Endothelial cells produce heparan sulfate (to activate antithrombin III), thrombomodulin (for activation of protein C), plasminogen activators (to induce fibrin degradation), and TFPI (to inhibit tissue factor activity). In addition, these cells also produce prostacyclin (PGI$_2$) which inhibits platelet activation by raising platelet cAMP levels and endothelial derived relaxing factor (EDRF; NO) which inhibits platelet activation through a cGMP dependent mechanism. When this antithrombotic continuum of cells is interrupted by vascular injury, platelets adhere to the exposed subendothelial tissues.

Following adhesion, platelets become activated. In this activation process, there is a morphologic change in the platelet, with pseudopod formation observed. This brings about a change in the conformation of the glycoprotein IIb/IIIa receptor on the platelet surface which allows for fibrinogen binding [105]. Fibrinogen binding serves as a bridge which links individual platelets into larger aggregates. An increase in cytosolic calcium levels leads to activation of internal platelet enzymes with the subsequent release of platelet granule contents. The formation of these platelet aggregates is the process of primary hemostasis, the first step to arrest blood loss.

The release of platelet granule contents leads to further platelet activation and aggregation and an activation of coagulation. Most of the known aggregating agents cause release of the platelet storage granule contents. These agonists include thrombin, ADP, collagen, TXA_2, platelet activating factor, serotonin, epinephrine, immune complexes, and fibrinogen [105]. Thrombin is the most potent aggregating agent, capable of causing platelet aggregation without any contribution from thromboxane A_2 or ADP [105]. Serotonin and epinephrine do not induce aggregation on their own, but synergistically promote aggregation induced by other agents [27, 58, 124].

Platelet membranes contain a variety or receptors for the various agonists including the thrombin receptor, the TXA_2 receptor, $5-HT_2$ receptors, and α_2-adrenergic receptors. In addition, a number of glycoproteins present on the membrane serve as receptors for collagen (GP Ia/IIa), fibrinogen (GP IIb/IIIa), von Willebrand factor (GP Ib), and fibronectin (GP IIb/IIIa) [27, 58, 124]. A high molecular weight chondroitin sulfate proteoglycan has been shown to be released from the surface of the platelet during the aggregation process. This proteoglycan contains homopolymers of 4-O chondroitin sulfate which inhibit ADP induced aggregation of platelets.

Activated platelets also provide a procoagulant surface on which several reactions of the coagulation cascade take place. Unstimulated platelets provide only a minimally effective surface on which the "tenase" and prothrombinase complexes can assemble [36, 138, 140]. This is due to the bilayer partitioning of various phospholipids. In unstimulated platelets, the outer leaflet of the membrane consists of mostly phosphatidylcholine while the inner leaf contains most of the phosphatidylserine. Two mechanisms have been proposed for maintaining this distribution [116, 132]. When platelets are stimulated to release their granular contents, the procoagulant phospholipids are brought to the surface as the granules fuse to the membranes [140]. This expression of phosphatidylserine on the outer leaflet along with factor V release from the α-granule greatly accelerates the formation of thrombin [62, 95, 136].

Platelet activation leads to the formation of platelet derived microparticles derived from the platelet surface. These microvesicles typically account for 25 to 30 % of platelet procoagulant activity and factor V binding sites [116, 126].

Role of platelet integrins

A number of the glycoproteins on the surface of the platelet belong to the superfamily of adhesive protein receptors known as integrins. Integrins are α/β heterodimer protein complexes which are present on the surface of adherent cells of most species [16, 29, 84]. These integrins mediate cell-cell and cell-matrix interactions involved in a diverse number of biologic functions [61, 128]. Integrins are divided into subfamilies based on the identity of the β-subunit. The first two subfamilies of integrins, the VLA complexes and the Leu-Cams, are found on white cells and mediate various leukocyte aggregation responses [3, 53]. Platelets contain two members of the third subfamily of integrins, glycoprotein IIb/IIIa or P-selectin and the vitronectin receptor [19, 25, 75, 139].

Integrins function by interacting with a number of extracellular glycoprotein ligands such as fibronectin, laminin, collagen, vitronectin, fibrinogen, and von Willebrand's factor [18]. Integrins are capable of binding several ligands and the nature of the ligand specificity is not known.

Platelet membranes contain five integrin-like receptors which are involved in the formation of the primary hemostatic plug. These include VLA-2, VLA-5, VLA-6, glyco-protein IIb/IIIa, and the vitronectin receptor. Of these, GP IIb/IIIa is the most abundant. VLA-2 (GPIa/IIa) is the binding site for collagen on the platelet surface. VLA-5 and VLA-6 are responsible for the binding to vitronectin and laminin, respectively [54, 108]. The extent to which these receptors contribute to platelet adhesion *in vivo* is not known. The physiologic function of the vitronectin receptor is not known.

Platelet aggregation requires that platelets become activated by at least one platelet agonist, the presence of functional GPIIb/IIIa molecules and the presence of at least one GPIIb/IIIa ligand [122]. Lack of GPIIb/IIIa complexes leads to the cogenital bleeding disorder known as Glanzmann's thrombasthenia. In nonactivated platelets, GPIIb/IIIa is capable of binding only immobilized fibrinogen. Platelet activation allows plasma-borne adhesive proteins to bind to GPIIb/IIIa complexes [64]. The activation of the IIb/IIIa complex occurs by an unknown mechanism though the number of receptors on the membrane is not altered by activation [107]. Fibrin polymers bind to the activated GPIIb/IIIa complexes and anchor the platelet plug in place.

Recent studies have shown that the binding of ligands to GPIIb/IIIa also activates a number of cellular processes important for platelet stimulation including the synthesis of 3-phosphorylated phosphatidylinositols, the release of arachidonic acid, and the increase in plasma calcium levels. Stimulation of these processes allows for bidirectional signaling between the intracellular and extracellular compartments.

Role of leukocytes

Leukocytes typically express minimal amounts of procoagulant activity in the unstimu-lated state [30]. Cytokines such as interleukin-1 (IL-1) and tumor necrosis factor (TNF) can elicit the expression of tissue factor on endothelial and mononuclear cells [23]. Monocyte procoagulant activity is also induced by endotoxin, the complement system, phorbol esters, prostaglandins, and a number of other agonists [32]. Procoagulant activity associated with leukocytes is not limited to the expression of tissue factor. Several mono-cyte/macrophage derived procoagulant activities have been characterized. These include tissue factor [44, 91, 117], factor VII [24, 90], and factor XIII (137). In addition, some mono-cytes and macrophages have been shown to express functional factor V/Va [11] and to possess binding sites for factor X [1]. The factor Xa binding site on leukocytes has been shown to be the integrin CD11b/CD18 [1]. Not only does this integrin bind factor X, but it also proteolytically activates factor X to Xa, allowing for initiation of coagulation on the surface of the monocytes and neutrophils [2]. Monocytes have also been shown to contain a receptor for the factor IXa/VIII complex which allows the reactions of the intrinsic pathway of coagulation to take place on the surface of the monocyte [92].

Prothrombin has been shown to be efficiently activated on the cell surface of monocytes and lymphocytes [134, 135]. As with platelets, the prothrombinase activity on monocytes is increased with activated monocytes as compared to the non-activated cells [112].

It has been stated that when coagulation takes place on the surface of leukocytes, it "... assumes the aspects of a broad inflammatory mechanism, directly influencing cellular motility and adhesion, phagocytosis, cell-cell communication, and normal or deregulated cellular growth" [2]. Fibrin formation not only forms the basis for a blood clot, but can also serve to limit the inflammatory response. In addition, products of the coagulation process such as thrombin, fibrinopeptides, and fibrin degradation products have chemotactic and mitogenic properties [106, 120, 123].

Studies have indicated that leukocytes play a critical role in activation of coagulation in patients with septicemia and in animal models of acute lung injury [22, 101]. One study has presented direct evidence indicating the role of tissue factor expression on activated endothelial cells on *in vivo* thrombogenesis [99].

Role of the endothelium

The endothelium plays a relatively important role in the modulation of overall coagulation, fibrinolytic, and platelet dependent processes. Endothelial cells are reactive to various physiologic and pathologic states and release various mediators which modulate plasmatic processes. The role of endothelial function in mediating the overall coagulation process can be summarized by the following:

- Regulation of thrombin function by binding to thrombomodulin.
- Release of fibrinolytic mediators in the regulation of the fibrinolytic system.
- Release of prostaglandin derivatives in the control of platelet function and vascular hemodynamics.
- Release of nitric oxide, TFPI, and other substances to mediate various functions.

Under normal conditions, endothelial cells play a regulatory role in balancing the cellular and plasmatic reactions. However, in pathologic states, such as ischemia and occlusive states (thrombotic or restenotic), endothelial function changes markedly with endothelial cells producing various substances which mediate the pathologic changes. Some of these functions are summarized in the following:

- Release of tissue factor to initiate the clotting process.
- Release of PAI to inhibit the fibrinolytic response.
- Generation of procoagulant proteins and von Willebrand's factor to activate thrombogenesis.

It is, therefore, important to consider the endothelium as a major player in the overall regulation of hemostasis.

Synopsis on the mechanisms of blood coagulation

The process of blood coagulation is no longer considered to be a simple transformation of fibrinogen to fibrin by the action of thrombin. Rather, this remarkably complex process is a result of several transformations which are mediated by enzymes, activators, inhibitors, and cellular contributors. The process of coagulation contributes significantly to thrombogenesis; however, it is no longer considered to be the sole event. The role of platelets, leukocytes, and endothelial cells has gradually accepted to be crucial in the overall regulation of thrombogenesis.

Surgical intervention, in particular during a cardiovascular procedure, inflicts a major stimulus for coagulation through the release of large amounts of tissue factor, enzyme, and platelet activation from the extracorporeal circulation and endothelial distress resulting in a procoagulant environment. This necessitates the use of anticoagulant and antithrombotic agents to keep blood coagulation under control. The understanding of the activation processes as led to the development of newer approaches to inhibit the coagulation process. Furthermore, the physiologic means, such as hypothermia and blood salvage techniques, have added to the restoration approaches during cardiovascular surgical procedures. Endogenous inhibitors such as antithrombin III, protein C, and TFPI have also played a major role in the control of thrombigenesis. Thus, endogeneous regulatory mechanisms have been crucial in controlling the thrombotic process both during and after surgical procedures. Alternate anticoagulant drug development will continue to provide us new drugs to control the coagulation process.

Newer aspects of anticoagulant and antithrombotic therapy

Overview

Thrombosis is clearly the most common cause of death in the United States. About two million individuals die each year from an arterial or venous thrombosis or the consequences thereof. About 80 to 90 % of all causes of thrombosis can now be defined with respect to cause. Of these, over 50 % of all patients harbor a congenital or acquired blood coagulation protein or platelet defect which caused the thrombotic event. It is obviously of major importance to define those individuals harboring such a defect [40] as this allows appropriate antithrombotic therapy to decrease risks of recurrence [42] determine length of time the patient must remain on therapy for secondary prevention, and [41] allow for testing of family members in those harboring a blood coagulation protein or platelet defect which is hereditary (about 50 % of all coagulation and platelet defects mentioned above). Aside from mortality, significant additional morbidity occurs from both arterial or venous thrombotic events, including, but not limited to paralysis (non-fatal thrombotic stroke), cardiac disability (repeated coronary events), loss of vision (retinal vascular thrombosis) and fetal waste syndrome (placental vascular thrombosis), stasis ulcers and other manifestations of postphlebitic syndrome, etc.

The incidence of DVT in the USA is about 159 per 100,000 or about 398,000 per year. A definable etiology can be found in 80 to 90 % of these patients which allows for effective therapy to be delivered and allows for the other advantages of defining the blood caogulation protein or platelet defects mentioned above, to be instituted.

The overall incidence of PE in the USA is about 139 per 100,000 or about 347,000 cases per year based on clinical data; the incidence of fatal PE in the USA based on autopsy data is 94 per 100,000 or 235,000 deaths per year. The same scenario as that for DVT prevails for PE. If the PE is not fatal, every attempt should be made to define the blood coagulation or platelet defect.

About 1.5 million individuals in the USA will have an acute myocardial infarction per year; 50 % will be fatal and 50 will be a premature event. Thus, there are about 750,000 deaths from coronary artery thrombosis per year. Of these coronary thrombotic events, 67 % of patients harbor a coagulation blood protein or platelet defect leading to thrombosis. Fifty percent of these coagulation protein or platelet defects will be hereditary, thus, emphasizing the importance of defining the presence and type of defect in survivors of acute myocardial infarction. Defining the defect will also allow one to optimize antithrombotic therapy for secondary prevention.

Cerebrovascular thrombosis (CVT) occurs in over 1.5 million individuals yearly in the USA, of these 66 % suffer death or severe permanent paralysis. In those suffering CVT, including transient cerebral ischemic attacks (TIA's), small stroke syndrome (SSS), and frank thrombotic stroke, at least 30 % harbor a blood coagulation protein or platelet defect causing thrombosis. Like the disorders discussed above, the need for defining the presence or abscence and type of defect is of obvious importance.

Although the incidence of retinal arterial or venous thrombosis is unclear and death does not occur, significant visual morbidity is a major problem. Like CVT, about 30 % of individuals sustaining retinal vascular thrombosis harbor a blood coagulation protein or platelet defect; reasons for defining these are obvious as for the other disorders discussed. Thrombosis therefore represents the leading cause of death and disability throughout the world. Antithrombotic and anticoaguolant drugs, therefore, represent an important class of drugs with a major impact on healthcare.

The pathophysiology of thrombotic events is multicomponent and involves blood, vascular system, and target sites. The process of thrombogenesis is depicted in Fig. 1. Initially, vascular injury results in the localized alterations of the vessels, generation of tissue factor, and subsequent activation of platelets. Activated cells mediate several direct

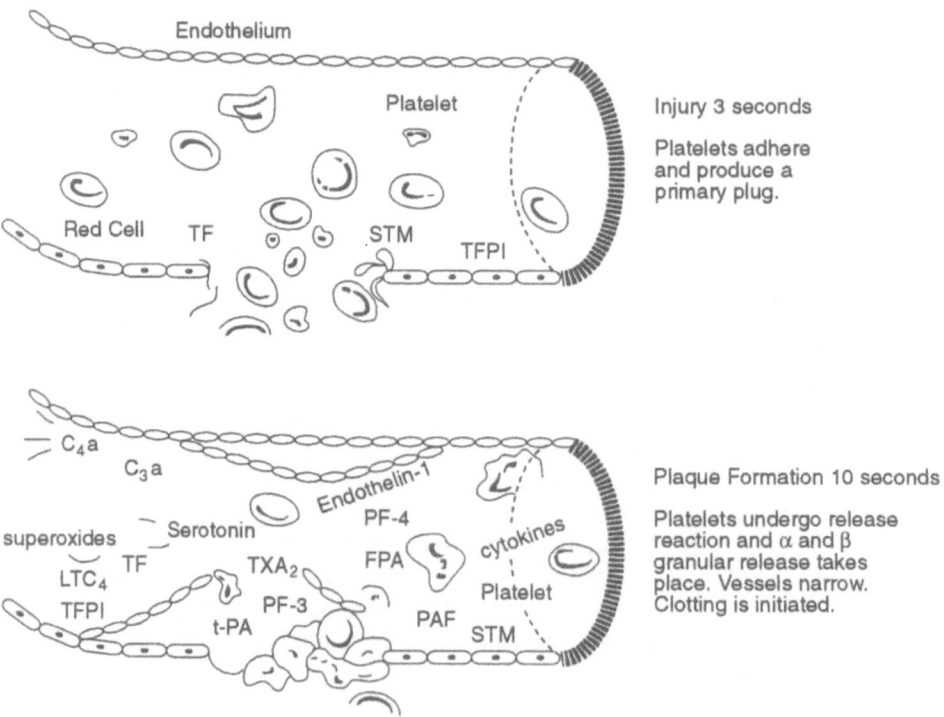

Fig. 1. Blood and vascular activation process resulting in thrombogenesis. Vascular damage, cell activation, and related products contribute to the development of thrombus and vascular constriction. Antithrombotic drugs are capable of targeting single or multiple sites in the control of thrombogenesis.

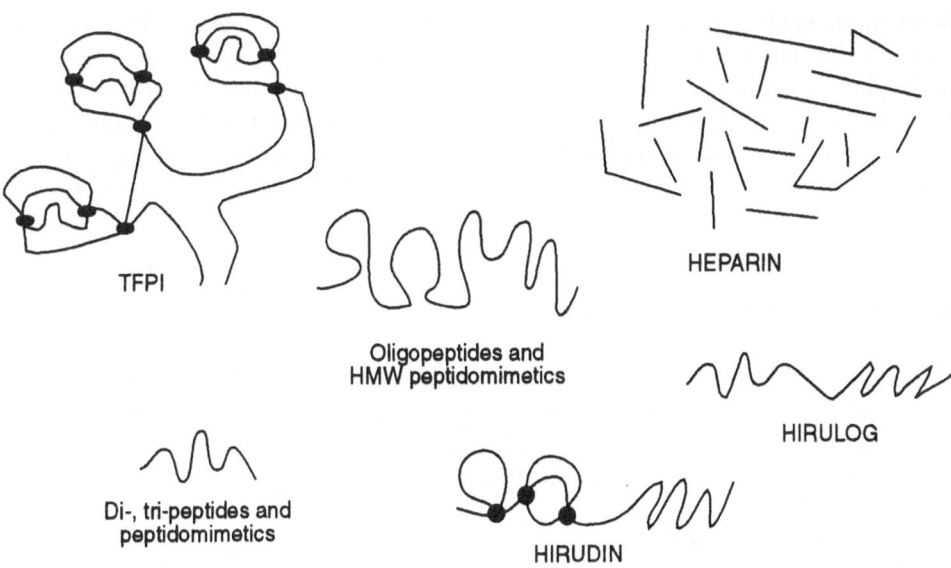

Fig. 2. A diagrammatic illustration of the structural diversity in anticoagulant drugs. These drugs represent protein, peptides, nucleic acids, carbohydrates, and synthetic heterocyclic agents.

or signal transduction induced processes resulting in the activation of platelets. Cellular activation also results in the release of various mediators which amplify vascular spasm and the coagulation process. Drugs that target various sites of the activation process can be developed to control thrombotic events. Because of the coupled pathophysiology, a single drug may not be able to target these sites to produce therapeutic actions. Furthermore, many of these mediators produce localized actions at cellular and subcellular levels. The feedback amplification process also plays an important role in the pathology of these disorders. This understanding has led to the concept of polytherapy in the management of thrombotic disorders.

The newer developments in antithrombotic drugs are rather significant. Many advanced techniques to develop antithrombotic drugs are used at the present time. Advances in biotechnology and separation techniques have also contributed to the development of newer antithrombotic drugs [40–42]. These drugs may prove to have a better efficacy in the control of thrombogenesis and its treatment. Drugs and devices, which have been or are being developed, are based on newer concepts.

It can be appreciated that antithrombotic drugs represent a wide spectrum of natural, synthetic, semi-synthetic, and biotechnology produced agents with marked differences in chemical composition, physicochemical properties, biochemical actions, and pharmacologic effects. Fig. 2 depicts the molecular diversities in the structure of various classes of new anticoagulant drugs. These represent proteins, peptides, carbohydrates, and synthetic oligosaccharides. Besides the structural heterogeneity, each of these agents also shows distinct functional properties.

The endogenous actions of the antithrombotic drugs are remarkably complex. It is no longer valid to assume that an antithrombotic drug must produce an anticoagulant action in blood as the conventional heparin and oral anticoagulants. Many of the drugs do not produce any alteration of blood clotting parameters, yet they are effective therapeutic agents because of their interactions with the various elements of the vasculature and other

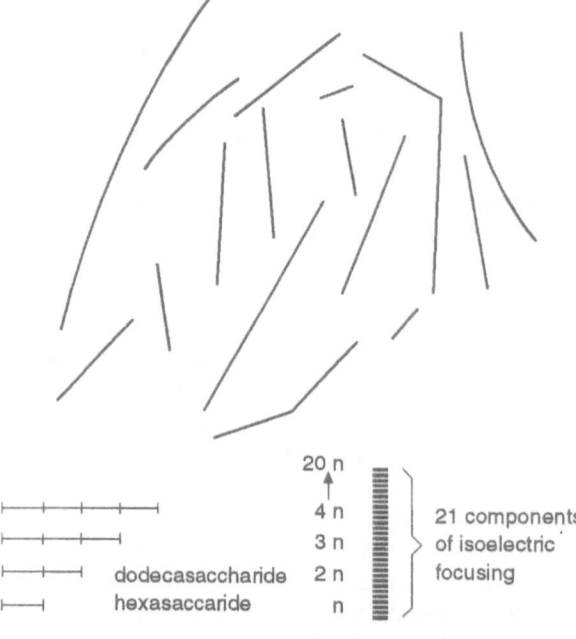

blood components. Another perspective is that several of these agents require endogenous transformation to become active products. Therefore, it becomes important to rely on the pharmacodynamic actions of these agents rather than on their in vitro characteristics to assess potency of efficacy of the product. Hematologic modulation plays a key role in the mediation of the antithrombotic actions of these drugs involving red cells, white cells, platelets, and blood proteins. This is particularly true for the case of trauma induced thrombotic disorders where multiple processes are involved in thrombogenesis.

Newer applications of unfractionated heparin

Unfractionated heparin (UFH) is primarily used as an anticoagulant for both the therapeutic and surgical indications. Usually beef lung and porcine mucosal derived products are available for these indications. The unfractionated heparins have been recently used for the following additional therapeutic uses:

- management of unstable angina
- adjunct to chemotherapeutic agents
- adjunct to anti-inflammatory drugs
- modulatory agent for growth factors
- treatment of hemodynamic disorders

The unfractionated heparins are heterogeneous in nature, as depicted in Fig. 3. Based on the origin, the molecular weight of these anticoagulant drugs varies. The beef lung heparin preparations are usually of higher molecular weight, in contrast to the porcine mucosal heparin. However, the charge density and other characteristics, such as the affinity to ATIII is similar for both preparations. Several newer pharmacological effects,

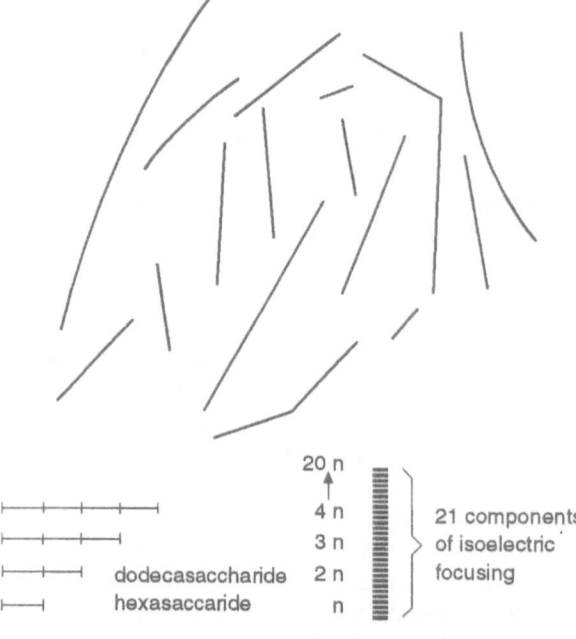

Fig. 3. A diagrammatic illustration of the molecular heterogeneity in unfractionated heparin. Beside compositional variation, heparin exhibits functional heterogeneity in terms of its interaction with endogeneous proteins and cells. The antithrombotic and anticoagulant effects of heparin are based on its polypharmacologic actions.

independent of the anticoagulant effects, have been described. These include glycosylation mediated functional modulation of macromolecules, growth factor modulation, release of endothelial products and interactions with various endogenous sites.

Chemical modification of unfractionated heparin, such as desulfation, deamination, and coupling with various agents, has resulted in products of non-anticoagulant nature with selective actions on enzymes and cellular receptors. Thioxyloside derivatives have also been reported to produce oral antithrombotic actions in animal models. However, relatively larger dosages are needed to produce these effects. These heparin derivatives are currently tested for such indications as sepsis, viral infections, and the treatment of proliferative disorders.

The development of low molecular weight heparins

The development of low molecular weight heparin (LMWH) has added a new dimension to the clinical management of thrombotic disorders. These agents have revolutionized the prophylaxis of post-surgical thrombosis [59, 109]. More recently these drugs have been used for the treatment of trauma related thrombosis. In particular, their effects on platelets are minimal in comparison to heparin. Thus, these agents are of value in platelet compromised patients.

For the past few decades, heparin has been widely used for the prevention of post-operative thromboembolism [56, 60]. However, there are several adverse side-effects associated with the use of heparin such as bleeding, heparin induced thrombocytopenia, heparin induced thrombosis [70, 125], and osteoporosis [45]. In addition, the regimen of prophylactic heparin used in the prevention of deep venous thrombosis (DVT) is tedious, requiring 2 to 3 daily injections because of the limited bioavailability and short half-life of heparin when administered subcutaneously.

The many clinical problems associated with heparin led several investigators to study the structure of heparin and to identify the active component(s) of this agent. The observation that only low molecular weight heparins are absorbed after subcutaneous administration has led to the development of LMWHs. As shown in Fig. 4, the bioavailability of LMWH components is much greater than for unfractionated heparin. Experimental studies revealed the first LMWH had a subcutaneous bioavailability of

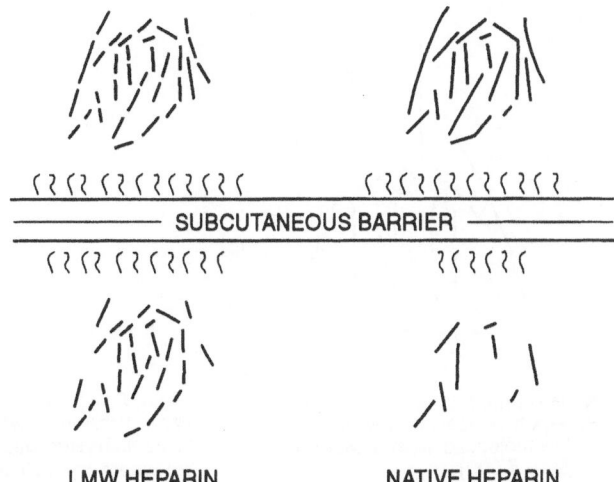

Fig. 4. Bioavailability of heparin and LMWH after subcutaneous administration. The subcutaneous barrier only allows the absorption of lower molecular weight components of heparin. This observation as one of the major factors in the development of LMWHs.

SUBCUTANEOUS BARRIER

LMW HEPARIN

NATIVE HEPARIN

about 90 % compared to 15 to 25 % for unfractionated heparin [8]. Furthermore, these agents exhibit a much longer biologic half-life in contrast to heparin [41]. Thus, LMWH preparations could be administered with a single daily injection making them easy to administer as a prophylactic agent. Eight LMWHs have already been approved for the prophylaxis of thrombosis in the European community. Several of these LMWHs are under clinical trials in the US. One was approved in 1993 for use in post-orthopedic surgery prophylaxis of DVT.

Low molecular weight components in unfractionated heparins were identified long before the development of clinically effective agents. However, because of technologic problems, they were not made available for clinical use. The very first LMWH was obtained by a fractionation method [41]. However, this method only yielded a limited amount of the active product and was cost prohibitive. During the past decade, different chemical and enzymatic processes have been developed to obtain LMWHfrom the parent UFH. The depolymerization process for the production of LMWH is shown in Fig. 5. Such

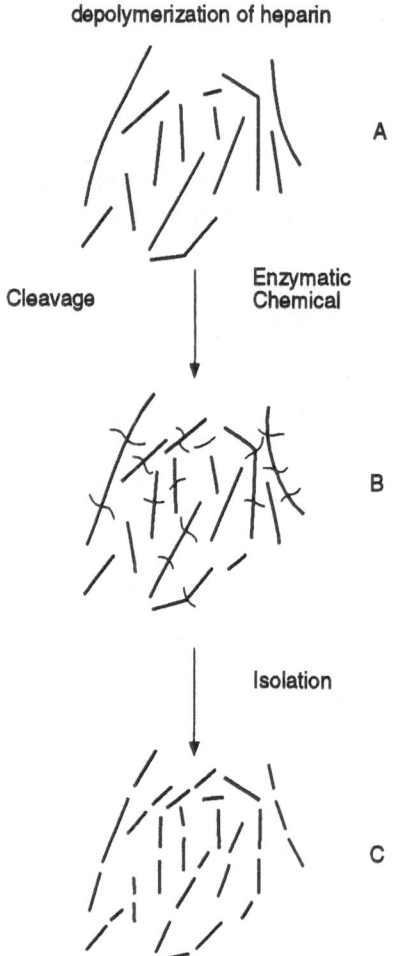

depolymerization of heparin

A

Cleavage   Enzymatic
                  Chemical

B

Isolation

C

A. native heparin (Mr = 17.000)
B. depolymerization process
C. low molecular weight heparin
   (Mr = 5.000)

Fig. 5. A diagrammatic illustration of the manufacturing process for LMWHs. Unfractioned heparin of porcine or bovine origin is depolymerized by chemical or enzymatic digestion in controlled conditions. The degree of depolymerization is adjusted to obtain LMWH of varying weight.

methods as chemical degradation, enzymatic depolymerization, and γ-radiation cleavage can be used to produce the LMWHs.

Recent studies have shown that the individual LMWHs obtained from each process exhibit chemical and pharmacological differences [41]. Such differences may influence the clinical outcome especially in the case of higher dosage use for treatment of cardiovascular indications. No clinical data on the differential pharmacologic preferences of these agents is available at this time.

In the past, LMWHs have been used for the postsurgical prophylaxis of DVT. However, these agents are now also used in the treatment of pre-existing events utilizing both the subcutaneous and intravenous (Breddin, personal communication) routes of administration.

In some of the randomized studies in which LMWHs have been compared with UFH in patients undergoing abdominal surgery a significant decrease in DVT was observed in patients receiving LMWHs compared with UFH [11, 17, 37, 46]. There was no statistical difference in efficacy observed between the two treatments in the other studies [9, 21, 49]. In most studies there was no significant difference between the observed bleeding effects of the LMWHs and UFH. In all of these studies, LMWH was given as a single daily dose while UFH was administered 2 or 3 times daily. The results of these studies suggest that LMWHs are effective and well tolerated in patients undergoing general surgery. The advantage of LMWHs over heparin was primarily in the reduced number of injection per day.

The most extensively studied method of prophylaxis of DVT in orthopedic patients in recent years has been with LMWH. Evidence that this treatment is both effective and safe is quickly accumulating.

Several randomized trials using venography or ^{125}I fibrinogen uptake as the endpoint have also been analyzed. Four studies compared LMWH with dextran. In two of these studies there was no significant difference between the LMWH and the dextran groups. However, in the other two studies, LMWH was more effective than dextran. The different results obtained in these studies is probably due to the different dosages selected for dextran as well as the difference in the dosages and composition of the different LMWHs. Two other studies compared LMWH with placebo. In one study, a difference in the incidence of DVT was found, but in the other study there was no significant difference.

Many surgeons and physicians around the world now appreciate that a large number of cases of venous thromboembolism, particularly those following surgery, can be avoided by correct use of prophylaxis. With additional education and with the introduction of newer and more efficacious agents, it should become routine for all patients undergoing surgery to be assessed for their risk of venous thrombosis and protected accordingly.

Of the many drugs used as prophylactic antithrombotic agents, heparin has a long history as therapy for both DVT and pulmonary emboslim (PE). Many studies have shown that in moderate and high risk patients, heparin can prevent postoperative DVT and PE [34, 59, 77, 89]. Now, with the introduction of LMWHs, these benefits can be had together with easier dosing and potentially less risk of bleeding.

Many surgeons still, however, harbor fears and doubts about using thromboprophylaxis. One of the most common fears is that of bleeding. There are still some surgeons who are not convinced that the benefits of prophylaxis outweigh the risks.

Available clinical data suggests that LMWHs can be safely substituted for low dose heparin. To validate this, several comparative trials throughout the world on low dose heparin and LMWHs are in progress. In several European clinical trials, the efficacy of LMWHs in the prevention of post-surgial DVT has now been proven, and these agents are considered to be the drug of choice for this indication [11, 68, 76].

When used for prophylactic treatment (subcutaneous), most LMWHs mediate their actions in a similar manner; however, their efficacy and tolerability profiles differ markedly as discussed above, and the recommended dosages for the various products differ. Because of the differences between products, such practices as standardization by a single in vitro assay and assignment of single INN designation are deemed invalid for LMWHs as a group. The individualized agent approach to all LMWHs has recently been adopted by the World Health Organization (WHO), US Food and Drug Administration (FDA), and the Scientific and Standardization Subcommittee of the International Society of Thrombosis and Hemostasis (ISTH). The recognition of the individuality of each of the LMWHs is extremely important to avoid excessively high or low doses of a product. Dose finding studies are essential and will have a major impact on the prophylactic and therapeutic acceptance of LMWHs.

Having satisfactorily passed their first step in clinical use, LMWHs are now being applied to other clinical situations. LMWHs are moving into the area of established DVT and therapeutic treatment of thrombosis LMWHs may be therapeutic alternatives to heparin in some, but not all patients who develop a sensitivity to heparin or who develop heparin-induced thrombocytopenia. At optimal dosages, these agents produce antithrombotic effects, but whether they have fewer adverse effects than standard heparin may vary with the product and is unproven for many of them. LMWHs have proven to be equally effective as heparin in general surgery and orthopedic surgery [37, 49, 71].

More recently, LMWHs are being used for specific indications such as percutaneous transluminal coronary angioplasty (PTCA), as adjuncts to thrombolytic agents in disseminated intravascular coagulation (DIC) and the hypercoagulable state. A recent study has reported on the inhibition of cellular proliferation after experimental balloon angioplasty by LMWH in rabbits [48]. There are several other indications such as the treatment of cardiovascular disorders where these agents may also prove to be useful.

LMWHs have been used in isolated areas as anticoagulants during cardiovascular bypass surgery procedures. However, a relatively larger amount of LMWH is needed to produce comparable anticoagulant responses during the surgical procedure. Furthermore, it is rather difficult to antagonize the effect of these agents with conventional protamine usage. Thus, their use in cardiovascular surgical indications requires additional clinical studies. Currently, LMWHs are undergoing clinical trials in the management of thrombotic and ischemic stroke. It has been suggested that the use of LMWHs reduces the risk of thrombosis and improves the quality of life in patients who suffered thrombotic stroke.

Recombinant and synthetic antithrombin drugs

Thrombin is known to play a crucial role in the overall thrombotic events leading to both arterial and venous thrombosis [39]. Beside the transformation of fibrinogen to fibrin, this enzyme is claimed to mediate the activation of platelets and macrophages and produces on-site vascular effects leading to ischemia and vascular contraction. Furthermore, this enzyme is also linked with cellular proliferation and related events leading to restenosis. Thus, the development of agents which can solely target this enzyme is considered to be an important approach in providing newer drugs for the treatment of venous and arterial thrombosis. A list of the currently available thrombin inhibitors and their clinical development status is summarized in Table 1.

One of the building blocks used to develop synthetic inhibitors is arginine with optimal C and/or N-terminal modifications. Many of these agents have been found to be highly

Table 1. Developmental status of site directed thrombin inhibitors

Agents	Chemical Nature	Developmental Status
Hirudin and its analogues	Recombinant protein	Developed for both arterial and venous thrombosis
Hirulogs	Synthetic bifunctional oligopeptides	Several clinical studies are completed; additional studies are planned in various indications
Peptidomimetics	Synthetic heterocyclic derivatives (argatroban, inogatran, napsagatran)	Phase II clinical development in the USA; used in Japan
Peptides and their derivatives	Peptide arginals (efegatran)	Phase II clinical development
Aptamers	DNA and RNA derived oligonucleotides with thrombin-binding domains (defibrotide)	Preclinical stage; limited animal data available
Plasma derived antithrombin	Protein and their recombinant equivalent products	Antithrombin (AT-III) is currently used. HC-II is still in developmental status
Transition state peptide analogues	Oligopeptides and synthetic organic agents (boronic acid derivatives)	Preclinical screening is being completed

toxic due to inhibition of butyl cholinesterase [55]. After further modifications an isomer called argatroban (MD805 or MCI9038) has been generated as a selective reversible inhibitor of thrombin (K_i = 0.019 μM) [55]. It acts by directly inhibiting thrombin and preventing it from acting in the coagulation and fibrinolytic system [86,129]. Argatroban is effective in preventing thrombus formation in various animal models at low concentrations (~ 1 μM) [55, 86]. This compound is being tested clinically for several indications [74, 87]. Another promising low molecular weight (439 Da) reversible peptidomimetic thrombin inhibitor, Inogatran, is currently being developed by Astra Hässle Ab (Sweden). Phase I clinical studies (Ki = 15 nM) and have shown the half-life of this agent to be about 1 hour [130].

A series of tripeptide aldehydes containing arginine have been developed as the first reversible peptide thrombin inhibitors. The prototype compound to be synthesized is D-Phe-Pro-Arg-H (GYKI-14166) [6], which although a very selective and potent inhibitor of thrombin, is very unstable in neutral aqueous solution where it cyclizes and is inactivated. In order to achieve compounds that are both stable and specific for thrombin, a series of N-alkyl derivatives have been synthesized (a basic amino terminus promotes thrombin specificity) and from this series the methyl derivative D-MePhe-Pro-Arg-H (GYKI 14766) [7] has been found to be as potent and selective reversible inhibitors of thrombin as the prototype aldehyde. One of these agents, Efegatran® (D-MePhe-Pro-Arg-H), was developed by Eli Lilly and studied briefly in clinical trials for prevention of reocclusion during interventional cardiovascular procedures.

With the availability of molecular biology techniques, it has become possible to produce pharmaceutical quantities of a recombinant equivalent of hirudin, a potent antithrombin agent which was originally isolated from the medicinal leech, *Hirudo medicinalis* [85]. This anticoagulant is a 65 amino acid protein which is much stronger in producing its anticoagulant effects than heparin. Furthermore, it does not require any endogenous factors for producing its effects. A comparison of this new anticoagulant and heparin is given on Table 2.

Although r-hirudin is a stronger antithrombin agent than heparin, the thrombin generation pathways in the coagulation cascade appear to be inhibited only under certain conditions. Thus, a very high dose of r-hirudin as compared to heparin may be needed for effective antithrombotic activity as only one target site can be inhibited. By inhibiting thrombin, the bioregulatory actions of thrombin such as protein C activation, the release of t-PA and cellular function may also be inhibited.

Table 2. Comparison of R-hirudin and heparin

R-Hirudin	Heparin
Monocomponent protein with single target (thrombin)	Polycomponent drug with multiple sites of action
Thrombin-mediated amplification of coagulation is effected only under certain conditions	Thrombin and factor Xa feedback amplification of clotting is affected
	Fibrinolysis and platelet function is affected
No known interactions with endothelium other than blocking thrombin-thrombomodulin mediated activation of protein C	Significant interactions with endothelium; Both physical and biochemical modulation of endothelial function
Shorter half-life via i.v. route	Short half-life via i.v. route
Functional bioavailability is variable and dependent on the structure of r-hirudin	Functional bioavailability is 20–30 %; LMWHs are better absorbed
Endogenous factors (PF4, FVIII) do not alter its antithrombotic action	Marked modulation by endogenous factors; Several factors may alter the anticoagulant actions
Relatively inert proteins not altered by metabolic processes	Transformed by several enzyme systems which reduce its anticoagulant actions
Information on cellular uptake and depot formation is not presently known	Significant cellular uptake and depot formation

A synthetic analogue of hirudin, namely Hirulog (Biogen USA), has also been developed and tested in various clinical trials [83]. This agent represents a completely synthetic anticoagulant whose anticoagulant actions are comparable to heparin. However, it does not require any plasmatic factors for its anticoagulant actions. Currently, this anticoagulant is being evaluated in various indications such as in the management of unstable angina and interventional cardiology related occlusive phenomenon.

Site-directed antithrombin agents such as recombinant hirubin, hirulog, and synthetic tripeptides are currently undergoing various phases of clinical trials. These agents were initially developed with the premise that sole targeting of thrombin may be the most important step in the development of anticoagulants and antithrombotic drugs to treat thrombotic and cardiovascular disorders [63, 133]. It is nearly five years that these agents have undergone clinical trials. The primary focus of these trials has been in cardiovascular areas such as pretreatment of ischemic heart disorders, anticoagulation during coronary angioplasty, treatment of post-interventional abrupt closure and late reocclusion (restenosis), and adjunct usage during thrombolysis. In heparin compromised patients, these new anticoagulants may be useful.

Several peptidomimetic antithrombin agents are also currently in clinical development for both cardiovascular and therapeutic indications. These include argatroban (Mitsubishi, Japan), inogatran (Astra, Sweden), and napsagatran (Roche, Switzerland). The results of some of these clinical trials are expected later this year. In addition, many other antithrombin agents are in active preclinical development at this time. Of the various peptide derived antithrombin agents, efegatran (Eli Lilly, USA) is the only agent which is currently developed for cardiovascular indications.

Some of the thrombin inhibitors also possess direct vasodilatory effects, independent of their activity on thrombin. These effects are believed to be mediated through metabolic products containing guanidino groups which result in increased nitric oxide generation. Depending on the specific indication for which the thrombin inhibitor is developed, this vascular effect may be desirable. Nevertheless, this type of effect should be investigated and considered.

Although several reports on the experimental use of these antithrombin agents have been made available on their use in cardiovascular surgery in animal models, only isolated reports of human studies are available [111]. Since a known antagonist to neutralize the effects of antithrombin agents is not available, concerns over the use of these agents have been expressed [33]. Currently, no pharmacologic antagonists exist for hirudin or any of the other direct thrombin inhibitors, making the managing of precipitated hemorrhagic effects problematic. Current hirudin reversal strategies employed include prothrombin complex concentrate to neutralize the circulating antithrombin agents or dialysis to remove an antithrombin agent from the blood. Strategies that are under development of effective neutralizing agents are production of mutant thrombin molecules that are devoid of clotting activity but for which antithrombin agents retain a high affinity, thus, saturating circulating levels of these agents.

Current clinical trends also point to polypharmacologic approaches for the treatment and management of cardiovascular disorders. Combination modalities of anticoagulants with other drug classes such as antiplatelet and fibrinolytic drugs has been employed. While clinically developed thrombin inhibitors are reportedly specific for thrombin inhibition, these agents exhibit interactions with other drugs. Antiplatelet drugs such as aspirin and ticlopidine have additive or synergistic actions when used in conjunction with thrombin inhibitors. Similar interactions would be expected when thrombin inhibitors would be used with heparin, LMWHs or antithrombin III concentrates. On the other hand, adjunct usage of thrombin inhibitors with thrombolytic agents, depending on the dose, could result in facilitation of thrombolysis or, if the thrombin inhibitor dose is high in thrombolytic compromise. Some of these agents may also directly inhibit activated protein C, or inhibit activated protein C formation by neutralizing thrombo-modulin bound thrombin [63]. Furthermore, thrombin inhibitors may neutralize the coagulant actions of factor VIIa and prothrombin complex concentrates. Therefore, it is imperative that the interactions of thrombin inhibitors are well studied and considered when designing drug combination protocols for clinical applications, as such interactions may have both safety and efficacy implications.

Plasma derived inhibitors

Several inhibitors of plasmatic origin have been identified as important inhibitors of the coagulation process including antithrombin III (ATIII), protein C, tissue factor pathway inhibitor (TFPI) and heparin cofactor II. Of these inhibitors, ATIII is the only agent which has been developed for commercial purposes. Patients with hereditary thrombophilia due to a classic deficiency of ATIII can be treated with ATIII concentrate. In addition patients with disseminated intravascular coagulation (DIC), renal insufficiency, post-surgical thrombosis, thermal injury and trauma, which are associated with a decrease of ATIII in proportion to the degree of illness/injury, can also be treated [72].

Recently ATIII concentrates have been used successfully for prophylaxis using continuous infusion for the bone marrow transplant (BMT) associated toxicity [96]. Organ dysfunction during BMT has also been treated with ATIII concentrate [47]. In the same report ATIII was stated to have a major impact on both medical and economic outcomes of BMT [47]. In patients with ATIII treatment hospital duration and hospital cost were significantly decreased.

Protein C concentrates have only been used in preclinical settings. TFPI is also currently under development for clinical use.

Factor Xa inhibitors

Currently, factor Xa targeting is one of the major focuses of drug development. The factor Xa inhibitor strategy was actually derived, in part, from heparin. The LMWHs have higher anti-Xa activity than anti-thrombin activity, whereas heparin has equal factor Xa and thrombin inhibitory activities. Indirect evidence of the validity of the hypothesis that factor Xa inhibition is important for the control of thrombogenesis is given by the efficacy of LMWHs which contain a large proportion of molecules with high antifactor Xa activity [26]. Pharmacologic development has now separated these two properties so that solely antifactor Xa or anti-thrombin agents are available.

The first development of factor Xa inhibitors was met with less interest than thrombin inhibitors. These early inhibitors had low affinity to factor Xa, low selectivity, and low potency [51, 127]. Because of the increase in enzymatic activity of the coagulation cascade once the prothrombinase complex is formed, a potent factor Xa inhibitor is required to have an extremely high affinity for the enzyme. The first factor Xa inhibitors did not fulfill this requirement.

Potent factor Xa inhibitors have several potential advantages. Factor Xa is in the common pathway of both the intrinsic and extrinsic systems, playing a central role in the coagulation pathway, so it is a logical focus of drug development for the control of thrombosis. Factor Xa is formed at an earlier stage than thrombin, and the procoagulant effect of factor Xa is strongly amplified by the prothrombinase complex. Factor Xa has no known activity other than as a procoagulant, as opposed to thrombin which has multiple activation roles at various plasmatic and cellular levels (patelets, endothelial cells, other cells), not the least of which is activation of the protein C inhibitor pathway. Inhibition of protein C by a thrombin inhibitor would lead to a reduced formation of activated protein C, an important natural anticoagulant.

Since factor Xa has relatively slow activation kinetics, as opposed to thrombin, effecting its function should result in easier management of the balance between the therapeutic and bleeding effects of a drug. From recent clinical trials thrombin inhibitors have exhibited a relatively narrow safety/efficacy margin which could lead to an overdose of the therapeutic dose with a resultant bleeding complication [4, 151]. Because of their different mechanism of action, factor Xa inhibitors are expected to have a better efficacy/safety profile than thrombin inhibitors.

Factor Xa inhibitors are structurally diverse ranging from peptides to proteins to heparin sacchridic sequences [66, 67]. They can be either naturally derived, recombinant or synthetic in origin. Molecular size differs between the inhibitors, as does specificity and kinetics of factor Xa inhibition. The targeted binding site on factor Xa can differ between the inhibitors; they can be direct binding to factor Xa or indirect via a cofactor such as ATIII. Binding to the enzyme can be either reversible or irreversible. The protein

Table 3. Factor Xa Inhibitors

Agent	Chemical Nature	Source	Developmental Status
Direct Inhibitors			
Yagin	Medicinal leech protein (85 a.a.)	Animal derived	Terminated
Antistasin	Mexican leech protein (119 a.a.)	Recombinant	Terminated
TAP	Tick protein (60 a.a.)	Recombinant	Pre-clinical
NAP-5	Hookworm protein	Recombinant	Pre-clinical
TFPI	Human protein	Recombinant	Pre-clinical
DX-9065a	Propanoic acid derivative	Synthetic	Phase II clinical trials
SEL 2711	Pentapeptide produced by combinatorial chemistry	Synthetic	Pre-clinical
YM-60828			Pre-clinical
Indirect Inhibitors			
Heparin pentasaccharide	Oligosaccharide; requires binding to AT	Synthetic	Phase II clinical trial

inhibitors have limitations due to their size which limits access to factor Xa bound within clots, and, furthermore, they tend to be immunogenic, can carry viral or animal contaminants, and can become limited in supply.

Because of the structural differences, the primary mechanism of action, i.e., direct or indirect acting on factor Xa as well as other attributes, differs with the various agents. The factor Xa inhibitors that are in development are shown in Table 3. Only a few of these agents are currently undergoing clinical trials.

The factor Xa inhibitors presently under clinical development are a diverse class of new antithrombotic agents with direct and indirect mechanisms of inhibition. The penta-saccharide represents a synthetic oligosaccharide which requires the endogeneous cofactor ATIII for its activity. TAP is a low molecular weight peptide with direct inhibitory activity, whereas DX-9065a is a synthetic organic compound of lower molecular weight and direct inhibitory actions. DX-9065a is less specific than TAP. NAP-5, TFPI, and several new agents also seem promising.

Despite differences in their mechanisms of action and in vitro activities, penta-saccharide, DX-9065a and TAP have been shown to be effective antithrombotic agents in experimental models of venous thrombosis, coronary artery occlusion, arterial thrombolysis and acute reocclusion, restenosis after angioplasty, dialysis, and DIC. Pentasaccharide has also demonstrated measurable antithrombotic effects in human trials. Both TAP and DX-9065a produce measurable in vitro anticoagulant effects. In contrast, pentasaccharide does not produce an anticoagulant effect by the typical clot based assays. Thus, with factor Xa inhibitors there is not necessarily a correlation between current lab assays and antithrombotic efficacy as there is with heparin.

Factor Xa inhibitors vary in their efficacy to inhibit factor Xa depending on molecular size, access to clot bound factor Xa, access to prothrombinase bound factor Xa, specificity and kinetics of inhibition. It is probably the inhibition of clot bound factor Xa that relates to the prolongation of the aPTT as observed with some of the factor Xa inhibitors and, therefore, the inability to inhibit clot bound factor Xa that relates to a lack of aPTT prolongation by other agents. DX-9065a with a relatively lower molecular weight may be more effective in the inhibition of clot bound factor Xa than TAP or pentasaccharide.

In contrast to thrombin inhibitors, the factor Xa inhibitors are devoid of bleeding effects even at supra-therapeutic levels, which in the case of heparin are responsible for bleeding. Thus, a dissociation between the bleeding and antithrombotic responses is clearly evident for both DX-9065a and pentasaccharide.

There are potential advantages for factor Xa inhibitors over thrombin inhibitors, particularly a higher safety margin in prophylactic regimens and less frequent dosing requirements. With the development of factor Xa inhibitors it needs to be assured that the maximum benefit of factor Xa inhibitors has been achieved, be it in prophylactic or therapeutic use (i.e., in the choice of the clinical pathology, dose of drug, dosing regimen, etc. when establishing clinical trials). It is likely that each drug will have a role in specific clinical indications and that one drug will not be optimal for all thrombotic situations. How and where they are used clinically and how they will compete with LMW heparins and direct thrombin inhibitors remain to be determined.

The limited data available on factor Xa inhibitors is favorable and thus warrants additional investigations to demonstrate the relative inhibitory profile of these agents in thrombotic and cardiovascular indications. The future holds promise for finding effective factor Xa inhibitors and their challenge to the widely accepted thrombin hypothesis.

Antiplatelet drugs in development

Antiplatelet drugs such as aspirin and propionic acid derivatives have been convention-ally used to manage platelet mediated thrombotic disorders such as peripheral arterial occlusive disorders thrombotic stroke and coronary artery diseases. Newer generation antiplatelet drugs such as ticlopidine and clopidogrel have been introduced for the management of stroke [115]. More recently, these two antiplatelet drugs have been tested for other indications. While these drugs are useful, they only inhibit certain activation processes. None of these agents are capable of producing inhibition of tissue factor and thrombin mediated activation of platelets. Direct thrombin inhibitors, such as hirudin [39], may be useful in targeting tissue factor and coagulation activation processes where platelet activation is mediated by thrombin. It is therefore clear that different sites of activation are independently responsible for activating platelets in the mediation of thrombotic events related to platelets. Knowing this, glycoprotein IIb/IIIa (GpIIb/IIIa) antagonists, thromboxane A_2 receptor blockers, thromboxane synthase inhibitors, synthetic cyclooxygenase inhibitors, prostacyclin analogues, and 5-HT_2 receptor blockers have been developed.

Fig. 6 shows a diagrammatic illustration of the sites of action of various anticoagulant and antithrombotic drugs on platelets. As can be seen, different drugs have different sites of action on the platelet activation process. Platelet receptor modulators, (GPIIb/IIIa, TxA_2, ADP), cyclooxygenase inhibition and inhibition of the thrombin mediated function of platelets are some of these sites.

The GpIIb/IIIa receptor targeting drugs are claimed to act on the final common path-ways for platelet activation by various activating processes [110]. The interaction of fibrinogen with GPIIb/IIIa sites is partly mediated by the arginine-glycine-aspartic acid

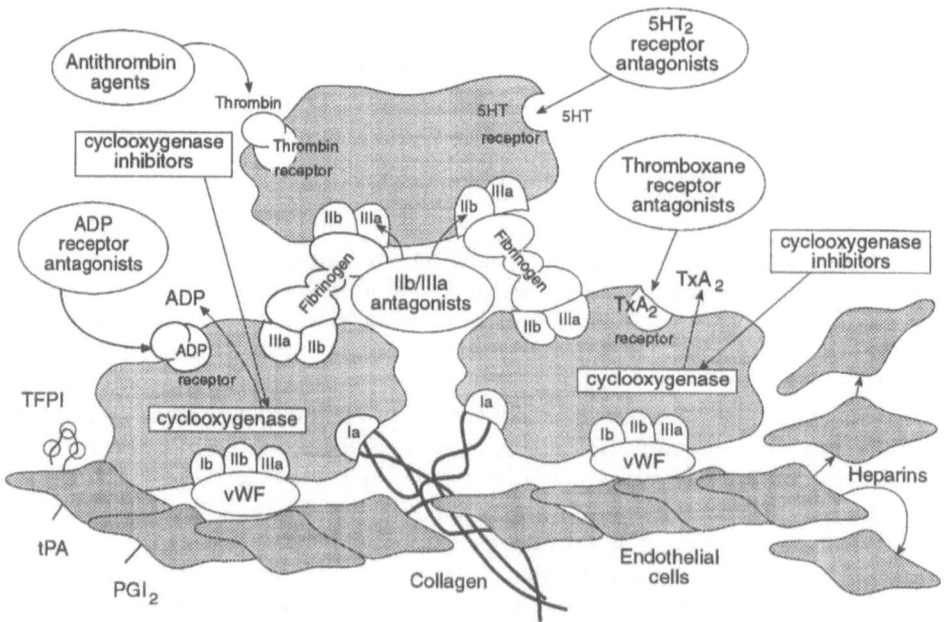

Fig. 6. Pharmacologic target sites of the antiplatelet actions of various anticoagulant and antithrombotic drugs. Receptors enzymes and other membrane sites are targeted by these drugs.

(RGD) recognition site [107]. Several synthetic peptides and peptidomimetic agents have been developed to target this site in order to prevent the aggregation of platelets [114]. FAB fragment Monoclonal fab fragment antibodies, such as 7E3 (ReoPro®) [94] have been clinically tested. ReoPro® has recently been approved by the US FDA for the prevention of post-PTCA restenosis. More recently, a fragment of a humanized monoclonal antibody against the GpIIb/IIIa site has also been identified (YM-337). The use of monoclonal antibodies as therapeutic agents may have some limitations such as immunogenicity, lack of reversibility, and non-availability by subcutaneous or oral route. Thus, the development of analogues of RGD or modification of the RGD sequence is considered more practical, safe, and cost-effective.

The pharmacological data on each of these drugs is primarily obtained in experimental settings where the effects of these agents are solely investigated in platelet function. Non-platelet mediated effects on cells have not been taken into account in the clinical development of these agents. It is conceivable that some of these effects may also contribute to their overall clinical effects. Furthermore, very little is known on the drug interactions of these agents. For proper development of these agents, valid preclinical pharmacologic data and information on drug interactions may be crucial.

Defibrotide and related agents

Aptamers are oligonuleotides (double or single stranded DNA, or single stranded RNA) which act directly on proteins to inhibit disease processes. Thirty two such aptamers have been recently isolated as inhibitors of thrombin with binding affinities in the range of 20–200 nM [15]. One of the most potent thrombin aptamers has been found to interact with thrombin's anion binding exosite, so that it competes with substrates that interact with that specific site, such as fibrinogen and thrombin platelet receptors [79, 104]. Another recent development in the area of oligonucleotide inhibitors of thrombin has been the isolation of two RNAs that bind thrombin with high affinity (Kd in the nM

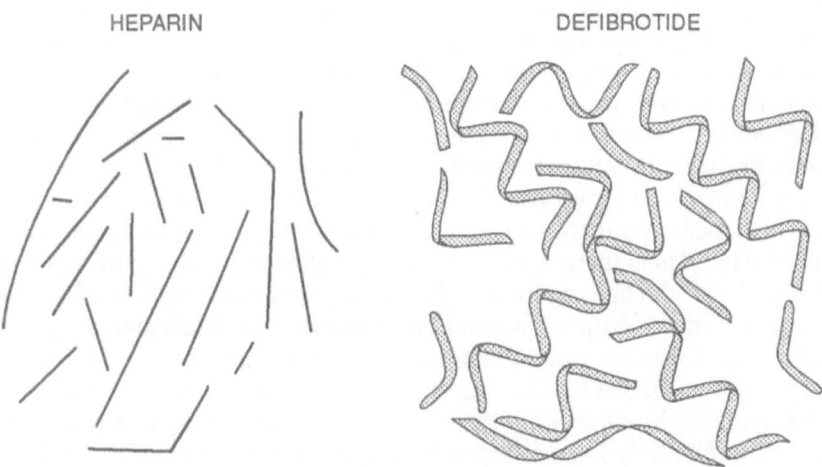

Fig. 7. A comparison of the molecular heterogeneity in unfractionated heparin and defibrotide. Both drugs are polycomponent and exhibit an apparent mean molecular weight of 15 KDA. While heparin is composed of sulfated mucopolysaccharide chains, defibrotide is composed of single stranded nucleic acid (DNA fragments). Both drugs produce polypharmacological effects and are capable of targeting multiple sites in blood and vasculature.

range). These oligonucleotides have been shown to inhibit fibrinogen clotting in an *in vitro* test [73].

Defibrotide is a polydeoxyribonucleotide derived drug of mammalian origin. Like heparin, this agent is also heterogeneous and is composed of nucleic acid strands ranging in molecular weight from 2,000 to 30,000 [38]. The mean molecular weight of this agents is around 17,000. This product is obtained from mammalian tissues such as lung and spleen. Fig. 7 shows a comparison of the heterogeneous nature of defibrotide and heparin. Like heparin, this agent is composed of several molecular components, whose molecular weight ranges from 2–50 KDA.

Despite the fact that defibrotide does not produce any systemic anticoagulant effects after intravenous injection, this agent is found to produce dose and time dependent antithrombotic effects in a stasis thrombosis model [38]. Defibrotide has been found to contain nucleotide sequences capable of producing direct antithrombin actions [18]. The antithrombotic mechanism by which defibrotide mediates its actions include endothelial modulation, increase in cAMP and TFPI release. Most interestingly, this agent produces its antithrombotic action without producing any systemic anticoagulant effects. It has therefore been used for the management of peripheral vascular disease and different microangiopathic disorders.

Summary and Conclusion

The current management of thrombotic and vascular disorders has been strongly influenced by the introduction of several new drugs and the optimal use of physical devices. One of the major impacts in the management of thrombotic disorders has been the LMWHs. Not only are these agents being used for prophylaxis, but recent studies have shown their efficacy in the treatment of established thromboembolic disorders. Other developments in the clinical use of LMWHs include the management of coronary syndromes, in pregnancy, pediatrics, transplant associated vasculopathy, and in cancer.

Dermatan sulfate and heparan sulfate have provided disappointing results to date, the synthetic heparin pentasaccharide, which acts via the inhibition of factor Xa, has been successfully used in angioplasty and is presently undergoing clinical trial for the prophylaxis of venous thrombosis in orthopedic surgical patients.

Although synthetic and recombinant thrombin inhibitors have been widely studied as adjuncts to thrombolytic therapy, in the management of unstable angina and other cardiovascular indications, for safety reasons their development has been slowed. Despite this, thrombin inhibitors have shown promise in the prevention of post-surgical venous thrombosis in orthopedic patients and they are useful anticoagulants for heparin compromised patients. Thus, these agents are being evaluated for the anticoagulant management of patients with heparin induced thrombocytipenia. Recombinant hirudin and a synthetic peptidometic drug, argatroban, are in an extensive developmental phase for HIT patients for anticoagulation of thrombosis, for anticoagulation during cardiologic interventional procedures, and as the anticogulant in cardiac surgery. The initial clinical trials with other synthetic thrombin inhibitors such as efegatran and inogatran have been rather disappointing. Similarly the development of oral thrombin inhibitors has been rather unsuccessful.

An aggressive developmental approach is in the antiplatelet drug area. In particular, numerous GP IIb/IIIa inhibitors are currently under investigation. The GP IIb/IIIa targeting antibody fab fragment, ReoPro®, has been approved for limited indications such as the management of high risk patients for angioplasty. Numerous synthetic GP IIb/IIIa inhibitors are being developed for both intravenous and oral use. However, marked variations in absorption and safety considerations represent important developmental issues which require further investigations. While these drugs may be useful in arterial thrombosis, their value in venous thrombosis is not yet proven. In addition, to the GP IIb/IIIa inhibitors, ADP receptor blockers such as ticlopidine and clopidogrel have provided impressive results in the management of thrombotic events during interventional cardiovascular procedures. The CAPRIE trial for the management of stroke and other arterial events has shown a superior effect of clopidogrel in comparison to aspirin in the overall outcome of patients where combined events are considered.

Combination modalities for the management of arterial and venous thrombosis are currently being explored. While these modalities provide an increase in the efficacy, safety considerations are of crucial importance. Aspirin is commonly used with various anticoagulants. Many other antiplatelet drugs, such as ticlopidine, are also being combined with heparin, hirudin, GP IIb/IIIa inhibitors, and aspirin itself.

Several other approaches to antithrombotic drug development are in both pre-clinical and clinical investigations with only limited data available at this time. These include factor Xa inhibitors, thrombomodulin, activated protein C, tissue factor pathway inhibitor (TFPI), PAI inhibitors, and protease nexin.

References

1. Altieri DA (1993) Coagulation assembly on leukocytes in transmembrane signaling and cell adhesion. Blood 81 (3): 569–79
2. Altieri DC, Edgington TS (1998) The saturable high affinity association of factor X to ADP-stimulated monocytes defines a novel function of the Mac-1 receptor. J Biol Chem 263: 7007–15
3. Anderson DC, Springer TA (1987) Leukocyte adhesion deficiency: An inherited defect in the Mac-1, LFA-1, and P150 glycoproteins. Annu Rev Med 38: 175–94
4. Antman EM for the TIMI 9B Investigators (1996) Hirudin in acute myocardial infarction. Thrombolysis and thrombin inhibition in myocardial infarction. (TIMI) 9B trial. Circulation 94: 911–921
5. Bach R, Konigsberg W, Nemerson Y (1998) Human tissue for contains thioester linked palmitate and stearate on the cytoplasmic half cystine. Biochemistry 27: 4227–31
6. Bajusz S, Széll E, Bagdy D, Barabas E, Horvath E, Dioszegi M, Fittler Z, Szabo G, Juhasz A, Tomori E, Szilagyi G: Highly active and selective anticoagulants D-Phe-Pro-Arg-H, a free tripeptide aldehyde prone to spontaneous inactivation, and its stable N-methyl derivative, D-MePhe-Pro-Arg-H. J Med Chem 33: 1729–35, 1990
7. Bajusz S, Barabás E, Széll E, Bagdy D (1975) Peptide aldehyde inhibitors of the fibrinogen-thrombin reaction. In: Meienhofer J (ed) Peptides – Chemistry, Structure and Biology. Ann Arbor Sci. Publ. Inc. Ann Arbor, MI. pp 603–8
8. Bara L, Billaud E, Gramond G, Kher A, Samama M (1985) Comparative pharmacokinetics of low molecular weight heparin (PK 10169) and unfractioned heparin after intravenous and subcutaneous administritation. Thromb Res 39: 631–636
9. Baumgartner A, Jacot N, Moser G, Krahenbuhl B (1989) Prevention of postoperative deep vein thrombosis by one daily injection of low molecular weight heparin and dihydroergotamine. Vasa 18 (2): 152–156
10. Bennett J (1991) Integrin structure and function in hemostasis and thrombosis. Annals N.Y. Acad Sci 614: 214–28
11. Bergqvist D, Mätzsch T, Burmark US, Frisell J, Guilbaud O, Hallböök J, Horn A, Lindhagen A, Ljungër H, Ljungström KG, Onarheim H, Risberg B, Törngren S, Örtenwall P (1988) Low molecular weight heparin given the evening before surgery compared with conventional low-dose heparin in prevention of thrombosis. Br J Surg 75 (9): 888–891
12. Bevers EM, Rosing J, Zwaal RFA (1985) Development of procoagulant binding sites on the platelet surface. In: Westweek J, Scully MF, McIntyre DE, Kakkar VV (eds) Mechanisms of Stimulus Response Coupling in Platelets, Plenum Press, NY pp 359–72
13. Biffoni M, Paroli E (1991) Complement in vitro inhibition by a low sulfate chondroitin sulfate (Matrix). Drugs Under Exp Clin Res 17 (1): 35–9
14. Blomback B, Vestermark A (1958) Isolation of fibrinopeptides by chromatography. Arkiv Kemi 12: 173–82

15. Bock LC, Griffin LC, Latham JA, Vermaas EH, Toole JJ (1992) Selection of single-stranded DNA molecules that bind and inhibit human thrombin. Nature 355 (6360): 564–6

16. Bogaert TN, Brown N, Wilcox M (1987) The Drosophila PS2 antigen is an invertebrate integrin that, like the fibronectin receptor, becomes localized to muscle attachments. Cell 51: 929–40

17. Borris LC, Hauch O, Jorgensen LN, Lassen MR (1990) Enoxaparin versus dextran 70 in the prevention of post-operative deep vein thrombsis after total hip replacement. A Danish multicenter study. Preceeding of the Danish Enoxaparin Symposium, Feb 3, 1990

18. Bray F, Schror K (1994) Isolation and identification of aptamers from defibrotide that act as thrombin antogonists in vitro. Biochem Biophys Res Com 200 (2): 933–937

19. Bray PF, Rosa JP, Johnston JI, Shin DT, Cook RG, Lau C, Kan YW, McEver RP, Shuman MA(1987) Platelet glycoprotein IIb. Chromosomal localization and tissue expression. J Clin Invest 80: 1812–7

20. Brittis PA, Canning DR, Silver J (1992) Chondroitin sulfate as a regulator of neuronal patterning in the retina. Science 225 (5045): 733–6

21. Caen JP (1988) A randomized double-blind study between a low molecular weight heparin Kabi 2165 and standard heparin in the prevention of deep vein thrombosis in general surgery. A French multicenter trial. Thromb Haemost 59 (2): 216–220

22. Car BD, Suyemoto M, Neilsen NR, Slauson DO (1991) The role of leukocytes in the pathogenesis of fibrin deposition in bovine acute lung injury. Am J Pathol 138 (5): 1191–98

23. Carlsen E, Flatmark A, Prydz H (1988) Cytokine-induced procoagulant activity in monocytes and endothelial cells. Further enhancement by cyclosporine. Transplantation 46: 575–80

24. Chapman HA, Allen CL, Stone OL, Fair DS (1985) Human alveolar macrophages synthesize factor VII in vitro. Possible role in interstital lung disease. J Clin Invest 75: 2030–37

25. Cheresh DA, Spiro RC (1987) Biosynthetic and functional properties of an Arg-Gly-Asp directed receptor involved in human melanoma cell attachment to vitronectin, fibrinogen, and von Willebrand factor. J Biol Chem 262 (36): 17703–11

26. Clagett GP, Anderson Jr FA, Heit J, Levine MN, Wheeler HB. Prevention of venous thromboembolism. Chest 108 (4) (Suppl): 312S–334S

27. Coller B (1992) Platelets in cardiovascular thrombosis and thrombolysis. In: Fozzard UA, Haber E, Jennings RB, Katz AM and Morgan HE. The Heart and Cardiovascular System 2nd ed. Raven Press, New York, pp 219–73

28. Davie EW, Ratnoff OD (1964) Waterfall sequence for intrinsic blood clotting. Science 145: 1310–2

29. DeSimone DW, Hynes RO (1988) Xenopus laevie integrins. Structural conservation and evolutionary divergence of integrin beta. J Biol Chem 263 (11): 5333–40

30. Drake TA, Morissey JH, Edgington TS (1989) Selective expresion of tissue factor in human tissues. Am J Pathol 134: 1087–97

31. Edgington TS, Mackman N, Brand K, Ruf W (1991) The structural biology of the expression and function of tissue factor. Thromb Haemost 66: 67–79

32. Edmunds LH (1995) HIT, HITT and desulfatohirudin: look before you leap. J Thorac Cardiovasc Surg 110 (1): 1–3

33. Edwards RL, Rickles FR (1992) The role of leudocytes in the activation of blood coagulation. Semin Hematol 29 (3): 202–12

34. Eriksson BI, Zachrisson BE, Teger-Nilsson AC, Risberg B (1988) Thrombosis prophylaxis with low molecular weight heparin in total hip replacement. Br J Surg 75 (11): 1053–1057

35. Esmon CT (1993) Cell mediated events that control blood coagulation and vascular injury. Annu Rev Cell Biol 9: 1–26

36. Esmon CT (1989) The roles of protein C and thrombomodulin in the regulation of blood coagulation. J Biol Chem 264: 4743–61

37. European Fraxiparin Study Group (1988) Comparison of low molecular weight heparin and unfractionated heparin for the prevention of deep vein thrombosis is patients undergoing abdominal surgery. Br J Surg 75: 1058–1063

38. Fareed J, Walenga JM, Hoppensteadt DA, Kumar A, Ulutin O, Cornelli U (1988) Pharmacologic profiling of defibrotide in experimental models. Semin Thromb Hemost 14: 27–37

39. Fareed J, Walenga JM, Hoppensteadt D, Pifarre R (1991) An objective perspective on recombinant hirudin A new anticoagulant and antithrombotic agent. Blood Coag Fibrinol 2: 135–147

40. Fareed J, Walenga JM, Pifarre R (1992) Newer approaches to the pharmacologic management of acute myocardial infarction. Cardiac Surgery: State of the Art Reviews 6 (1): 101–111

41. Fareed J, Walenga JM, Hoppensteadt D, Racanelli A, Coyne E (1989) Chemical and biochemical heterogeneity in low molecular weight heparins: Implications for clinical use and standardization. Semin Thromb Hemost 15: 440–463

42. Fareed J, Bacher P, Messmore HL, Walenga JM, Hoppensteadt DA, Strano A, Pifarre R (1992) Pharmacological modulation of fibrinolysis by antithrombotic and cardiovascular drugs. Prog Cardiovas Dis 6: 379–398

43. Gailani D, Broze GJ (1991) Factor XI activation in a revised model of blood coagulation. Science 253: 909–12

44. Gregory SA, Morissey JH, Edgington TS: Regulation of tissue factor gene expression in the monocyte procoagulant response to endotoxin. Mol Cell Biol 9: 2752–55

45. Griffith GC, Nichols G Jr, Asher JD, Flanagan B (1965) Heparin osteoporosis. J Am Med Assoc 193: 85–88

46. Haas S, Stemberger A, Fritsche HM, Welzel D, Wolf H, Lechner F, Blumel G (1987) Prophylaxis of deep vein thrombosis in high risk patients undergoing total hip replacement with low molecular weight heparin plus dihydroergotamine. Arzneimittel-Forschung 37 (7): 839–843

47. Haire WD, Stephens LC, Ruby EI (1996) Antithrombin III (AT3) treatment of organ dysfunction during bone marrow transplantation (BMT) – results of a pilot study. Blood 88 (10) (Suppl 1): 456a

48. Hanke H, Oberhoff M, Hanke S, Hassenstein S, Kamenz J, Schmid KM, Betz E, Karsch KR (1992) Inhibition of cellular proliferation after experimental balloon angioplasty by low molecular weight heparin. Circulation 85: 1548–1556

49. Hartl P, Brucke P, Dienstl E, Vinazzer H (1990) Prophylaxis of thromboembolism in general surgery Comparison between standard heparin and Fragmin. Thromb Res 57 (4): 577–584

50. Haskel EJ, Torr SR, Day KC, Palmier MO, Wun TC, Sobel BE, Abendschein DR (1991) Prevention of arterial reocclusion after thrombolysis with recombinant lipoprotein associated coagulation inhibitor. Circulation 84 (2): 821–7

51. Hauptmann J, Kaiser B, Nowak G, Stürzebecher J, Markwardt F (1990) Comparison of the anticoagulant and antithrombotic effects of synthetic thrombin and factor Xa inhibitors. Thromb Haemost 63: 220–223

52. Hemker HC, Kessels H (1991) Feedback mechanisms in coagulation. Haemostasis 21: 189–96

53. Hemler ME, Crouse C, Takada H, Sonnenberg A (1988) Multiple very late antigen (VLA) heterodimers on platelets. Evidence of distinct VLA-2, VLA-5 (fibrinogen receptor) and VLA-6 structures. J Biol Chem 263 (16): 7660–5

54. Hemler ME, Ware CF, Strominger JL (1988) Characterization of a novel differentiation antigen complex recognized by a monoclonal antibody (A-1A5): unique activation specifies molecular forms in stimulated T cells. J Immunol 131: 334–40

55. Hijikata-Okunomiya A, Okamoto S (1992) A strategy for a rational approach to designing synthetic selective inhibitors. Sem Thromb Hemost 18 (1): 135–149

56. Hirsh J, Levine M (1987) The development of low molecular weight heparins for clinical use. In: Verstraete M et al. (eds) Thrombosis and Haemostasis, pp. 425–448, Leuven University Press, Leuven

57. Holmsen H (1987) Platelet secretion. In: Colman RW, Hirsh J, Marder VJ, Salzman EW (eds) Hemostasis and Thrombosis. Lippincott, Philadelphia, p 606

58. Hourani SMO, Cusack NJ (1991) Pharmacological receptors on blood platelets. Pharmacol Rev 43: 243–98

59. Hull R, Raskob G, Pineo G (1992) Subcutaneous low molecular weight heparin compared with continuous intravenous heparin in the treatment of proximal vein thrombosis. N Eng J Med 326 (15): 975–982

60. Hull R, Delmore T, Carter C, Hirsh J, Genton E, Gent M, Turpie G, McLaughlin D (1983) Adjusted subcutaneous heparin versus warfarin sodium in the long-term treatment of venous thrombosis. N Eng J Med 306: 954–958

61. Hynes RO (1987) Integrins: a family of cell surface receptors. Cell 48: 549–54

62. Ittyerah TR, Rawala R, Colman RW (1981) Immunochemical studies of factor V of bovine platelets. Eur J Biochem 120: 235–41

63. Iyer L, Fareed J (1996) Recombinant hirudin: a perspective. Exp Opin Invest Drugs 5 (5): 469–494

64. Jackson SP, Yuan Y, Schoenwaelder SM, Mitchell CA (1993) Role of the platelet integrin glycoprotein IIb-IIIa in intracellular signalling. Thromb Res 71: 159–68

65. Jurkiewicz E, Panse P, Jentsch KD, Hartmann H, Hunsmann G (1989) In vitro anti-HIV-1 activity of chondroitin polysulfate. AIDS 3 (7): 423–7

66. Kaiser B, Hauptmann J (1994) Factor Xa inhibitors as novel antithrombotic agents: Facts and perspectives. Cardiovascular Drug Reviews 12 (3): 225–236

67. Kaiser B (1997) Factor Xa versus factor IIa inhibitors. Clin Appl Thrombosis/Hemostasis 3 (1): 16–24

68. Kakkar VV, Murray WJG (1985) Efficacy and safety of low molecular weight heparin (CY 216) in preventing postoperative venous thrombo-embolism A cooperative study. Br J Surg 72: 786–791

69. Kaplan KL (1981) Platelet granule proteins: localization and secretion. In: Gordon AS (ed), Platelet in Biology and Pathology vol. 5. Elsevier, Amsterdam, p 77

70. Kelton JG (1986) Heparin induced thrombocytopenia. Haemostasis 16: 173–186

71. Koppenhagen K, Adolf J, Matthes M, Troster E, Roder JD, Haas S, Fritsche HM, Wolf H (1992) Low molecular weight heparin and prevention of postoperative thrombosis in abdominal surgery. Thromb Haemost 67 (6): 627–630

72. Kowal-Vern A, Gamelli RL, Walenga JM, Hoppensteadt D, Sharp-Pucci M, Schumacher HR (1992) The effect of burn wound size on hemostasis: A correlation of hemostatic changes to the clinical state. Journal of Trauma 33 (1): 50–57

73. Kubik MF, Stephens AW, Schneider D, Marlar R, Tasset D (1994) Highaffinity RNA ligands to human α-thrombin. Nucleic Acids Research 22 (13): 2619–2626

74. Kumon K, Tanaka K, Nakajima N, Naito Y, Fijuta T (1984) Anticoagulation with a synthetic thrombin inhibitor after cardiovascular surgery and for treatment of disseminated intravascular coagulation. Crit Care Med 12: 1039–1043

75. Lam SC, Plow EW, D'Souza SE, Cheres DA, Frelinger AL, Ginsberg MH (1989) Isolation and characterization of a platelet membrane protein related to the vitronectin receptor. J Biol Chem 264: 3742–9

76. Levine MN, Hirsh J (1988) An overview of clinical trials with low molecular weight heparin fractions. Acta Chirur Scand 154 (543): 73–39

77. Leyvraz PF, Richard J, Bachmann F, Van Melle G, Treyvaud JM, Livio JJ, Candardjis G (1983) Adjusted versus fixed subcutaneous heparin in the prevention of deep vein thrombosis after total hip replacement. N Eng J Med 309: 954–958

78. Lindahl AK, Sandset PM, Abildgaard U (1992) The present status of tissue factor pathway inhibitor. Blood Coag Fibrinol 3: 439–49

79. Macaya RF, Schultze P, Smith FW, Roe JA, Feigon J (1993) Thrombinbinding DNA aptamer forms a unimolecular quadruplex structure in solution. Proc Natl Acad Sci USA 90: 3745–3749

80. MacFarlane RG (1964) An enzyme cascade in the blood clotting mechanism and its function as a biochemical amplifier. Nature 202: 498–9

81. Mann KG, Jerry RJ, Krishnaswamy S (1988) Cofactor proteins in the assembly of blood clotting enzyme complexes. Annu Rev Biochem 57: 915–56

82. Mann KG, Nesheim ME, Church WR, Haley P, Krishnaswamy S (1990) Surface-dependent reactions of the vitamin K-dependent enzyme complexes. Blood 76: 1–16

83. Maraganore JM, Bourdon P, Jablonski J, Ramachandran KL, Fenton JW 2nd: Design and characterization of hirulogs. A novel class of bivalent peptide inhibitors of thrombin. Biochemistry 29: 7095–7101

84. Marcantonio EE, Hynes RO (1988) Antibodies to the conserved cytoplasmic domain of the integrin beta 1 subunit react with proteins in vertebrates, invertebrates and fungi. J Cell Biol 106 (5): 1765–72

85. Markwardt F, Fink G, Kaiser B, Klocking HP, Nowak G, Richter M, Sturzebecher J (1988) Pharmacological survey of recombinant hirudin. Pharmazie 43: 202–207

86. Maruyama I (1990) Synthetic anticoagulants. Jpn J Clin Hematol 31: 776–781

87. Matsuo T, Kario K, Kodama K, Okamoto S (1992) Clinical applications of the synthetic thrombin inhibitor, Argatroban (MD-805). Sem Thromb Hemost 18 (2): 155–160

88. Matsushima T, Nakashima Y, Suganp M, Tasaki H, Kuroiwa A, Koide O (1987) Suppression of atherogenesis in hypercholesterolemic rabbits by chondroitin 6-sulfate. Artery 14 (6): 316–37

89. Matzsch T, Bergqvist D, Fredin H, Hedner U (1988) Safety and efficacy of a low molecular weight heparin (Logiparin) versus dextran as prophylaxis against thrombosis after total hip replacement. Acta Chirur Scand 543: 80–84

90. McGee MP, Devlin R, Saluta G, Koren H (1990) Tissue factor and factor VII messenger RNAs in human alveolar macrophages: Effects of breathing ozone. Blood 75: 122–27

91. McGee MP, Li LC (1991) Functional difference between intrinsic and extrinsic coagulation pathways. Kinetics of factor X activation on human monocytes and alveolar macrophages. J Biol Chem 266: 8079–85

92. McGee MP, Wallin R, Devlin R, Rothberger H (1989) Identification of mRNA coding for factor VII protein in human alveolar macrophages. Cogaulant expression may be limited due to postribosomal processing. Thromb Haemost 61: 170–4

93. McVey JH (1994) Tissue factor pathway. Bailliere's Clin Haemat 7 (3): 469–84

94. Mickelson JK, Simpson PJ, Cronin M, Homeister JW, Laywell E, Kitzen J, Lucchesi BR (1990) Antiplatelet antibody [7E3 f (ab')₂] prevents rethrombosis after recombinant tissue-type plasminogen activator-induced coronary artery thrombolysis in a canine model. Circulation 81: 617–627

95. Miletich JP, Jackson CM, Majerus PW (1977) Interaction of coagulation factor Xa with human platelets. Proc Natl Acad Sci USA 74: 4033–36

96. Morris CL, Lutes R, Gruppo RA, Hashmi R, Harris R, Sambrano J, Morris JD (1996) Prophylactic continuous infusion (CI) antithrombin III (AT-III) for prevention of regimen related toxicity (RRT) following bone morrow transplantation (BMT). Blood 88 (10) (Suppl 1): 117a

97. Morrissey JH, Mack BG, Neuenschwander PF, Comp PC (1993) Quantitation of activated factor VII levels in plasma using a tissue factor mutant selectively deficient in promoting factor VII activation. Blood 81: 734–44

98. Naito K, Fujikawa K (1991) Activation of human blood coagulation factor XI independent of factor XII: Factor XI is activated by thrombin and factor XIa in the presence of negatively charged surfaces. J Biol Chem 266: 7353–8

99. Nawroth P, Handley D, Esmon C, Stern DM (1986) Interleukin 1 induces endothelial cell procoagulant while suppressing cell surface anticoagulant activity. Proc Natl Acad Sci USA 83: 3460–64

100. Nemerson Y (1988) Tissue factor and haemostasis. Blood 71: 1–8

101. Okajima K, Yang WP, Okabe H, Inoue M, Takatsuki K (1991) Role of leukocytes in the activation of intravascular coagulation in Patients with septicemia. Am J Hematol 36: 265–71

102. Okamoto M, Mori S, Endo H (1994) A protective action of chondroitin sulfate proteoglycans against neuronal cell death induced by glutamate. Brain Res 637 (1–2): 57–67

103. Osterud B, Rapaport SI (1977) Activation of factor IX by the reaction product of tissue factor and factor VII: additional pathway for initiating blood coagulation. Proc Natl Acad Sci USA 74: 5260–4

104. Paborsky LR, McCurdy SN, Griffin LC, Toole JJ, Leung LLK (1993) The single-stranded DNA aptamer binding-site of human thrombin. J Biol Chem 268: 20808

105. Packham MA (1994) Role of platelets in thrombosis and hemostasis. Can J Physiol Pharmacol 72: 278–84
106. Perdue JF, Lubenskyi W, Kivity E, Sonder SA, Fenton JW (1981) Protease mitogenic response of chick embryo fibroblasts and receptor binding/processing of human α-thrombin. J Biol Chem 256: 2767–76
107. Philips DR, Charo IF, Scarborough RM (1991) GPIIb-IIIa the responsive integrin. Cell 65: 359–62
108. Phillips DR, Chaio IF, Scarborough RM (1991) GPIIB/IIIa: The responsive integrin. Cell 65: 359–62
109. Pischel KD, Bluestein HH, Woods VL (1988) Platelet glycoproteins Ia, Ic and IIa are physicochemically indistinguishable from the very late activation antigens adhesion related proteins of lymphocytes and other cell types. J Clin Invest 81: 505–13
110. Prandoni P, Lensing A, Buller H, Carta M, Cogo A, Vigo M, Casara D, Ruol A, ten Cate JW (1992) Comparison of subcutaneous standard low-molecular weight heparin with intervenous standard heparin in proximal deep-vein thrombosis. Lancet 339: 441–445
111. Pytele R, Pierschbacher MS, Ginsberg MH, Plow EF, Ruoslathi E (1986) Platelet membrane glycoprotein IIb/IIIamember of a family od RGD specific adhesion receptors. Science 231: 1559–1562
112. Riess FC, Lower C, Seelig C, Bleese N, Kormann J, Muller-Berghaus G, Potzsch B (1995) Recombinant hirudin as a new anticoagulant during cardiac operations instead of heparin: Successful for aortic valve replacement in man. J Thorac Cardiovasc Surg 110: 265–267
113. Robinson RA, Worfolk L, Tracy PB (1992) Endotoxin enhances expression of monocyte prothrombinase activity. Blood 79: 406–16
114. Rothberger H, McGee MP (1984) Generation of coagulation factor V activity by cultured rabbit alveolar macrophages. J Exp Med 160: 1880–90
115. Ruggeri ZM, Houghton RA, Russel SR, Zimmerman TS (1986) Inhibition of platelet function with synthetic peptide designed to be high affinity antagonist of fibrinogen binding to platelets. Proc Natl Acad Sci USA 83: 5708–12
116. Saltiel E, Ward A (1987) Ticlopidinea review of its pharmacodynamic and pharmacokinetic properties and therapeutic efficacy in platelet dependent disease states. Drugs 34: 222–62
117. Sandberg H, Bode AP, Dombrose FA, Hoechli M, Lentz BR (1985) Expression of coagulant activity in human platelets: Release of membranous vesicles providing platelet factor 1 and platelet factor 3. Thromb Res 39: 63–79
118. Schwartz BS, Levy GA, Curtiss LK, Fair DS, Edgington TS (1981) Plasma lipoprotein induction and suppression of the generation of cellular procoagulant activities in vitro. Two procoagulant activities are produced by peripheral blood mononuclear cells. J Clin Invest 67: 1650–58
119. Scully MF, Ellis V, Seno N, Kakkar VV (1986) The anticoagulant properties of mast cell product chondroitin sulfate E. Biochem Biophys Res Comm 137 (1): 15–22
120. Scully MF (1992) The biochemistry of blood clotting: The digestion of a liquid to form a solid. Essays in Biochem 27: 17–36
121. Senior RM, Skogen WF, Griffin GL, Wilner GD (1986) Effects of fibrinogen derivatives upon the inflammatory response. J Clin Invest 77: 1014–19
122. Shainoff JR, Dardik BN (1979) Fibrinopeptide B and aggregation of fibrinogen. Science 204 (4389): 200–2
123. Shattil SJ, Bennett JS (1981) Platelets and their membranes in hemostasis: Physiology and patho-physiology. Ann Intern Med 94 (1): 108–18
124. Shavit R, Kahn A, Wilner G, Fenton JW (1992) Monocyte chemotaxis: Sheffield WP, Brothers AB, Wells MJ, Haiton MWC, Clarke BJ and Blajchman MA. Molecular cloning and expression of rabbit antithrombin III. Blood 79 (9): 2330–9.
125. Siess W (1989) Molecular mechanisms of platelet activation. Physiol Rev 69: 58–178
126. Silver D, Kapsch D, Tosi E (1983) Heparin induced thrombocytopenia, thrombosis and haemorrhage. Ann Surg 198: 301–305
127. Sims PJ, Wiedmer T, Esmon CT, Weiss HJ, Shattil SJ (1989) Assembly of the platelet prothrombinase complex is linked to vesiculation of the platelet plasma membrane. J Biol Chem 264: 17049–57
128. Stürzebecher J, Stürzebecher U, Vieweg H, Wagner G, Hauptmann J, Markwardt F. Synthetic inhibitors of bovine factor Xa and thrombin. Comparison of their anticoagulant efficiency. Thromb Res 54: 245–252
129. Takada Y, Strominger JL, Hemler ME (1987) The very late antigen family of heterodimers is part of a super-family of molecules in adhesion and embryogenesis. Proc Natl Acad Sci USA 84 (10): 3239–43
130. Tamao Y, Yamamoto T, Hirata T, Kinugasa M, Kimumoto M (1986) Effect of argipidine (MD-805) on blood coagulation. Jpn Pharmacol Ther 14: 869–74
131. Teger-Nilsson A, Eriksson U, Gustafsson D, Bylund R, Fager G, Held P (1995) Phase I studies on Inogatran, a new selective thrombin inhibitor. J Am Col Cardiol 117A–118A
132. The Global Use of Strategies to Open Occluded Coronary Arteries (GUSTO) IIb Investiators A compari-son of recombinant hirudin with heparin for the treatment of acute coronary syndromes. N Engl J Med 335 (11): 775–82
133. Tilly RHJ, Senden JMG, Comfurius P, Bevers EM, Zwaal RFA (1990) Increased aminophospholipid translocase activity in human platelets during secretion. Biochim Biophys Acta 1029: 188–90
134. Topol EJ (1995) Novel antithrombotic approaches to coronary artery disease. Am J Cardiol 76 (6): 27B–33B
135. Tracy PB, Rorhbach MS, Mann KG (1983) Functional prothrombinase complex assembly on isolated monocytes and lymphocytes. J Biol Chem 258: 7264–7

136. Tracy PB, Eide LL, Mann KG (1985) Human prothrombinase complex assembly and function on isolated peripheral blood cell populations. J Biol Chem 260: 2119–24
137. Tracy PB, Nesheim ME, Mann KG (1992) Platelet factor Xa receptor. Meth Enzymol 215: 329–60
138. Weisberg LJ, Shin DT, Conkling PR (1987) Identification of normal human peripheral blood monocytes and liver as sites of synthesis of coagulation factor XIII alpha chain. Blood 70: 579–82
139. Wiedmer T, Esmon CT, Sims PJ (1986) Complement proteins C5b-9 stimulate procoagulant activity through platelet prothrombinase. Blood 68: 875–80
140. Zimrin AB, Eisman R, Vilaire G, Schwartz E, Bennett JS, Poncz M (1988) Structure of platelet glycoprotein IIIa. A common subunit for two different membrane receptors. J Clin Invest 81 (5): 1470-5
141. Zwaal RFA, Bevers EM, Comfurius P, Rosing J, Tilly RHJ, Verhallen PFJ (1989) Loss of membrane phospholipid asymmetry during activation of blood platelets and sickled red cells; mechanisms and physiological significance. Mol Cell Biochem 91: 23–31

W. Jeske · D. A. Hoppensteadt · R. Pifarre · J. M. Walenga · J. Fareed (✉)
Loyola University
Medical Center
2160 South First Avenue
USA - Maywood, ILL 60153

Low molecular weight heparins –
Pharmacological principles and indications in clinical practice

J. Harenberg

Summary The pharmacological effects of low molecular weight heparins are characterized by an increased inhibition of factor Xa and decreased inhibition of thrombin of the coagulation cascade in comparison to unfractionated heparins. After administration into the circulation blood, levels are sustained twice as long as for unfractionated heparin on factor Xa inhibition leading to a biological half-life of 2 h after intravenous administration and of 4 h after subcutaneous administration. The clearance of LMW heparins is decreased and the area under the activity time curve is increased more than 2-fold compared to unfractionated heparin. The effects on bleeding time and hemorrhage are decreased in animal models.

In postoperative medicine LMW heparins once daily (o.d.) have a higher efficacy as low dose unfractionated heparin three times daily (t.e.d.). In medical bedridden hospitalized patients LMW heparin o.d. is as effective and probably safer than unfractionated heparin t.e.d. Heparin-induced thrombocytopenia type II occurs less frequently. Treatment of recent deep venous thrombosis is performed more effectively and safely using low molecular weight heparins. So far, there is no sufficient evidence for different efficacies of LMW heparins in these indications. The efficacy and safety of low molecular weight heparins is currently proven in patients with cerebral ischaemia and unstable angina.

Key words Low molecular weight heparin – prophylaxis of thromboembolism – heparin-induced thrombocytopenia – cerebral ischaemia – unstable angina

Introduction

Initially, low molecular weight heparins were developed due to the fact that they inhibit more potently the serine protease factor Xa compared to unfractionated heparin and that they effect less potently thrombin, the last key enzyme of the coagulation cascade. Thus, the equilibrium of the low molecular weight heparins is shifted more towards an inhibition of the early phase in contrast to unfractionated heparin inhibiting more potently the endstage of the coagulation cascade. The inhibition of thrombin by heparin has been attributed to bleeding complications, whereas the inhibition of low doses of heparin or low molecular weight heparin has been attributed to mediate the antithrombotic effects of low doses of these anticoagulants. Accordingly, the inhibition of the early stage of the coagulation system has been assumed to mediate the antithrombotic effects of heparins, whereas the inhibition of the endstage of the coagulation cascade has been attributed to mediate the bleeding complication of heparins. Thus, it was supposed, that low molecular weight heparin may have advantages over unfractionated heparin by inhibiting more potently the early phase of the coagulation cascade and to a lower extent the ultimate protease of the coagulation cascade at low as well as at high dosages (Fig. 1) [10].

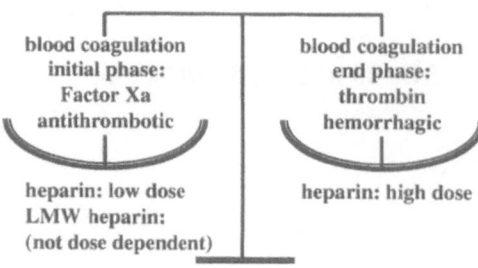

Fig. 1. Rationale for development of low molecular weight heparins: low doses of heparin and LMW heparin at every dosage inhibit the initial phase of the coagulation cascade, mainly factor Xa. The antithrombotic effect of all heparins at low dosages as well as of high dose low molecular weight heparin is explained in this way. The inhibition of the end-stage of the coagulation system through thrombin occurs only at high doses of heparin. Hemorrhagic side effects of heparin are explained by inhibition of this last enzyme in the coagulation cascade.

Pharmacokinetic and pharmacodynamic investigations of low molecular weight heparins have demonstrated an increased half-life on factor Xa in comparison to unfractionated heparin. The half-life was twice as long after intravenous as well as after subcutaneous administration of various low molecular weight heparins (Fig. 2). More

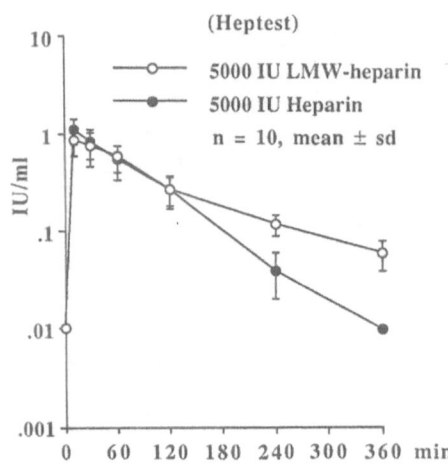

Fig. 2. Factor Xa inhibition of low molecular weight heparin is twice as long as for unfractionated heparin, as measured by factor Xa specific test systems (n = 10 volunteers, mean ± SD, half-life 2 h versus 2 h)

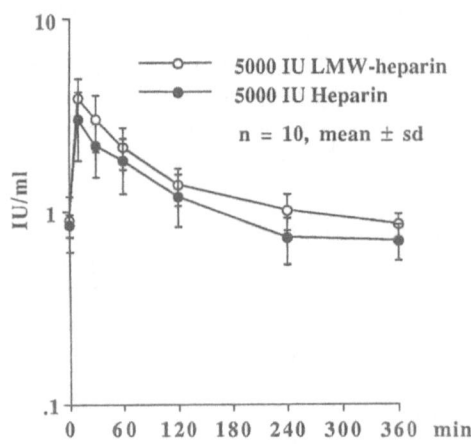

Fig. 3. The inhibitor of the extrinsic pathway, named tissue factor pathway inhibitor, is released by heparin as well as by LMW heparins. The effect of LMW heparins seems to be somewhat higher compared to unfractionated heparin. Half-lives are 60 min for both compounds on TFPI release (n = 10 volunteers, mean ± SD)

recently, the inhibition of the extrinsic pathway by the lipoprotein named tissue factor pathway inhibitor (TFPI) was demonstrated to be released by heparins as well as by low molecular weight heparins (Fig. 3). Thus, heparins have been shown to inhibit not only the intrinsic system of the coagulation cascade through antithrombin III, but also the extrinsic system by tissue factor pathway inhibitor. The inhibition of the extrinsic pathway is maintained by low molecular weight heparins through the release of TFPI [2].

The anticoagulant effects of heparins and low molecular weight heparins can be neutralized by protamine. On a weight basis of 1 : 1 the inhibition of heparins or low molecular weight heparins on aPTT, thrombin and TFPI are completely antagonized by protamine in vitro and in vivo. However factor Xa inhibition of low molecular weight heparins is neutralized to about 50 % by protamine in contrast to unfractionated heparin, being completely antagonized [9, 10]. Bleeding effects of heparin and low molecular weight heparins are antagonized by protamine [21]. Antithrombotic effects of heparin or low molecular weight heparins are not seen any more after administration of protamine [8].

Postoperative medicine

Low molecular weight heparins have been demonstrated to effectively reduce the incidence of pulmonary embolism and deep venous thrombosis in orthopaedic and abdominal surgery. The effect is about twice as potent as for low dose heparin, i.e., $3 \times 5,000$ IE heparin subcutaneously per day (Fig. 4) [18].

Heparin-induced thrombocytopenia type II

In postoperative medicine heparin-induced thrombocytopenia type II has been demonstrated to occur less frequently with low molecular weight heparin. In about 3 % of patients in orthopaedic surgery thrombocytopenia and thrombosis occurred during prophylaxis of thromboembolism with low dose heparin. In contrast, no patient on low molecular weight heparin developed thrombocytopenia or thrombosis in this study [25]. However, antibodies against heparin/platelet factor 4 complex were detected in about

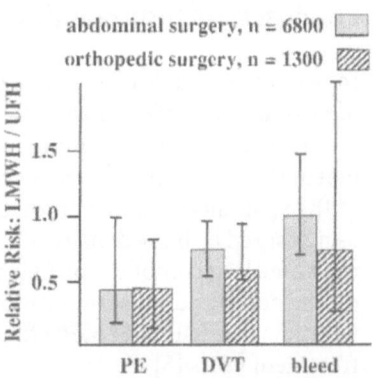

Fig. 4. Relative risk of the development of pulmonary embolism (PE), deep venous thrombosis (DVT) or bleeding complications (bleed) of low molecular weight heparin (LMWH) compared to unfractionated heparin (UFH) in abdominal and orthopedic surgery (data obtained from reference 18). The ratio LMWH/UFH demonstrates an about 50 % reduction of the incidence of PE in patients receiving LMW heparin for prophylaxis of thromboembolism in these indications.

15 % of patients during prophylaxis with unfractionated heparin and in about 3 % of patients during prophylaxis with low molecular weight heparin. The specificity of the test system and the clinical relevance of these laboratory data remain unclear so far.

Prophylaxis of thromboembolism in outpatients without or with surgery

The incidence of thromboembolic complications in patients with plaster casts ranges from 5–10 %. Prophylaxis of thromboembolism has been performed in several settings using different low molecular weight heparins. The incidence of thromboembolic complications during the period of immobilization with a plaster cast was reduced ranging from 0 to 4 %, depending on the screening method used for detection of venous thrombosis [12, 14, 22, 26].

Recently, after discharge of patients with total hip replacement deep venous thrombosis was observed in 10–20 %. Low molecular weight heparins reduced the incidence of DVT in these patients by about 50 % during a treatment period of 4 weeks [2, 3, 20]. Thus, prolonged prophylaxis of thromboembolism significantly reduced DVT in patients with an immobilizing plaster cast and after elective hip replacement for a period up to 4 weeks after discharge from hospital in several prospective, randomized double-blind studies.

Hospitalized medical patients

Prophylaxis of thromboembolism in hospitalized medical patients was an increased risk for thromboembolism due to immobilization, cardiac insufficiency, malignancy, or other concomitant diseases has been compared using low molecular weight heparin o.d. versus unfractionated heparin t.e.d. The equivalence of low molecular weight heparin has been demonstrated in a total of 3 studies in about 3,000 patients [1, 6, 15]. The safety of low molecular weight heparins was higher compared to unfractionated heparin with regard to local erythemas, local pruritus, local hematomas, decrease of antithrombin III, and increase of liver enzymes [6].

Prophylaxis of recurrent thromboembolism

In patients with side effects to oral anticoagulants low molecular weight heparins may be of advantage. Warfarin has been studied against Enoxaparin in about 200 patients. The recurrence of thromboembolism was equivalent in both treatment groups, whereas bleeding complications were more frequent in patients with oral anticoagulant treatment (19). In patients receiving unfractionated heparin osteoporosis occurred more frequently as measured by bone density compared to low molecular weight heparin [17]. In patients with bleeding complications on oral anticoagulants, i.e., with intracerebral bleeding or esophageal bleeding complications, low molecular weight heparin was effectively used with low incidences of side effects and only 1 recurrence of thromboembolism in 250 treatment years [5].

Table 1. Incidence of recurrent venous thromboembolism, hemorrhage or mortality, and duration of hospital stay of patients receiving low molecular weight heparin subcutaneously or unfractionated heparin by aPTT-controlled intravenous infusion for treatment of recent deep venous thrombosis

n =	LMWH 1009	UFH 1012
Recurrent VTE (%)	5.3	5.8
Haemorrhage (%)	2.2	1.9
Mortality (%)	6.0	7.1
Hospital days (mean)	1.1 – 6.4	6.5 – 9.4

Treatment of recent DVT

Three studies have been finished with the aim of demonstrating the efficacy and safety of twice daily 1 mg/kg body weight low molecular weight heparin subcutaneously in comparison to continuous intravenous aPTT-controlled unfractionated heparin. Recurrence of venous thromboembolism after 3 or 6 months was similar in both treatment groups as well as the incidence of hemorrhage. The mortality rate was 6 % in patients receiving low molecular weight heparin groups and 7 % in patients receiving unfractionated heparin. The hospital stay was reduced from about 7 to about 2 days in patients receiving low molecular weight heparin. A total of about 2,000 patients were included in the 3 studies (Table 1) [13, 16, 24].

Analyzing the various low molecular weight heparins, which have been compared to unfractionated heparin for treatment of thromboembolism, some differenced between the clinical efficacy and safety can be seen; however, the number of patients is too small to give some conclusion on the clinical relevance (Table 2). So far, the conclusion of these comparisons is that s.c. low molecular weight heparins are better, but not different between each other for treatment of DVT compared to i.v. unfractionated heparin.

The daily dosage of low molecular weight heparins may be given at once or as half daily dose twice daily for treatment of DVT. Two studies are currently available, aiming to demonstrate the equivalence of once versus twice daily low molecular weight heparin for treatment of DVT in comparison to continuous intravenous aPTT-adjusted heparin. The 2 studies included more than 1,200 patients and recurrent venous thromboembolism and major bleeding and mortality were not different, when LMW heparin was given once or

Table 2. Analysis of the risk reduction of low molecular weight heparin or heparin on the incidence of mortality 3–6 months after treatment for recent DVT with various low molecular weight heparins. No significant differences can be verified so far for the different low molecular weight heparins

Compound		LMWH/	UFH	RR	p
Nadroparin	n	20/361	32/355	40	0.07
	%	5.5	9	– 5 to 66	
Tinzaparin	n	6/213	15/219	59	0.07
	%	2.8	6.8	– 1 to 83	
Enoxaparin	n	13/314	20/320	35	0.23
	%	4.1	6.2	– 8 to 35	
Dalteparin	n	16/322	8/339	– 110	0.07
	%	5.0	2.4	nd	

Table 3. Comparison of the treatment of recent DVT using 1 daily subcutaneous injection of full dose low molecular weight heparin versus twice daily subcutaneous injection using half the daily dose. One study has compared these regimes with aPTT-controlled intravenous heparin. The incidences of recurrent venous thromboembolism (VTE), major bleeding complications, and mortality are given

Dosage	Ref.		Once	Twice 1/2	Heparin
LMWH 1	(23)	n =	316	335	–
LMWH 2	(24)	n =	300	300	300
All		616	635	300	
Rec. VTE		(%)	3.4	4.6	4.3
Major bleed		(%)	2.3	3.0	5.0
Mortality		(%)	2.6	3.6	3.0

twice daily (Table 3) [4, 23]. As seen so far, slight advantages of the once daily adminis-tration cannot lead to a positive conclusion. However, the data demonstrate the equal efficacy and safety of the once daily high dose LMW heparin administration in comparison to twice dosing for treatment of DVT.

A German consensus of the Gesellschaft für Thrombose und Hämostaseforschung concluded that subcutaneous shigh dose low molecular weight heparin is as effective and safe as continuous intravenous aPTT-adjusted heparin for treatment of recent DVT. However, data are not sufficient to support treatment of DVT on outpatient basis or to reduce the hospital stay using LMW heparins [7, 8].

LMW heparin in acute ischaemic stroke

In patients with acute ischaemic stroke high dose intravenous aPTT-adjusted heparin is one of the main treatment regimes. However, bleeding complications or secondary cerebral hemorrhage in the ischaemic area are the main complications and limitations of this treatment. A dose finding study of low molecular weight heparin has demonstrated the efficacy and safety of increasing doses in the treatment of acute ischaemic stroke on top of 100 mg acetyl salicylicacid o.d. Increasing dosage of LMW heparin up to 4,000 IU twice daily subcutaneously, the disability over 3 months and the incidence of death was lower as compared to lower daily dose of low molecular weight heparin and compared to placebo. Surprisingly, the cerebral hemorrhagic complications significantly decreased with increasing doses of low molecular weight heparin (11). Several studies are currently undertaken to substantiate these findings and to finalize dose finding studies.

LMW-heparin in unstable angina

The administration of unfractionated heparin during unstable angina has several limitations. Low molecular weight heparins are currently investigated in this indication. The ESSENCE study, the TIMI 11a study, the FRISC and the FRIC study demonstrate the reduction of combined endpoints, i.e. incidence of myocardial infarction, incidence of death, incidence of aortacoronary bypass operation, and incidence of ischaemic episodes are reduced up to 4 weeks, if low molecular weight heparins are given twice daily in high dosages in the acute phase of unstable angina. Various studies are actually undertaken to validate the long-term effect of low molecular weight heparins in patients with unstable angina.

Conclusion

The improved biological properties of low molecular weight heparins lead to a higher safety with special regard to a lower incidence of heparin-induced thrombocytopenia type II. Proven indications of low molecular weight heparins are the various postoperative situations. New clinical indications which have not yet approved in many countries by the local authorities are prolonged prophylaxis in outpatients with immobilizing plaster casts, after elective hip replacement, and in medically bedridden inpatients. New indications for low molecular weight heparins, which are currently being investigated, are prophylaxis of recurrent thromboembolism, treatment of recent thromboembolism, acute ischaemic stroke, and unstable angina.

References

1. Bergmann JF, Neuhart E (1996) A multicentric randomized double-blind study of enoxaparin compared with unfractionated heparin in the prevention of venous thromboembolism disease in elderly in-patients bedridden for an acute medical illness. Thromb Haemostas 76: 529–534
2. Bergqvist D, Benoni G, Björgell O, Fredin H, Hedlundi U, Nicolas S, Nilsson P, Nylander G (1996) Low-molecular-weight heparin (Enoxaparin) as prophylaxis against venous thromboembolism after total hip replacement. N Engl J Med 335: 696–700
3. Dahl OE, Andreasson G, Aspelin T, Müller C, Mathiesen P, Nyhus S, Abdelnoor M, Solhaug JH, Arnesen H (1997) Prolonged thromboprophylaxis following hip replacement surgery – Results of a double-blind, prospective, randomised, placebo-controlled study with Dalteparin (Fragmin®). Thromb Haemostas 77: 26–31
4. Fiessinger JN, Charbonnier BA, Sixma JJ, Wenzel E (1997) Comparison of once daily with a twice daily subcutaneous nadroparin calcium regimen in the treatment of deep vein thrombosis. The FRAXODY study. Thromb Haemost suppl: 1582, Abstr
5. Harenberg J, Huhle G, Piazolo L, Giese CH, Heene DL (1997) Long-term anticoagulation of outpatients with adverse events to oral anticoagulants using low-molecular-weight heparin. Semin Thromb Hemost 23: 167–172
6. Harenberg J, Roebruck P, Heene DL on behalf of the Heparin Study in Internal Medicine Group (1996) Subcutaneous low-molecular-weight heparin versus standard heparin and the prevention of thromboembolism in medical inpatients. Haemostasis 26: 127–139
7. Harenberg J, Schmitz-Huebner U (1997) Therapie der Beinvenenthrombose mit niedermolekularen Heparinen. Dtsch Ärztebl 94: 2257–2260
8. Harenberg J, Schmitz-Huebner U, Breddin K, Haas S, Heinrich F, Heinrichs CH, Kienast J, Roebruck P, Theiss W, Wenzel E (1997) Treatment of deep vein thrombosis with low-molecularweight heparins: A consensus statement of the Gesellschaft für Thrombose- und Hämostaseforschung (GTH). Semin Thromb Hemost 23: 91–96
9. Harenberg J, Siegele M, Dempfle CE, Stehle G, Heene DL (1993) Protamine neutralization of the release of tissue factor pathway inhibitor activity by heparins. Thromb Haemostas 70: 942–943
10. Harenberg J, Stehle G, Augustin J, Zimmermann R (1989) Comparative human pharmacology of low molecular weight heparins. Semin Thromb Hemost 15: 414–423
11. Kay R, Wons SW, Yu YL, Chan YW, Tsoi TH, Ahuja AT, Chan FL, Fong KY, Law CB, Wong A, Woo J (1995) Low-molecular-weight heparin for the treatment of acute ischaemic stroke. N Engl J Med 333: 1588–1593
12. Kock HJ, Schmit-Neuerburg KP, Hanke J, Rudofsky G, Hirche H (1995) Thromboprophylaxis with low-molecular-weight heparin in outpatients with plaster-cast immobilization of the leg. Lancet 346: 459–461
13. Koopman MMW, Prandoni P, Piovella F, Ockfort PA, Brandjes DP, Van der Meer J, Gallus AS, Simonneau G, Chesterman CH, Prins MH et al. (1996) Treatment of patients with proximalvein thrombosis with intravenous unfractionated heparin in hospital compared with subcutaneous low-molecular-weight heparin out of hospital or with early discharge. N Engl J Med 334: 682–687

14. Kujath P, Spannagel U, Habscheid W, Schindler G, Weckbach A (1992) Thrombosis prevention in outpatients with lower limb injuries. Dtsch Med Wochenschr 117: 6–10
15. Lechler E, Schramm W, Flosbach CW (1996) The venous thrombotic profile of a low-molecular-weight heparin (enoxaparin). The Prime Study Group. Haemostasis 26 (suppl. 2): 49–56
16. Levine M, Gent M, Hirsh J, Leclerc J, Anderson D, Weitz J, Ginsberg JS, Turpie AG, Demers C, Kovacs M (1996) A comparison of low-molecular-weight heparin administered primarily at home with unfractionated heparin administered in the hospital for proximal deepvein-thrombosis. N Engl J Med 334: 677–681
17. Monreal M, Lafoz E, Olive S, del Rio L, Vedia C (1994) Comparison of subcutaneous unfractionated heparin with a low molecular weight heparin (Fragmin) in patients with venous thromboembolism and contra-indications to coumarin. Thromb Haemostas 71: 7–11
18. Nurmohamed MT, Rosendaal FR, Büller HR, Dekker E, Hommes DW, Vanderbroucke JP, Briet L (1992) Low molecular weight heparin versus standard heparin in general and orthopaedic surgery: a meta-analysis. Lancet 340: 152–156
19. Pini M, Manotti C, Pattacini C, Quintavalla R, Poli T, Tagliaferri A, Dettori AG (1994) Low molecular weight heparin versus warfarin in the prevention of recurrences after deep vein thrombosis. Thromb Haemostas 72: 191–197
20. Planes A, Vochelle N, Darmon Y, Fagola M, Bellaud M, Huet Y (1996) Risk of deep-venous thrombosis after hospital discharge in patients having undergone total hip replacement: Double-blind randomised comparison of enoxaparin versus placebo. Lancet 348: 224–228.
21. Racanelli A, Fareed J (1992) Ex vivo activity of heparin is not predictive of blood loss after neutralization by protamine. Thromb Res 67: 263–273
22. Reilmann H, Weinberg AM, Forster EE, Happe B (1993) Thromboseprophylaxe bei ambulanten Patienten. Orthopäde 22: 117–120
23. Spiro TE (1997) A multicenter clinical trial comparing once and twice-daily subcutaneous enoxaparin and intravenous heparin in the treatment of acute deep vein thrombosis. Thromb Haemost 1997; suppl: 1527, Abstr.
24. Charbonnier BA, Fiessinger JN, Banga JD, Wenzel E, d'Azemar P, Sagnard L. Thromb Haemost (1998) Comparison of a once daily with a twice daily subcutaneous how molecular weight heparin regimen in the treatment of deep vein therombosis 79: 897–901
25. Warkentin TH, Levine MN, Hirsh J, Horsewood P, Roberts RS, Gent M, Kelton JG (1995) Heparin-induced thrombocytopenia in patients treated with low molecular weight heparin or unfractionated heparin. N Engl J Med 332: 1330–1335
26. Zagrodnick J, Kaufner HK (1990) Ambulante Thromboembolie-prophylaxe in der Traumatologie durch Selbstinjektion von Heparin. Unfallchirurg 93: 331–333.

J. Harenberg (✉)
Professor of Medicine
I. Dept. of Medicine
Faculty of Clinical Medicine Mannheim, University of Heidelberg
Theodor-Kutzer-Ufer
68167 Mannheim, Germany

Heparin-induced thrombocytopenia

N. A. Cicco, G. Gerken, M. Frey, H. Just

Summary Heparin-induced thrombocytopenia (HIT), next to bleeding complications, is the most important side-effect of heparin therapy in cardiac patients and the most frequently found thrombocytopenia induced by medication. Two types of HIT are distinguished on the basis of both severity of disease, and pathophysiology: type I HIT is an early, transient, clinically harmless form of thrombocytopenia, due to direct heparin-induced platelet aggregation. Thromboembolic complications are usually not seen. No treatment is required. A normalization of platelet count even if heparin is continued is a usual observation. Type II HIT is more severe than type I HIT and is frequently complicated by extension of preexisting venous thromboembolism or new arterial thrombosis. The thrombocytopenia is caused by a pathogenic heparin-dependent IgG antibody (HIT-IgG) that recognizes as its target antigen a complex consisting of heparin and platelet factor IV. Type II HIT should be suspected when the platelet count falls to less than 100,000 per cubic millimeter or less than 50 % of the base line value 5 to 15 days after heparin therapy is begun, or sooner in a patient who received heparin in the recent past. The clinical diagnosis of type II HIT can be confirmed by several sensitive assays. In cases of type II HIT, heparin must be stopped immediately. However, if the patient requires continued anticoagulant therapy for an acute event such as deep venous thrombosis, substitution of an alternative rapid-acting anticoagulant drug is often needed. In the authors experience Danaparoid sodium, a low-sulfated heparinoid with a low cross-reactivity (10 %) to heparin, can be regarded as an effective anticoagulant in patients with type II HIT. Preliminary experiences with intravenous recombinant hirudin are also encouraging and suggest that this direct thrombin inhibitor will emerge as a valuable alternative treatment for patients who suffer from HIT.

Key words Thrombocytopenia – heparin – thromboembolism – anticoagulants – hirudin

Introduction

Hematological abnormalities are frequent complications of drugs used to treat cardiac disorders. Anemias may be of the aplastic or immunohemolytic type. A reduction in circulating neuthrophils as well as thrombocytopenia may be secondary to depression of the marrow, or due to immune mechanisms causing peripheral cellular destruction. For example, thiazide diuretics directly suppress megakaryocyte production [41], whereas thrombocytopenia caused by amrinone is related to peripheral destruction of platelets [3]. Although many other drugs have been reported to cause thrombocytopenia (Table 1), this review will focus on heparin-induced thrombocytopenia (HIT) because of the following reasons: (1) heparin is a mainstay in the prevention and treatment of thromboembolic disorders of the venous and arterial circulatory systems and is the anticoagulant of choice for extracorporeal procedures; (2) HIT, next to bleeding complications, is the most important side-effect of heparin therapy in cardiac patients, (3) the most frequently found thrombocytopenia induced by medication, and (4) an allergic drug reaction with

Table 1. Cardiac medications inducing thrombocytopenia

antihypertensives	captopril
	hydralazine
anticogulants	heparin
diuretics	thiazides
antiarrhythmics	digitoxin
	phenytoin
	procainamide
	quinidine
phosphodiesterase	inhibitors
	amrinone

a unique clinical profile: thrombocytopenia plus associated thrombotic events. That a patient's risk for thrombosis increases despite a decrease in circulating platelets and while treated with heparin is one of the most intriguing paradoxes in clinical medicine [36]. Recently, there have been important advances in our knowledge of the pathophysiology, clinical features, diagnosis, and treatment of this serious adverse effect.

Definition

HIT is commonly described as two syndromes (Table 2), although the clinical distinction is often unclear [15, 51]. The first, sometimes designated Type I, occurs during the first few days of heparin treatment with platelet counts seldom less than 100×10^9/liter, is transient, and may resolve even with continuation of heparin. The patients usually remain asymptomatic [51].

In contrast, most clinical studies of HIT define the second form of HIT (Type II) that typically occurs several days after institution of heparin, but sooner in patients recently exposed to the anticoagulant [38], and has more severe implications, according to the following criteria: (1) a decrease in platelet counts to values below 150×10^9/L (or 100×10^9/L) in patients who originally had normal platelet counts (or a greater than 50 % decrease from the admission value); (2) exclusion of other causes of thrombocytopenia (liver failure, sepsis, disseminated intravascular coagulation, aplastic anemia); (3) the presence of thrombotic complications; (4) normalization of platelet counts within several days of discontinuation of heparin.

Table 2. Definitions

	HIT Type I	HIT Type II
onset	soon after starting heparin	5 to 14 days after starting heparin
platelet count	seldom $< 100 \times 10^9$/L	$< 100 \times 10^9$/L or > 50 % decrease
complications	none	thromboembolic events
incidence	approximately 10 %	0.5 – 5 %

History and incidence

Thrombocytopenia was first reported as a transient side effect of heparin therapy in normal individuals more than three decades ago [26]. A possible association of heparin therapy and arterial embolism was first suggested in 1958 by Weismann and Robin [75]. In 1964, Roberts et al. [57] reported 11 cases of peripheral arterial emboli occurring in patients being treated with heparin. These investigators were the first to suggest an immunological etiology. Between 1969 and 1974 severe heparin-associated thrombocytopenia was recognized in five patients, some with evidence of thrombosis [56] or disseminated intravascular coagulation [40]. In 1973, Rhodes et al. [56] were able to identify a heparin-dependent IgG antibody as being responsible for the platelet aggregation. In the first prospective study in 1974 to 1975, thrombocytopenia was documented in 16 of 52 treated patients [8, 9]. This remarkable observation stimulated more prospective clinical studies evaluating HIT in patients receiving heparin with a reported incidence ranging from 0 % to 30 % [14–61]. This wide variation may be attributed to several factors: (1) type of heparin used: heparin isolated from beef lung appeared to cause thrombocytopenia more often than heparin from pork intestinal mucosa in some studies, reaching statistical significance in two [7–55]. A recent overview of pooled data from the literature estimated an incidence of 1.1 % for porcine and 2.9 % for bovine heparin [61]. (2) Route of administration: the frequency of thrombocytopenia among patients treated with prophylactic subcutaneous heparin is very low [18]. Thrombocytopenia more commonly occurs in patients receiving high doses of heparin for treatment of thromboembolism [46], although HIT has also been reported in patients receiving heparin flushes of indwelling intravenous catheters in doses as low as 100 U/day [23] and in patients with heparin-coated pulmonary artery catheters [43]. (3) Heparin preparation: the risk of developing thrombocytopenia is likely to be higher in patients treated with standard unfractionated heparin than in those receiving low molecular weight heparins [70]. The definition of thrombocytopenia, the patient populations studied and the varying quality of the studies might also have contributed to the variability among different studies. According to recent reviews [71], the overall frequency of HIT is 5 %. Severe thrombocytopenia, with platelet counts of less than 50×10^9/liter, occurred in 1% of these patients. Arterial and venous thrombosis, with potentially severe and fatal complications, have been estimated to occur in as many as 20 % of patients with HIT although accurate determination of the incidence is quite difficult and may vary with the population being studied. Many prospective studies suggest that thrombotic events during heparin administration are relatively uncommon; however, they include patients with early thrombocytopenia (i.e., within 4 days of heparin use), even though these do not represent patients with (immune) heparin-induced thrombocytopenia. Thus, the frequency of HIT could have been overestimated, and the associated risk of thrombosis underestimated. Furthermore sudden thrombotic events such as myocardial infarction, peripheral arterial thrombosis, stroke, and pulmonary emboli are often not initially recognized as a complication of heparin because of the patient's underlying illness.

Pathophysiology

Our understanding of the pathogenesis of HIT has increased considerably in recent years. Current evidence suggests that Type I HIT results from the direct proaggregating action of heparin on platelets [11, 17, 28, 59], leading to increased platelet sequestration in the

Table 3. Possible explanation for high risk of thrombosis in heparin-induced thrombocytopenia

- platelet activation by HIT-IgG
- endothelial cell activation by HIT-IgG
- induction of procoagulant platelet-derived microparticles by HIT-IgG
- formation of antibodies to the heparin domaine that bind to ATIII
- heparin neutralization by platelet factor IV released from activated platelets
- increased platelet Fc-receptors
- underlying risk for thrombosis

spleen or increased clearance of aggregated platelets by the reticuloendothelial system. The immunologic type of HIT (type II) is defined by the presence of pathogenic heparin-dependent antibodies that are specific not for heparin but for complexes formed between heparin and platelet factor IV, a basic heparin-binding protein normally present in platelet alpha granules that is secreted in response to activating stimuli. A multimolecular complex between HIT-IgG and heparin/platelet factor IV is formed on the surface of circulating platelets. The Fc portions of the IgG antibodies interact with the platelet Fc receptors [37], leading to platelet activation and subsequent release of additional platelet factor IV. Newly released platelet factor IV binds to free heparin, and the antibody forms more immune complexes, establishing a cycle of platelet activation and leading to increased removal of activated platelets/platelet microaggregates from the circulation. Platelet Fc receptors may play a key role in regulating the degree of thrombocytopenia in these patients. Platelets from different individuals vary significantly in the number of Fc receptors carried on their surfaces [39, 58, 67], and their expression can be increased after activation of platelets with an agonist such as thrombin. Even more intriguing, however, is the finding that patients with acute inflammatory illnesses also have a three- to five-fold increased platelet Fc receptor expression, which may place them at greater risk for HIT. Moreover IL-6, a cytokine that mediates the acute-phase response, stimulates the production of larger platelets [12] that are more responsive to agonists [53]. Thus, platelets may be more vulnerable to interactions with heparin antibody complexes in the presence of acute inflammatory illness.

Although the induction of strong platelet activation by HIT-IgG is likely to be a major cause of thromboembolic complications, there are other factors that could explain the association with thrombosis (Table 3). In particular, the pathogenic antibodies, which can be either IgG or IgM, are also capable of activating endothelial cells [20, 68]. This is because endothelium is coated with heparin-like molecules (glycosaminoglycans) that like heparin can bind platelet factor IV (released in excess of the amount that can be neutralized by available heparin) to form complexes for which antibodies are specific. Such a binding to the endothelial cells may cause a generalized endothelial cell lesion with release of ristocetin-cofactor, tissue plasminogen activator, and tissue factor, resulting in an hypercoagulable state. Another potential etiology for thrombosis could be formation of antibodies to the heparin domain that binds to AT III, therefore reducing the AT III activity [63]. Evidence is also presented to indicate that antibodies associated with HIT induce the formation of platelet-derived microparticles having procoagulant activity.

Other factors such as local atherosclerosis, vascular injury from surgical procedures, venous stasis, and the aforementioned increased platelet Fc receptors may determine whether thrombosis will occur and the site of thrombosis.

Clinical syndromes

Two clinically distinct types of HIT have been described: in *type I HIT* the thrombo-cytopenia is mild with platelet counts not less than 50×10^9/liter, may begin soon after heparin is initiated, and may return to normal levels even while heparin is continued. The patients usually remain asymptomatic [51].

In contrast, the hallmark of *HIT type II* is a fall in the platelet count that begins five to eight days after institution of heparin, but sooner in patients previously exposed to the anticoagulant [26, 75] (especially, within the past month). Usually, the platelet count falls to below 100×10^9/liter, and the thrombocytopenia will not recover unless heparin is discontinued. After heparin withdrawal the platelet count rises to normal levels usually in 5–7 days. Occasionally, the platelet count may be normal, having dropped from a higher level [54]. Typically, patients have moderate thrombocytopenia (median nadir in the literature, approximately 50×10^9/liter) [72], which itself rarely provokes bleeding. However, the patients are threatened by the *thromboembolic complications* associated with HIT [17], usually distinct from the thrombosis for which heparin was initially given (Table 4).

They may present as arterial thrombosis which may cause ischemic injury to the legs or arms, stroke, acute myocardial infarction, and end-organ dysfunction, e.g., renal failure [10, 24, 64]. Venous thrombotic events, especially proximal deep vein thrombosis, are frequently extensive and complicated by recurrent pulmonary embolism [16, 47]. Some-times, arterial obstructions develop mainly in the microcirculation, leading to digital gangrene, transient global amnesia [73], respiratory distress syndrome [4], and skin necrosis [25]. Other unusual complications associated with type II HIT include multiple hepatic infarctions and hemorrhagic necrosis of the adrenal gland, i.e., adrenal infarction

Table 4. Clinical syndromes

⊕ arterial thrombosis	lower limb arteries cerebral arteries coronary arteries renal arteries
⊕ venous thrombotic events	proximal deep vein thrombosis pulmonary embolism
⊕ adrenal hemorrhagic infarction	
⊕ involvement of the microcirculation	digital gangrene transient global amnesia ARDS
⊕ disseminated intravascular coagulation	

Table 5. Laboratory techniques

⊕ functional assays (platelet activation) C^{14}-serotonin release platelet aggregation platelet derived microparticles (flow cytometry)
⊕ antigen assay enzyme-linked immunosorbent assay (ELISA)

caused by adrenal vein thrombosis, followed by hemorrhage into the gland. Thrombosis frequently occurs at multiple sites [10], and arterial and venous thrombosis may be present together [47]. Some patients present with disseminated intravascular coagulation [9] and others will have thrombosis in the absence of thrombocytopenia. This may be due to the rapid onset of the thrombotic manifestation or to increased platelet production. Clinical conditions that increase the risk of thrombosis in patients with HIT are sepsis, recent cardiovascular surgery, and atherosclerotic vascular disease.

Common denominators for these patients are high levels of circulating cytokines such as IL-6, pre-existing endothelial damage due to invasive procedures, and activated platelets; all of which promote arterial and venous thromboembolism in the presence of heparin immune complexes.

Resistance to the anticoagulant effect of heparin is sometimes observed in patients who develop HIT with or without thrombosis, but this is a non-specific finding also described in patients who do not have HIT.

Diagnosis

Thromboembolic vessel occlusions associated with HIT can produce severe morbidity and mortality with an estimated mortality rate of about 30 % in patients with HIT and thrombosis and a 20 % risk of leg amputation. Thus, every effort should be made to ensure prompt diagnosis. In clinical practice HIT should be suspected and tests should be done immediately on any patient receiving any form of heparin who becomes thrombocytopenic or develops an unexplained significant decrease in platelet counts (i.e., > 40 %) even though levels remain above 150×10^9/liter. Moreover, if heparinized patients show increasing requirements of heparin to maintain adequate anticoagulation, or develop any new or recurrent thromboembolic event despite heparin therapy, HIT should be considered and a platelet count must be performed. An apparent thrombocytopenia due to platelet clumping in vitro can be excluded by examination of the peripheral smear. After the thrombocytopenia is confirmed, the diagnosis of HIT should be made on the basis of platelet counts less than 100×10^9/liter on 2 consecutive days [6] in the absence of any other potential etiology for the thrombocytopenia.

If laboratory assays for heparin-dependent antibodies are available, they may provide supportive information. Two diagnostic approaches have been described for the detection of heparin-dependent platelet antibodies: (1) functional assays, and (2) antigen assays (Table 5). In the former, patient serum plus heparin are incubated with platelets from healthy donors and an aggregation or secretion response of the platelets is measured. A test widely used for the laboratory diagnosis of HIT is the platelet aggregation test, which measures HIT serum-induced platelet aggregation in the presence of a therapeutic concentration of heparin. This assay is technically simple and can be

Table 6. r-Hirudin

- potent, direct and specific inhibitor of the enzymatically active site of thrombin
- not dependent on cofactors
- neutralizes both free and clot-bound thrombin
- no known interaction with endothelium
- no major allergic reactions
- more uniform anticoagulation effect than heparin
- dose adjustment necessary in patients with compromised renal function

performed quickly. However, the amount of platelet aggregation may vary among different healthy donors [19, 74], and some platelets from normal donors appear completely unresponsive [19, 35]. Another well-characterized assay is the two-point ^{14}C-serotonin release assay described by Sheridan et al. [62], which measures the release of radioactive serotonin from washed platelets when they are activated by type II HIT serum in the presence of therapeutic heparin concentrations (0.1 U/ml). Recently, developed modifications of this assay that avoid the requirement for radioactive tracers have been described [30, 45]. However, platelet aggregation and platelet release tests seem to be 10-fold less sensitive than antigen assays, based on the detection of heparin-induced antibodies using preformed immobilized heparin/platelet factor IV complexes as the target antigen in an enzymelinked immunosorbent assay (ELISA) [2, 29, 69].

This assay is now commercially available and is routinely performed at our institution. On the other hand a possible disadvantage of this assay is that some patient sera (perhaps 5–10 %) may test falsely negative using this test. This is apparently because antibodies other than those reactive with heparin/platelet factor IV complexes could play a role in the pathogenesis of HIT. For example, heparin-associated antibodies that induce platelet aggregation but fail to react in HIT-ELISA have been described [29] as well as antibodies that react directly with heparin [1]. For these reasons the initial diagnosis of HIT should be made on a clinical basis. Although assays for heparin-dependent antibodies are not necessary for the initial management of thrombocytopenic patients, they are useful to confirm a clinical diagnosis of HIT retrospectively, to determine if re-exposure to heparin can occur during a surgical procedure, or to identify antibodies that are crossreactive with low molecular weight heparin or heparinoid.

Prevention

Frequent performance of platelet counts in patients on heparin is the most important preventive measure. The incidence of type II HIT may be decreased by using shorter courses of heparin therapy with concomitant initiation of a vitamin K antagonist [34] and the increasing use of low molecular weight heparin [33]. These compounds consist of heparin fragments that react with Antithrombin III (AT III) to inhibit activated Factor X (Factor Xa), but not Thrombin (Factor IIa).

Low molecular weight heparin is less capable than unfractionated heparin of activating resting platelets [5], and it binds less well to platelet factor IV [42]. Thus, it might be expected that low molecular weight heparin would be less likely to cause HIT than standard heparin. Actually, a recent study by Warkentin et al. [70] suggests that patients receiving prophylactic low molecular weight heparin after HIP surgery had a lower incidence of thrombocytopenia, thrombosis, and antibody formation than those receiving unfractionated heparin. However, in spite of this suggestive evidence low molecular weight heparins may have some cross-reactivity with heparin-dependent antibodies and are capable of causing HIT as well [44].

Therapy

In patients with type I HIT no specific treatment is required. A normalization of platelet count even if heparin is continued is a usual observation. However, differentiation from early type II HIT can be difficult. The decision to continue or to stop heparin should take into consideration the risk of extension or recurrence of the underlying thrombotic disease compared to the thrombocytopenia, as well as the knowledge that in most patients the thrombocytopenia will be mild and self-limited. On the other hand, thrombotic complications cannot be predicted in a given patient, and serious morbidity, often resulting in death, has been reported in 50 % of patients with HIT who develop thrombosis.

Thus, if there is any doubt and especially if the platelet count is less than 50×10^9/liter in the absence of any other potential etiology, our policy is to withdraw heparin immediately. However, if the patient requires continued anticoagulant therapy for an acute event such as deep venous thrombosis, substitution of an alternative rapid-acting anticoagulant drug is often needed.

Although low molecular weight heparins (LMW Hep) have been shown to cause HIT less readily than standard heparin, once a patient has developed HIT, the use of LMW Hep is associated with a high risk of persisting or recurring thrombocytopenia, progression of thrombotic complications, and even death. In fact, once a patient who takes standard heparin becomes sensitized, the heparindependent antibodies formed nearly always cross-react with LMW Hep causing platelet aggregation [31]. Therefore, LMW Hep cannot be recommended to treat HIT. In our opinion, one of the more viable alternatives at this time for the management of HIT is *Danaparoid sodium* (formerly, *Organ* 10172). This LMW heparinoid compound is a mixture of antithrombotic glycosaminoglycans, particularly low-sulfated heparan sulphate, dermatan sulphate, and chondroitin sulphate. Organ inhibits activated Factor X (Xa), thereby leading to reduced thrombin generation. Although small amounts of heparinlike substances (high-sulfated glycosaminoglycans), potentially cross-reactive with preformed heparin-dependent antibodies are present within Organ, the risk for in vivo cross-reactivity appears to be low (< 5 %) [48].

Although not completely safe, experiences with this drug in Europe, the USA, and Australia have shown encouraging results in the treatment of thrombotic events in patients with HIT [48, 52]. In our own small group of type II HIT patients (12 cases over 1 year treated with Organ) we could reproduce the favorable outcome reported in larger studies, even in patients with massive pulmonary embolism and extensive deep vein thrombosis. Bleeding complications were not observed. Thus, LMW heparinoids can be a valuable alternative treatment for patients who suffer from HIT and who require anticoagulation although the low cross-reactivity rate (5–10 %) with heparin-induced antibodies suggests that problems remain.

An ideal alternative to heparin would be a thrombinspecific inhibitor such as hirudin or its analogue hirulog. Hirudin is a 65 amino acid protein with a molecular weight of about 7000, derived from the leech Hirudo medicinalis that acts as a potent and selective inhibitor of thrombin (Table 6). Hirudin is currently synthesized using recombinant DNA technology (r-hirudin). Hirudin complexes with both the substrate recognition and catalytic sites of the thrombin molecule rendering it incapable of enzymatic activity. Since the fibrin binding site of the thrombin molecule is not involved in this reaction, both free and clot-bound thrombin are equally well inhibited by hirudin. Because of the specificity of the carboxy terminus binding to thrombin, hirudin does not inhibit other enzymes in the coagulation or fibrinolytic pathways.

The binding of hirudin to thrombin is not covalent. However, the dissociation rate is extremely slow, making hirudin an essentially irreversible inhibitor of thrombin. Circulating free hirudin is cleared by renal elimination and, thus, bears the risk of cumulation in patients with impaired renal function. Nonetheless, in view of its properties potential advantages of hirudin in the treatment of HIT could be the following: (1) no risk of cross-reactivity with HIT-IgG, (2) no inhibition by activated platelets, and (3) convenient therapy monitoring using Ecarin Clotting Time (ECT). Although these new synthetic thrombin inhibitors are not yet widely available, preliminary reports in a small number of patients suggest that hirudin and hirulog are effective and predictable anticoagulants for patients suffering from HIT and are free from adverse effects [13, 60].

Another option in the treatment of HIT include the administration of Ancrod; this defibrinogenating snake venom has been successfully used [22] in Canada and is available under compassionate use in the U.S. However, Ancrod does not inhibit thrombin generation and, therefore, is not a satisfactory alternative in the acute setting of HIT and thrombosis. Besides the use of alternative anticoagulants in patients with HIT and severe, life-threatening thromboembolic complications (e.g., massive pulmonary embolism with haemodynamic instability), thrombolytic agents have been successfully [21, 49] without significant bleeding complications, despite the presence of severe thrombocytopenia.

Surgical interventions may also be indicated, including placement of an inferior vena cava filter to prevent recurrent pulmonary emboli and embolectomy in patients with arterial thrombosis. Patients with HIT undergoing cardiac operations pose particularly difficult problems. For patients undergoing elective surgery, a possible option is to wait for the disappearance of the HIT-IgG. Alternatively, the antibody could be removed by plasmapheresis [50,66]. In patients who urgently need cardiac surgery, the best approach in our opinion is to use the LMW glycosaminoglycan Orgaran instead of heparin, provided the heparin-dependent antibody does not cross-react with the drug. Although the overall experience is limited, evidence could be presented that Orgaran might be a useful alternative for anticoagulation during extracorporeal circulation [48, 76]. Another option is the use of heparin for anticoagulation during surgery along with a prostacyclin-like drug (Iloprost) or aspirin to suppress the heparin-dependant antibody-induced platelet aggregation. Ancrod has also been used successfully in one patient in the setting of cardiac surgery [65]. Since HIT may develop from use of heparin during hemodialysis or acute renal failure may complicate HIT it is mandatory to find an adequate substitute for heparin for anticoagulation in these patients. In a clinical study of 45 patients receiving Orgaran for this purpose, the outcome was favorable [48], as well as in our small group of intensive care patients requiring continuous veno-venous hemofiltration.

Finally, therapy of severe thrombocytopenia may include administration of iv Immunoglobulin [27] or the use of plasmapheresis [50] as mentioned above. We suggest that platelet transfusions should be used with caution to treat patients with HIT. Although there are no reports of adverse events to platelet transfusions so far, their use in the presence of an antibody that may aggregate platelets could theoretically result in thrombosis, as has been described in thrombotic thrombocytopenic purpura [32].

References

1. Adams JG, Humphrey LJ, Zhang XC (1995) Do patients with heparin-induced thrombocytopenia syndrome have heparin specific antibodies? J Vasc Surg 21: 247–254
2. Amiral J, Bridey F, Dreyfus M (1992) Platelet factor 4 complexed to heparin is the target for antibodies generated in heparin-induced thrombocytopenia (letter) Thromb Haemost 68: 95–96
3. Ansell J, McCue J, Tiarks C (1981) Amrinone-induced thrombocytopenia. Blood 58 (Suppl 1): 187a
4. Asimacopoulos PJ, Athanasiadis I, McCathy JJ et al. (1994) Can heparin cause adult respiratory distress syndrome by a similar mechanism as heparin associated thrombocytopenia? Chest 105: 1266–1268
5. Barradas MA, Mikhailidis DP, Epemolu O et al. (1987) Comparison of the platelet pro-aggregatory effect of conventional unfractionated heparins and a low molecular weight heparin fraction (CY222). Br J Hematol 67: 451–7
6. Bell WR (1988) Heparin-associated thrombocytopenia and thrombosis. J Lab Clin Med 111: 600

7. Bell WR, Royall RM (1980) Heparin-associated thrombocytopenia: a comparison of three heparin preparations. N Engl J Med 303: 902–907
8. Bell WR (1976) Thrombocytopenia occuring during heparin therapy. N Engl J Med 295: 276
9. Bell WR, Tomasulo PA, Alving BA (1976) Thrombocytopenia occuring during the administration of heparin. A prospective study of 52 patients. Ann Intern Med 85: 155
10. Blanke H, Lesch M, Strauer BE (1987) Heparin-induced thrombopenia. D Med Wochen 12: 96–99
11. Brace LD, Freed J (1985) An objective assessment of the interaction of heparin and its fractions with human platelets. Semin Thromb Haemost 11: 190–198
12. Burstein SA, Downs T, Friese P et al. (1992) Thrombocytopoiesis in normal and sublethally irradiated dogs: Response to human interleukin-6. Blood 80: 420
13. Chamberlin JR, Lewis B, Leya F et al. (1995) Successful treatment of heparin-associated thrombocytopenia and thrombosis using Hirulog. Can J Card 11 (6): 511–4
14. Chong BH Heparin-induced thrombocytopenia. (1988) Blood Reviews 108–114
15. Chong BH, Pitney WR, Castaldi PA (1982) Heparin-induced thrombocytopenia: Association of thrombotic compliations with heparin-dependent IgG antibody that induces thromboxane synthesis and platelet aggregation. Lancet 2: 1246
16. Chong BH, Ismail F, Cade J et al. (1989) Heparin-induced thrombocytopenia: studies with a new low molecular weight heparinoid, Org 10172. Blood 73: 1592–1596
17. Chong BH (1995) Annotation: Heparin-induced thrombocytopenia. Br J Haematol 89: 431–439
18. Chong BH (1992) Heparin-induced thrombocytopenia. Austr N Zeal Journ Med 22: 145–152
19. Chong BH, Burgess J, Ismail F (1993) The clinical usefulness of the platelet aggregation test for the diagnosis of heparin-induced thrombocytopenia. Thromb Haemost 69: 344
20. Cines DB, Tomaski A, Tannenbaum S (1987) Immune endothelial-cell injury in heparin-associated thrombocytopenia. N Engl J Med 316: 581–589
21. Clifton GD, Smith MD (1986) Thrombolytic therapy in heparin-associated thrombocytopenia with thrombosis. Clin Pharm 5: 597–601
22. Demers C, Ginsberg JS, Brill-Edwards P et al. (1991) Rapid anticoagulation using Ancrod for heparin-induced thrombocytopenia. Blood 78: 2194–97
23. Doty JR, Alving BM, McDonnell DE et al. (1986) Heparin-associated thrombocytopenia in the neurosurgical patient. Neurosurg 19: 69
24. Feng WC, Singh AK, Bert AA et al. (1993) Perioperative paraplegia and multiorgan failure from heparin-induced thrombocytopenia. Ann Thor Surg 55: 1555–1557
25. Fowlie J, Stanton PD, Anderson JR (1990) Heparin-associated skin necrosis. Postgrad Med J 66: 573
26. Gollub S, Ulin AW (1962) Heparin-induced thrombocytopenia in man. J Lab Clin Med 59: 430
27. Grau E, Linares M, Olaso MA et al. (1992) Heparin-induced thrombocytopenia: response to intravenous immunoglobulin in vivo and in vitro. Am J Hematol 39: 312
28. Greinacher A (1995) Antigen generation in Heparin-induced thrombocytopenia: The non-immunologic type and the immunologic type are closely linked in their pathogenesis. Semin Thromb Haemost 21: 106–116
29. Greinacher A, Amiral J, Dummel V et al. (1994) Laboratory diagnosis of heparin-associated thrombocytopenia and comparison of platelet aggregation test, heparin-induced platelet activation test, and platelet factor 4/heparin enzyme-linked immunosorbent assay. Transf 34: 381–385
30. Greinacher A, Michels I, Kiefel V et al. (1991) A rapid and sensitive test for diagnosing heparin-associated thrombocytopenia. Thromb Haemost 66: 734–736
31. Greinacher A, Feigl M, Mueller-Eckhardt C (1994) Cross-reactivity studies between sera of patients with heparin-associated thrombocytopenia and a new low-molecular-weight heparin reviparin. Thromb Haemost 72: 644–5
32. Harkness DR, Byrnes JJ, Lian EC (1981) Hazard of platelet transfusion in thrombotic thrombocytopenic purpura. JAMA 246: 1931
33. Hull RD, Raskob GE, Pineo GF et al. (1992) Subcutaneous low-molecularweight heparin compared with continuous intravenous heparin in the treatment of proximal vein thrombosis. N Engl J Med 326: 975
34. Hull RD, Raskob JE, Rosenbloom D et al. (1990) Heparin for 5 days as compared with 10 days in the initial treatment of proximal venous thrombosis. N Engl J Med 322: 1260
35. Isenhart CE, Brandt JT (1993) Platelet aggregation studies for the diagnosis of heparin-induced thrombocytopenia. Am J Clin Pathol 99: 324
36. Kapsch D, Silver D (1995) Heparin-induced thrombocytopenia, thrombosis and haemorrhage. Arch Surg 116: 1423–1429
37. Kelton JG, Sheridan D, Santos A et al. (1988) Heparin-induced thrombocytopenia: Laboratory studies. Blood 72: 925–930
38. King DJ, Kelton JG (1984) Heparin-associated thrombocytopenia. Ann Intern Med 100: 536–540
39. King M, McDermott P, Schreiber AD (1990) Characterization of Fcgamma receptor on human platelets. Cell Immunol 128: 462–479
40. Klein HG, Bell WR (1974) Disseminated intravascular coagulation during heparin therapy. Ann Intern Med 80: 477

41. Kutti J, Weinfeld A (1968) The frequency of thrombocytopenia in patients with heart disease treated with oral diuretics. Acta Med Scand 183: 245

42. Lane DA, Pejler J, Flynn AM et al. (1986) Neutralization of heparin-related saccharides by histidine-rich glykoprotein and platelet factor 4. J Biol Chem 261: 3980-6

43. Laster JL, Nichols WK, Silver D (1989) Thrombocytopenia associated with heparin-coated catheters in patients with heparin-associated antiplatelet antibodies. Arch Intern Med 149: 2285

44. Lecompte T, Luo SK, Stieltjes N et al. (1991) Thrombocytopenia associated with low-molecular-weight heparin. Lancet 338: 1217

45. Lee DH, Warkentin TE, Hayward CPM et al. (1994) The development and evaluation of a novel test for heparin-induced thrombocytopenia (abstract). Blood 84 (Suppl l): 188a

46. Lepine-Martin M, Nichols WL, Heit Ja et al. (1997) Heparin-associated thrombocytopenia: Clinical and laboratory features of 54 patients tested for heparin-dependent platelet aggregation. Submitted for publication.

47. Leroy J, Lerclerc MH, Delahousse B et al. (1985) Treatment of heparin-associated thrombocytopenia and thrombosis with low-molecular-weight heparin (CY216). Sem Thromb and Haemost 11: 326-329

48. Magnani HN (1993) Heparin-induced Thrombocytopenia: An overview of 230 patients treated with Orgaran (Org 10172). Thromb Haemost 70: 554-561

49. Metha DP, Yoder EL, Appel J et al. (1991) Heparin-induced thrombocytopenia and thrombosis: Reversal with streptokinase: A case report and review of literature. Am J Hematol 36: 275-9

50. Nand S, Robinson JA (1988) Plasmapheresis in the management of heparin-associated thrombocytopenia with thrombosis. Am J Hematol 28: 204-6

51. Nelson JC, Lerner RG, Goldstein R et al. (1978) Heparin-induced thrombocytopenia. Arch Intern Med 138: 548

52. Ortel TL, Gockerman JP, Califf RM et al. (1992) Parenteral anticoagulation with the heparinoid Lomoparan (Org 10172) in patients with heparin-induced thrombocytopenia and thrombosis. Thromb Haemost 67: 292-6

53. Peng JP, Friese P, George JN et al. (1993) Alteration of platelet function in dogs mediated by interleukin-6. Blood 82

54. Phelan BK (1983) Heparin-associated thrombosis without thrombocytopenia. Ann Intern Med 99: 637

55. Powers PJ, Kelton JG, Carter CJ (1984) Studies of the frequency of heparin-associated thrombocytopenia. Thromb Research 33: 439

56. Rhodes GR, Dixon RH, Silver D (1973) Heparin-induced thrombocytopenia with thrombosis and hemorrhagic manifestations. Surg Gynecol Obstet 136: 409

57. Roberts B, Rosato FE, Rosato EF (1964) Heparin: A cause of arterial emboli? Surgery 55: 803

58. Rosenfeld SI, Ryan DH, Looney RJ et al. (1987) Human Fegamma receptors: stable inter-donor variations in quantitative expression on platelets correlates with functional responses. J Immunol 138: 2869-2873

59. Salzman EW, Rosenberg RD, Smith MH et al. (1980) Effect of heparin and heparin fractions on platelet aggregation. J Clin Invest 65: 64-73

60. Schiele F, Vuillemenot A, Kramarx P et al. (1995) Use of recombinant hirudin as antithrombotic treatment in patients with heparin-induced thrombocytopenia. Am J Hematol 50 (1): 20-5

61. Schmitt BP, Adelman B (1993) Heparin-associated thrombocytopenia: A critical review and a pooled analysis. Am Journ Med Science 305: 208-215

62. Sheridan D, Carter C, Kelton JG (1986) A diagnostic test for heparin-induced thrombocytopenia. Blood 67: 27-30

63. Shibata S, Harpel PC, Gharavi A et al. (1994) Autoantibodies to heparin from patients with antiphospho-lipid antibody syndrome inhibit formation of antithrombin III-thrombin complexes. Blood 83: 2532-2540

64. Singer RL, Mannion JD, Bauer TL et al. (1993) Complications from heparin-induced thrombocytopenia in patients undergoing cardiopulmonary bypass. Chest 104: 1436-1440

65. Teasdale SJ, Zulys VJ, Mycyk T et al. (1989) Ancrod anticoagulation for cardiopulmonary bypass in heparin-induced thrombocytopenia and thrombosis. Ann Thor Surg 48: 712-3

66. Thorp D, Canty A, Whiting J et al. (1990) Plasma exchange and heparin-induced thrombocytopenia. Prog Clin Biol Res 337: 521-22

67. Tomiyama Y, Kunicki TJ, Zipf TF et al. (1992) Response of human platelets to activating monoclonal antibodies: Importance of FcRII (CD 32) phenotype and level of expression. Blood 80: 2261-2268

68. Visentin GP, Ford SE, Scott JP et al. (1994) Antibodies from patients with heparin-induced thrombo-cytopenia/thrombosis are specific for platelet factor 4 complexed with heparin or bound to endothelial cells. J Clin Invest 93: 81-88

69. Visentin GP, Aster RH (1995) Heparin-induced thrombocytopenia and thrombosis. Curr Opin Hematol 2: 351-357

70. Warkentin TE, Levine MN, Hirsch J (1995) Heparin-induced thrombocytopenia in patients treated with lowmolecular-weight heparin or unfractionated heparin. N Engl J Med 332: 1330

71. Warkentin TE, Kelton JG (1991) Heparin-induced thrombocytopenia. Prog Hemost Thromb 10: 1

72. Warkentin TE, Kelton JG (1997) Interaction of heparin with platelets, including heparin-induced thrombocytopenia, in Bounameaux H (ed) Low-molecularweight heparins in prophylaxis and therapy of thromboembolic diseases. Series: Fundamental and clinical cardiology
73. Warkentin TE, Hirte HW, Anderson DR et al. (1994) Transient global amnesia associated with acute heparin-induced thrombocytopenia. Am J Med 97: 489–491
74. Warkentin TE, Hayward CPM, Smith CA et al. (1992) Determinants of donor platelet variability when testing for heparin-induced thrombocytopenia. J Lab Clin Med 120: 371
75. Weismann RE, Tobin RW (1958) Arterial embolism occurring during systemic heparin therapy. Arch Surg 76: 219
76. Wilhelm MJ, Schmid C, Kececioglu D et al. (1996) Cardiopulmonary bypass in patients with heparin-induced thrombocytopenia using Org 10172. Ann Thor Surg 61 (3): 920–4

N. A. Cicco (✉) · G. Gerken · M. Frey · H. Just
Abteilung Innere Medizin III
Kardiologie und Angiologie
Klinikum der Albert-Ludwigs-Universität
Hungstetter Str. 55
79106 Freiburg, Germany

New developments in the thrombolytic therapy of venous thrombosis

E. Seifried, W. Weichert

Summary Thrombolysis in deep venous thrombosis is indicated in acute thrombosis of the legs, because in most cases it is due to no or to minimal collateral flow with bad prognosis. Thrombolysis should not be used regularly in isolated thrombosis of the veins of the lower legs and in subclavia vein thrombosis. The aims in therapy of deep venous thrombosis are (1) reduction of fatal pulmonary embolism, (2) avoidance of progression and recurrence, and (3) avoidance of a postthrombotic syndrome. In contrast to heparin alone, thrombolysis has the advantage of high recanalization rates. With clinically used dosage regimens of streptokinase complete and partial recanalization rates are in the range of 60–70 % of primary occluded veins. According to pilotal and dose-finding studies, the results with rt-PA are in the same range. In a different approach, the thrombolytic substances are delivered in a locoregional type via a vein of the foot. There is some evidence from pilotal clinical trials that the comparable response rates are obtainable as with streptokinase in ultrahigh dosage combined with a lower incidence of bleeding complications and pulmonary embolism. Furthermore there is a need for prospective, randomized trials comparing therapy with rt-PA and heparins, especially low molecular heparin.

Key words Venous thrombosis – thrombolytic therapy – streptokinase – urokinase-rt-PA – locoregional thrombolysis

History and introduction

The fluidity of blood postmortem was first observed in the times of the Hippocratic school in the fourth century before Christ. An active fibrinolysin was postulated and the term "'fibrinolysis" coined by Dastre in 1893 [7]. An explanation that postmortem blood dissolved fibrinogen and fibrin in normal blood was given by Morawitz in 1905 [23]. From the end of the 19th century until today, investigators have tried to explain the functions of the fibrinolytic system. Its role in homeostasis has long been fully appreciated, but the potential of therapeutic manipulation of this system has only emerged in recent decades. The concept of dynamic equilibrium, proposed for the coagulation system by Astrup in 1958 [2], suggests a balance wherein fibrinolysis breaks down fibrin that is continously being deposited in the vascular system. This deposition is the result of continuing limited activation of the coagulation system superimposed on a background of fibrinolytic activity assuring fluidity of blood [29].

Surgery is a very important risk factor for deep-vein thrombosis and is responsible for more than one quarter of all thrombosis. Patients with symptomatic deep venous thrombosis have a high risk for recurrent venous thromboembolism that persists for many years. The postthrombotic syndrome occurs in almost one third of these patients during the 8 years after the first deep venous thrombosis [26]. In Western Germany 25000 people die of pulmonary embolism every year. Approximately one million patients suffer from the postthrombotic syndrome. Ulcus cruris patients alone cause costs of about 2.5 billion DM [18].

The aims in therapy of deep venous thrombosis are (1) reduction of fatal pulmonary embolism, (2) avoidance of progression and recurrence, and (3) avoidance of a postthrombotic syndrome.

Thrombolytic substances

The human fibrinolysis system is a proteolytic enzymatic process in the blood. Its purpose is to limit locally intravascular thrombotic processes and to reopen vessels closed by thrombosis.

The main enzyme of the fibrinolysis system is the active protease plasmin produced by activation of the inactive first step plasminogen by means of plasminogen activators via limited proteolysis [4, 29].

The reduction of fibrin by plasmin is a complex process that produces soluble chains clinically detectable as fibrin degradation products.

It is important to note that although fibrin is its main substrate other plasma molecules may be digested by plasmin. Digestion of circulating fibrinogen will result in an increased risk of bleeding. Under normal conditions, circulating plasmin inhibitors will prevent this otherwise disordered lytic action. However, therapy with a fibrinolytic agent that is dependent on plasminemia for its effect depletes these circulating inhibitors [29].

Thrombolytic therapy with plasminogen mimics and enhances physiological fibrinolysis. The following substances are presently available for clinical use: the nonphysiological thrombolytics streptokinase and APSAC (acylated plasminogen streptokinase activator complex), as well as the physiological plasminogen activators urokinase and tissue plasminogen activator (t-PA). Whereas the first three systematically activate the fibrinolytic system, t-PA possesses a relative fibrin selectivity. The fibrinselective active prourokinase and a recombinant mutant of t-PA with prolonged in vivo half-life have not yet been officially approved for the treatment of thromboembolic diseases but are being clinically tested [29].

Thrombolytic treatment

Streptokinase (SK)

Several controlled, randomized prospective studies have evaluated the effect of systemic lytic therapy with streptokinase (SK) (loading dose 250,000–600,000 IU/10–30 min, then 100,000 IU/h) compared to systemic anticoagulation in the treatment of deep vein thrombosis. Dissolution of deep vein thrombi with SK is faster and more complete than that seen with the heparin treatment. Complete lysis is seen on the average in 30 %, partial lysis in 39 % of the patients treated with SK, compared to 37 % (complete and partial lysis) of those treated with heparin alone [4]. Bleeding complications appear more frequently with thrombolytic therapy, occuring in close to 13 % of patients, compared to 4% of those treated with heparin [30]. Goldhaber et al. pooled results from 6 randomized studies in

Table 1a. Results of randomized trials of intravenous streptokinase versus heparin in phlebographically documented deep venous thrombosis: rates of thrombolysis

Author, year	Thrombolysis (%) Streptokinase	Thrombolysis (%) Heparin	Relative risk of thrombolysis
Robertson et al., 1968	7/8 (88)	3/8 (38)	2.3
Kakkar et al., 1969	6/10 (60)	2/10 (20)	3.0
Robertson et al., 1970	6/9 (67)	2/7 (29)	2.3
Tsapogas et al., 1973	10/19 (53)	1/15 (7)	7.9
Porter et al., 1975	13/24 (54)	8/26 (31)	1.8
Elliot et al., 1979	17/26 (65)	0/25 (0)	16
Pooled result			3.7

Table 1b. Randomized studies included in pooled analysis of major bleeding complications

Author	Proportion (%) in Streptokinase group	Proportion (%) in Heparin group	Relative risk of major bleeding
Robertson et al.	2/8 (38)	1/8 (12)	2.0
Porter et al.	4/24 (17)	1/26 (4)	4.3
Elliot et al.	2/25 (8)	0/25 (0)	2.0
Pooled result			2.9

which phlebography was used to confirm the diagnosis and to assess therapy. Thrombolysis was achieved 3.7 times more often among patients treated with SK than among patients treated with heparin (Table 1a). Only 3 studies allowed comparison of these drugs for major bleeding complications, which were 2.9 times greater with SK than with heparin (Table 1b) [10]. Similar results were reported by Ehringer and Minar [9].

Controversy exists as to the benefit of thrombolytic therapy in the treatment of deep vein thrombosis, primarily as it pertains to long-term outcome. Arnesen et al. reported the results of phlebographic evaluation at a mean of 6.5 years after treatment with either streptokinase (SK) or heparin in 35 patients. The evaluations were performed without knowledge of the initial therapy. Seven patients had phlebographically normal veins, and all belonged to the SK group.

This difference between the treatments groups was statistically significant (p < 0.01). At clinical examination, 13 of the 17 patients in the SK group had normal legs and 4 exhibited moderate posthrombotic changes. In contrast, 3 of the heparin-treated patients showed serious postthrombotic changes with open leg ulcers, and only 6 of 18 patients in this group had normal legs (Table 2) [1]. Eichlisberger et al. observed 223 patients, who

Table 2. Clinical evaluation of postthrombotic syndrome 6 years after a deep venous thrombosis – comparison Streptokinase versus Heparin

	Streptokinase group (%)	Heparin group (%)
Total no.	17	18
No signs (normal leg)	13 (76.5)	6 (33.3)
Moderate signs (edema, and/or varicosis veins, and/or pigmentation)	4 (23.5)	9 (50)
Serious signs (leg ulcer in addition)	0	3 (16.7)
Repeated DVT in the same leg during observation time	4*	3**
On permanent anticoagulation	1	1

*,** Moderate signs of postthrombotic syndrome, *n = 1, **n = 2

Table 3. Ultrahigh Streptokinase dosage (UHSK) versus continuance infusion Streptokinase – Results of the Nordbaden Multicenter Study on Lysis of Venous Thrombosis

	UHSK	Continuance – SK
IFP-C-score before lysis	4.55	4.2
IFP-C-score after lysis	2.41	2.93
Improvement	47 %	30 %
Duration of therapy	2.7 ± 0.6 series	3.7 ± 1.2 days

were reexamined 13 years after a deep venous thrombosis. The incidence of post-phlebitic syndrome in the group successfully thrombolysed with SK was significantly lower in patients with 3-level (calf, popliteal, and femoral) and 4-level (calf, popliteal, femoral, and pelvic) thrombosis in comparison to the group "only" anticoagulated or unsuccessfully thrombolysed (p = 0.01). Patients with complete and partial lysis also had less venous symptoms (for 3- and 4-level thrombosis p < 0.0001) [8].

With SK intermittent intravenous ultra-high doses (1.5 mill. U/h over 6 h), success rates are equal or better than with the conventional dose regime. Heinrich et al. demonstrated that ultra high dose SK treatment of deep venous thrombosis is more effective and produces less bleeding than conventional doses (Table 3) [13]. The time of treatment under ultrahigh doses is shorter and the handling is easier. However, contraindications to SK such as streptococcal infections and prior lysis with SK should always be kept in mind.

APSAC

In one study 13 patients with deep vein thrombosis were treated with BRL 26921 (5.5 mg 3x/d). A total lysis was demonstrated in 46 % and a partial lysis in 23 % of the patients [17].

Urokinase (UK)

Urokinase (UK) is used with different doses, at first with doses of about 100,000 U/h. There are no studies, which compared UK with heparin alone. The rates of recanalization are similar in comparison to the conventional SK therapy (Table 4) [32, 34, 36]. Figs. 1 and 2 show our results with UK from the Medizinische Universitätsklinik Ulm. The lysis rate was about 50 %, the complete rate 20 % [4].

Table 4. Thrombolytic therapy of deep pelvis-leg-vein thrombosis-comparison Streptokinase (SK) versus Urokinase (UK): rates of thrombolysis

Author, year	Number of patients	SK Complete (%)	Partial (%)	UK Complete (%)	Partial (%)
Trübestein et al., 1986 [32]	SK: 175	a)* 67	25	46	30
Non randomized	UK: 161	b)* 27	44	17	53
Zimmermann et al., 1985	SK: 19		79		75
Randomized	UK: 22				
Van de Loo et al., 1983 [34]	SK: 10				
Randomized	UK: 21	0	60	0	57

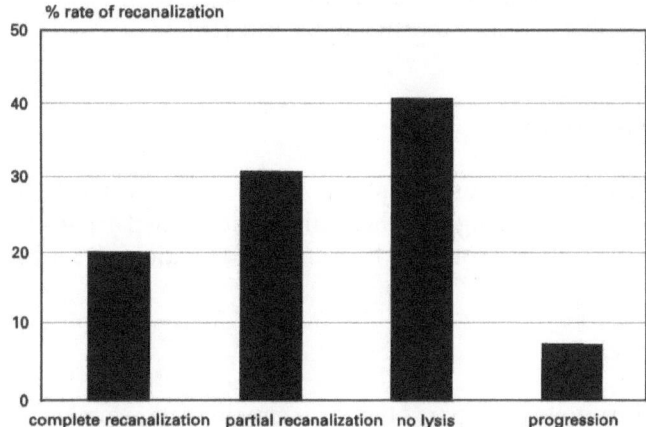

Fig. 1. Success rate after thrombolytic therapy of deep venous thromboses with Urokinase; results from the Medizinische Universitätsklinik Ulm 1983–1991; n = 64

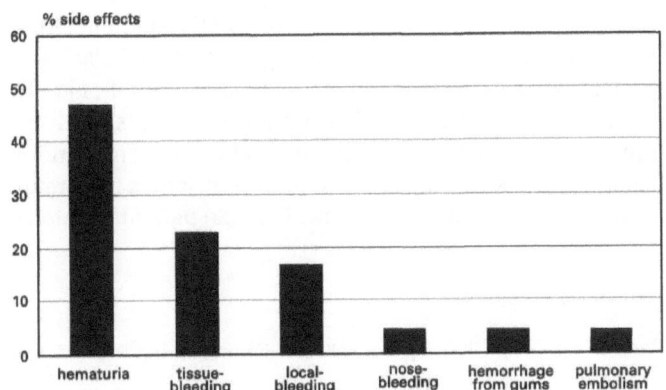

Fig. 2. Side effects during thrombolytic therapy of deep venous thromboses with Urokinase; results from the Medizinische Universitätsklinik Ulm 1983–1991; n = 64

Krzywanek treated 80 patients with acute venous thrombosis with streptokinase (SK) and/or urokinase (UK) with an intermittent ultrahigh dose regimen. Eleven patients received 0.5–1.5 mill. U SK/h for 6(–8) h. In 14 patients therapy was continued with UK in ultrahigh dosage because the primary results were unsatisfactory. 55 patients were treated with 0.5–1.5 mill. U UK/h for 5–8 h, together with low dose heparin. Depending on the results of control venographies, lytic series were repeated 1–8 times. The interval between two series was covered with heparin in adjusted dosage. The rates of complete and partial thrombolysis were 82% for SK, 86% for SK + UK, and 54.4% for UK (Table 5).

Table 5. Thrombolytic therapy of deep vein thrombosis – comparison of ultrahigh Streptokinase (UHSK), ultrahigh Urokinase (UHUK), and combination of UHSK and UHUK: rates of thrombolysis [16]

	Number of patients	Complete (%)	Partial (%)	No lysis (%)
UHSK	11	4 (36)	5 (46)	2 (18)
UHUK	55	12 (22)	18 (33)	25 (45)
UHSK–UHUK	14	6 (43)	6 (43)	2 (14)

Six serious spontaneous bleeding episodes occured under ultrahigh dose UK treatment, leading to discontinuation of therapy [16].

Prourokinase

In a first pilot study 15 patients were infused with 800,000 IU (5 mg)/h of prourokinase over 24 h (120 mg) together with unfractionated heparin. Two of the 11 evaluable patients (18 %) show a complete lysis and 8 of 11 patients (73 %) a partial lysis [22].

rt-PA

Turpie et al. compared two dosing regimes of recombinant tissue plasminogen activator (rt-PA) plus heparin vs. heparin alone in the treatment of acute proximal deep vein thrombosis in 83 patients. Of 12 patients who received 0.5 mg/kg rt-PA plus heparin over 4 h, 7 (58 %) had greater than 50 % lysis of the thrombus, compared with none of 12 who received placebo plus heparin (p = 0.02). Of 28 patients who received 0.5 mg/kg rt-PA over 8 h, repeated in 24 h, 6 (21 %) had greater than 50 % lysis, compared with 2 (7 %) of 30 patients who received placebo plus heparin (p = 0.11) [33].

Goldhaber et al. treated 65 patients; 36 patients received rt-PA alone, 17 patients rt-PA plus heparin, and 12 patients heparin alone. Patients randomly assigned to rt-PA received 0.05 mg/kg/h for 24 h via a perpheral vein, with a maximum dose of 150 mg. Complete or more than 50 % lysis occurred in 10 (28 %) patients treated with rt-PA, in 5 (29 %) patients

Table 6a. Thrombolytic therapy of deep venous thromboses with 4 rt-PA dosages – results of a multicenter study: rate of recanalization

rt-PA mg/kg/d	0.75	0.5	0.375	0.25
Number of patients	24	26	52	54
Complete (%)	29	23	15	9
Partial (%)	25	35	49	58
Thrombus reduction (%)	21	8	19	7
Unchanged (%)	25	34	17	26

Table 6b. Thrombolytic therapy of deep venous thromboses with 4 rt-PA dosages – results of a multicenter study: Marder Score (Total leg)

rt-PA mg/kg/d	0.75	0.50	0.375	0.25
Before therapy	23	28	22	26
After therapy	16	20	16	21
p-value <	0.001	0.001	0.001	0.001

Table 6c. Thrombolytic therapy of deep venous thromboses with 4 rt-PA dosages – results of a multicenter study: rate of safety

rt-PA mg/kg/d	0.75	0.5	0.375	0.25
Number of patients	27	27	54	56
Disruption of lysis because of bleeding (%)	44	26	15	8
Pulmonary embolism (%)	0	0	0	0
Fibrinogen	Unchanged	Unchanged	Unchanged	Unchanged

treated with rt-PA plus heparin, and no patients treated with heparin. No lysis occured in 16 (44 %) patients treated with rt-PA plus heparin and in 10 (83 %) patients who received heparin alone (p = 0.04) [11].

Bounameaux et al. treated 14 patients with rt-PA 0.25 and 15 patients with 0.5 mg/kg/ 24 h during 3–7 days in a randomized, multicenter, European (ETTT) trial. They concluded that the used low dosages cannot be recommended as a treatment for patients with deep venous thrombosis [3]. Apparently better results were obtained in a controlled prospective dose finding study by Zimmermann, Seifried et al. which compared 0.75, 0.5, 0.375 and 0.25 mg/kg/24 h. The recanalization rates increased with increasing dosages. The success rate due to the Marder score was comparable in all dosages (Tables 6a–c). However, the interruption of thrombolytic therapy because of bleeding including macrohematuria was with 44 % significantly higher in the 0.75 mg/kg/d group than in the 0.25 mg/kg/d group. The doses of 0.25–0.375 are apparently the best doses today [37].

Peripheral local lysis

Meyer presented an additional possibility for treatment of deep venous thrombosis, the peripheral local lysis. Hereby doses of up to 100,000 U of streptokinase or 300,000 U of urokinase per day are injected into a superficial vein of the forefoot. The patients remains in Anti-Trendelenburg position, the venous return through the superficial veins is blocked by mechanical compression, and the lytic agent diluted in 20 ml isotonic saline solution is directed into the deep venous branches by intermittent manual pressure of the foot. Twenty three patients were treated. The result of treatment according to clinical state and phlebographic control was judged excellent in 6 and good in 11 patients [21].

Cossio et al. compared 109 patients with acute deep vein thrombosis, treated with localized regional or systemic urokinase (initial dose 300,000 IU, maintenance dose 100,000 IU/h). With the help of localized regional therapy it was possible to achieve complete or partial thrombolysis in 64 % of all patients. The intravenous systemic route of application only achieved partial thrombolysis in 35 % of the cases [6].

Martin et al. compared 40 patients, treated with shortterm ultrahigh streptokinase (= UHSK) infusion either into the dorsalis pedis vein or with a systemic infusion. The distribution of side-effects was approximately identical in the two groups. The rates for total and partial thrombolysis in the systemic infusion group were 50 % and 10 %, respectively, compared with 30 % and 20 %, respectively, in the ipsipedal group [20].

Rudofsky and Timmermann treated 162 patients with 1–4 week old deep venous thrombosis with repeated regional application of 20 mg rt-PA during 4 h. 31–34 % of the patients showed a total lysis, 47–50 % a partial lysis, and 17–21 % a failure of lysis. Best results were achieved in single location thrombosis. Extended thrombotic occlusions of calf, popliteal, thigh, and pelvic veins could be recanalized in a lower percentage. Bleeding complications and other side effects are lower compared with systemic application of fibrinolytic therapy [27]. In another study, 137 patients with vein thrombosis were treated by Schwieder et al. with 20 mg of rt-PA for 4 h each day either locally via a dorsal pedal vein or systematically. The rates of recanalization were equal in both groups [28].

Jansen et al. compared 200 patients, treated with localized regional rt-PA (20, 30, 40 mg) or with systemic UHSK. With rt-PA it was possible to achieve complete lysis in 18 % and partial lysis in 39 %; with UHSK it was possible to achieve complete lysis in 41 % and partial lysis in 36 % of all patients. The rates of cerebral bleedings and necessitated blood transfusion was lower in patients treated with rt-PA [15].

Table 7. Thrombolytic therapy of deep venous thromboses with UHSK i.v. or rt-PA 20 or 40 mg loco-regional (Seifried et al. 1998)

	Alteplase 20 mg n = 212	Alteplase 40 mg n = 151	UHSK 9 Mio U n = 210
Success %	58.4	65.5	74.7
Failure %	41.5	34.5	25.2
Adverse events %	7.1	10.8	41.2

Success is defined as complete and partial recanalization; partial recanalization is defined as phlebographically documented flow. Thrombus reduction, no change or progression is defined as failure.

In a multicenter randomized study Seifried et al. compared 573 patients treated with systemic UHSK or with localized regional rt-PA at doses of 20 or 40 mg/6 h. Success rate was comparable in all three groups showin a higher rate of complete recanalisation rate after UHSK. A high rate of side effects including intolerability, fever, pain allergic reaction, bleeding complication, and pulmonary embolism was observed after UHSK.

One of 4 patients suffering from pulmonary embolism in this group died. After rt-PA no clinical pulmonary embolism was observed, (Table 7) [31].

In the PHLEFI study, 1498 patients were observed receiving different forms of fibrinolytic therapy as ultrahigh streptokinase and urokinase short-term therapy, streptokinase, urokinase and rt-PA long-term infusions and loco-regional (mainly rt-PA). The major factor for the rate of cerebral bleeding under fibrinolytic therapy was the age of the patient (0.354 % in patients under and 2.03 % in patients over 50 years) being higher in UHSK than in rt-PA treated patients. The major factor for pulmonary embolism was the site of the thrombosis (2.16 % with iliac, 0.701 % with femoral, none with popliteal, calf, and subclavian vein thromboses). The highest complete clearance rate achieved was 41.5% in patients treated with shortterm ultrahigh streptokinase therapy (Tables 8a and 8b) [19]. Concerning bleeding complication, the rate of fatal pulmonary embolism and other side effects rt-PA seems to be quite safe.

Table 8a. Results of fibrinolysis as a function of therapeutic regimen in 1324 patients [19]

Regimen	No. of patients	Complete clearance rate (%)	Partial clearance rate (%)	No clearance rate (%)
UHSK	733	41.5	42.8	15.7
SK	8	37.5	37.5	25.0
UHUK	20	20.0	35.0	45.0
UK	206	17.0	52.9	30.1
rt-PA	29	10.4	58.6	31.0
Loco-regional	146	23.3	45.9	30.8
Sequential	182	25.3	52.2	22.5
Total	1324	32.4	46.2	21.4

Table 8b. Rates of cerebral bleedings in 1498 patients who received fibrinolytic therapy and in 807 patients with UHSK treatment [19]

Age (years)	Thrombolysis (%)	UHSK (%)
10–29	0.49	0
30–49	0.28	0
50–69	1.60	1.44
70–89	3.83	3.81
Overall	1.40	1.24

A further possibility of local application of thrombolytic substances is the lysis-block technique. An oversystolic tourniquet is put on the thigh or upper arm. The substance is injected into a dorsal foot vein or forearm vein. By using this strictly local lysis with t-PA it was possible to remove 9 of 11 venous occlusions of v. femoralis or poplitea. However, the method is expensive. This procedure can probably be recommended for patients with contraindications for systemic lysis [12]. Hennigs et al. investigated ultrahigh dose SK lysis of deep venous thromboses modified by using an "ipsipedal" application technique and additional compression to the affected leg (141 patients). There was full recanalization of the thrombosed veins in 62.2 %, partial recanalisation in 32.2 %, and none in 5.6 % [14]. Mumme et al. found in vitro that the highest fibrinolytic activity was obtained at 40 °C. They recommend the regional hyperthermic perfusion of the leg with streptokinase using a heart-lung machine. This method is very expensive [24].

Benefit of lytic therapy

Caspary et al. tested prospectively how many patients in internal medicine are candidates for thrombolysis. A total of 62 patients were enrolled. Only eight patients were offered thrombolytic therapy, but 5 of them denied consent after having been comprehensively informed [5]. Thrombolysis in deep venous thrombosis is indicated in thrombosis of the legs, because in most cases it is due to no or to minimal collateral flow with bad prognosis. When an acute deep venous thrombosis is diagnosed with a proximal extension into the popliteal vein, thrombolytic therapy is clearly superior to heparin. Preferences of the patients or the values they attach to the possible outcomes of therapy must be considered. For every central nervous system bleeding with SK, 60 patients were spared mild postphlebitic syndrome and 7 were spared the severe syndrome [25]. Thrombolysis should not be used regularly in isolated thrombosis of the veins of the lower legs and in subclavia vein thrombosis (Table 9) [35].

Table 9. Therapeutic benefit of lysis therapy in patients with deep vein thromboses [35]

	No	Moderate	Clear	Very good
Age of patients				
< 50 years			+	
>50 years		+		
Life expectancy under 5–10 years	+			
Age of thrombosis				
1–7 days				+
8–14 days			+	
>14 days		+		
Location				
Pelvis		+		
Upper thigh			+	
Calf		+		
extended occlusion			+	

References

1. Arnesen H, Hoiseth A, Ly B (1982) Streptokinase or heparin in the treatment of deep vein thrombosis. Acta Med Scand 211: 65–68
2. Astrup T (1958) The haemostatic balance. Thromb Diath Haemorrh 2: 347–357
3. Bounameaux H, Banga JD, Bluhmki E, Coccheri S, Fiessinger JN, Haarmann W, Lockner D, Mahler F, Ninet J, Schneider PA, de Torrente A, van der Meer J, Verhaeghe R (1992) Double blind, randomized comparison of systemic continuous infusion of 0.25 versus 0.50 mg/kg/24 h of Alteplase over 3 to 7 days for treatment of deep venous thrombosis in heparinized patients: results of the European Thrombolysis with rt-PA in Venous Thrombosis (ETTT) Trial. Throm Haemost 67: 306–309
4. Breddin HK, Krzywanek HJ (1982) Die thrombolytische Behandlung tiefer Bein- und Beckenvenenthrombosen. Internist 23: 410–416
5. Caspary L, Creutzig A, Alexander K (1995) Wie häufig ist die Lysetherapie bei tiefer Becken-Bein-Venenthrombose indiziert? Medizinische Klinik 90: 618–622
6. Cossio JAJ, Ortin PM, Riera L, Reparaz L (1992) Erprobung einer neuen Methode in der lokoregionalen Behandlung mit Urokinase bei tiefer Venenthrombose. Phlebol 21: 119–122
7. Dastre A (1893) Fibrinolyse dans le sang. Arch Physiol Normale et Patholog 5: 661–663
8. Eichlisberger R, Frauchiger B, Widmer MT, Widmer LK, Jäger K (1994) Spätfolgen der tiefen Venenthrombose: ein 13-Jahres Follow-up von 223 Patienten. VASA 23: 234–243
9. Ehringer H, Minar E (1987) Die Therapie der akuten Becken-Bein-Venenthrombose. Internist 28: 317–335
10. Goldhaber SZ, Buring JE, Lipnick RJ, Hennekens CH (1984) Pooled analyses of randomized trials of streptokinase and heparin in phlebographically documented acute deep venous thrombosis. Am J Med 76: 393–397
11. Goldhaber SZ, Meyerovitz MF, Green D, Vogelzang RL, Citrin P, Heit J, Sobel M, Brownell-Wheeler H, Plante D, Kim H, Hopkins A, Tufte M, Stump D, Braunwald E (1990) Randomized controlled trial of tissue plasminogen activator in proximal deep venous thrombosis. Am J Med 88: 235–240
12. Heimig T, Martin M (1993) Lyseblocktechnik. Wiener Med Wochenschr 143: 185–186
13. Heinrich F, Heinrich U (1996) Ergebnisse der Nordbadischen Venen-Lyse-NBVL-Studie. Medizinische Klinik 91: 1–13
14. Hennigs S, Dembinski W, Kohl C, Loncarevic F (1996) Ultrahohe Streptokinaselyse tiefer Venenthrombosen bei ipsipedaler Applikation unter Kompressionsbedingungen. Phlebol 25: 26–37
15. Jansen W, Lepique C, Weidmann B, Franzen B, Becker K (1997) Effektivität und Nebenwirkungen der lokoregionalen Thrombolyse mit rt-PA im Vergleich zur intermittierenden hochdosierten Streptokinase-Therapie tiefer Beinvenenthrombosen. VASA Suppl 50: 5
16. Krzywanek HJ (1988) Vergleichende Untersuchungen zur intermittierenden fibrinolytischen Behandlung akuter Phlebothrombosen mit Streptokinase und Urokinase in ultrahoher Dosierung. Inn Med 15: 179–184
17. Marbet GA, Duckert F (1986) The development of thrombolytic treatment in venous thrombosis. Experience with SK-based regimes. VASA 15: 359–364
18. Marshall M (1986) Bedeutung tiefer Venenthrombosen im chirurgischen Krankengut. Med Klinik 81, Suppl III: 11–13
19. Martin M (1997) Results of the PHLEFI Study (PHLEbothrombosis-FIbrinolytic therapy): A prospective, multicenter study of the fate of 1498 patients receiving fibrinolytic therapy for deep vein thrombosis. International J of Angiology 6: 207–215
20. Martin M, Heimig Th, Fiebach BJO, Riedel Ch (1996) Fibrinolytic treatment with ultra-high streptokinase infusion via the dorsalis pedis vein offers no advantage over systemic infusion via the brachial vein in patients with deep vein thrombosis of the leg. VASA 25: 275–278
21. Meyer J. Die periphere lokale Lyse (PLL) (1990) Eine neue zusätzliche Behandlungsmöglichkeit bei tiefer Bein- und Beckenvenenthrombose – Bericht über 23 Patienten. Z Herz Thora Gefäßchir 4: 151–156
22. Moia M, Mannucci PM, Pini M, Prandoni P, Gurewich V (1994) A pilot study of pro-urokinase in the treatment of deep vein thrombosis. Thrombosis and Haemostasis 72: 430–433
23. Morawitz P (1905) Die Chemie der Blutgerinnung. Ergeb Physiologie, Biophysik und Psychophysik 4: 307–422
24. Mumme A, Kemen M, Homann HH, Zumtobel V (1993) Temperaturabhängigkeit der Fibrinolyse mit Streptokinase. Dtsch med Wschr 118: 1594–1596
25. O'Meara III JJ, McNutt RA, Evans AT, Moore SW, Downs M (1994) A decision analysis of streptokinase plus heparin as compared with heparin alone for deep-vein thrombosis. N Engl J Med 330: 1864–1869
26. Prandoni P, Lensing AWA, Cogo A, Cuppini S, Villalta S, Carta M, Cattelan AM, Polistena P, Bernardi E, Prins MH (1996) The long-term clinical course of acute deep venous thrombosis. Ann Intern Med 125: 1–7
27. Rudofsky G, Timmermann J (1993) Lokoregionale Thrombolysetherapie tiefer venöser Thrombosen. Z Kardiol 82, Suppl 2: 61–63
28. Schwieder G, Grimm W, Siemens HJ, Flor B, Hilden A, Gmelin E, Friedrich HJ, Wagner T (1995) Intermittent regional therapy with rt-PA is not superior to systemic thrombolysis in deep vein thrombosis (DVT) – a German multicenter trial. Thromb and Haemost 74: 1240–1243
29. Seifried E (1993) Das Fibrinolyse-System und seine Aktivatoren. Innere Medizin 48: 272–282
30. Seifried E (1993) Tiefe venöse Thrombosen – etablierte Behandlungsverfahren und neue Trends. Z Kardiol 82: 49–59

31. Seifried E. New developments in the acute treatment of venous thrombosis. Vortrag auf dem Kongreß, Acute pulmonary embolism – a challenge for hemostasiology, 21. 06. 1997, Gargellen 32. Trübestein G, Trübestein R, Wilgalis M, Popov S, Herder T (1986) Die fibrinolytische Therapie mit Streptokinase und Urokinase bei tiefer Venenthrombose. Med Klinik 81: 79–84
33. Turpie AGG (1989) Thrombolysis in deep vein thrombosis. In: Thrombolysis in Cardiovascular Disease. Julian et al. (eds) Marcel Dekker, New York, Basel, 397–408
34. Van de Loo JCW, Kriesmann A, Trübestein G, Knoch K, de Swart CAM, Asbeck F, Marbet GA, Schmitt HE, Servell AF, Duckert F, Theiss W, Ritz R (1983) Controlled multicenter pilot study of urokinase-heparin and streptokinase in deep vein thrombosis. Thromb Haemost 50: 660–663
35. Weichert W, Seifried E (1995) Fibrinolytika – Wer profitiert wann? Therapeutisch Umschau 52: 652–660
36. Zimmermann R, Epping J, Rasche R, Krzywanek HJ, Breddin HK, Rudolph T, Harenberg J, Gerhardt P, Roebruck P (1986) Urokinase- und Streptokinase-Therapie tiefer venöser Thrombosen. Ergebnisse einer multizentrischen, randomisierten Studie. In: 5. Gemeinsame Jahrestagung der Angiologischen Gesellschaft der Bundesrepublik Deutschlands, Österreichs und der Schweiz, Berlin. Demeter Gräfelfing 427–428
37. Zimmermann R, Seifried E, Schramm W, Haarmann W, Bluhmki E. rt-PA thrombolysis of deep vein thrombosis with different dosages, results of a prospective multicenter study (1991) XIIIth Congress of the International Society on Thrombosis and Haemostasis, Amsterdam, 30. 06. – 06. 07 Abstracts: 1132

Prof. Dr. med. E. Seifried (✉) · PD Dr. med. W. Weidert
Institut für Transfusionsmedizin
und Immunhämatologie
Blutspendedienst Hessen d. DRK
Sandhofstr. 1
D-60528 Frankfurt/M.

The risk of recurrent venous thromboembolic disease – implications for treatment

S. Eichinger, P. A. Kyrle, I. Pabinger, K. Lechner

Summary Patients with venous thromboembolism are at risk of recurrent thrombosis. Since this risk is particularly high within the first weeks and months after the acute event, intensive heparin treatment followed by oral anticoagulants for at least 3 to 6 months is generally recommended. After discontinuation of secondary thromboprophylaxis, the cumulative incidence of recurrence still remains high (approximately 20 % after 5 years).

Patients at risk of recurrence may be identified by evaluation of clinical and/or laboratory findings. Patients with cancer, the antiphospholipid antibody (APLA) syndrome, patients with antithrombin-, protein C- or protein S-deficiency, or patients with hyperhomocysteinemia are at an especially high risk of recurrent thrombosis. In patients with the factor V Leiden mutation or the G20210A variant in the prothrombin gene, data on the recurrence rate are currently controversial or unknown.

While a massive activation of coagulation and fibrinolysis is observed during and after an acute venous thromboembolic event, monitoring of coagulation activation markers, such as prothrombin fragment F1 + 2, has not proven helpful for prediction of recurrence.

Since the risks of secondary thromboprophylaxis (mainly bleeding) have to be weighed against the benefit in terms of prevention of recurrence, it is common practice to discontinue oral anticoagulants after 6 months. However, some patients have an increased risk of recurrence, and prolonged secondary thromboprophylaxis should be considered. Although randomized trials to compare different treatment modalities in patients at high risk of recurrence are currently lacking, we suggest that after a first or second venous thromboembolic event patients with cancer, with an APLA-syndrome, patients with type I antithrombin deficiency, patients with combined deficiencies and probably patients with hyperhomocysteinemia are candidates for secondary thromboprophylaxis beyond 6 months. The presence of factor V Leiden alone does not justify secondary thromboprophylaxis longer than 6 months.

Key words Venous thromboembolism – recurrence – treatment

Introduction

It is well-known that patients who have suffered from a venous thromboembolic event are at risk of recurrent thrombosis and that this risk is much higher than the risk to experience a first venous thrombosis. Only a few systematic studies on the incidence of recurrent venous thromboembolism and on thrombotic risk factors have been performed. Only recently, several groups including our own have addressed this issue in prospective trials.

The term "recurrence of venous thromboembolic disease" may have different meanings. It could mean that a patient with a history of a venous thrombosis develops a new venous thrombotic event at the initial site or in the contralateral leg. Recurrence might also occur at an unusual distant site in the venous system (portal, mesenteric, splenic or hepatic veins, cerebral sinus) and finally pulmonary embolism with or without recognizable new thrombus formation in the peripheral venous system may occur. In addition, patients who have a first venous thromboembolic event may also have an increased risk of arterial thrombosis due to the presence of an underlying abnormality which predisposes to both venous and arterial disease, such as in patients with the antiphospholipid antibody (APLA) syndrome. The pathogenesis and implications for treatment may be quite different in these various types of recurrences.

The risk of recurrence after the first venous thromboembolic event

The risk of recurrence is particularly high within the first weeks and months after a venous thromboembolic event. In several randomized studies it has been shown that initial intensive treatment with heparin followed by oral anticoagulants for at least 3 to 6 months is necessary to reduce the high risk of early recurrence [13, 15, 16]. However, when oral anticoagulants are stopped after 3 to 6 months, the risk of recurrent venous thrombosis still remains high. The incidence of recurrent venous thromboembolic events has recently been studied in several prospective trials. Prandoni et al. [12] found a 15.3 % cumulative incidence of recurrent venous thromboembolic event two years after discontinuation of oral anticoagulants after the first thromboembolic event. After 8 years the probability of recurrence increased to 30 %. We have performed a similar study and found a 20 % incidence of recurrence after five years (Fig. 1). The reasons for the different recurrence rates between these two studies are certainly due to different patient populations. In the study by Prandoni et al., a considerable number of patients with cancer or inherited inhibitor deficiencies have been included. These patients were excluded in our study (Table 1). Combining the results of these two studies, it can be assumed that at five years patients without cancer or an inherited inhibitor deficiency have a 20 % incidence of recurrent venous thrombosis.

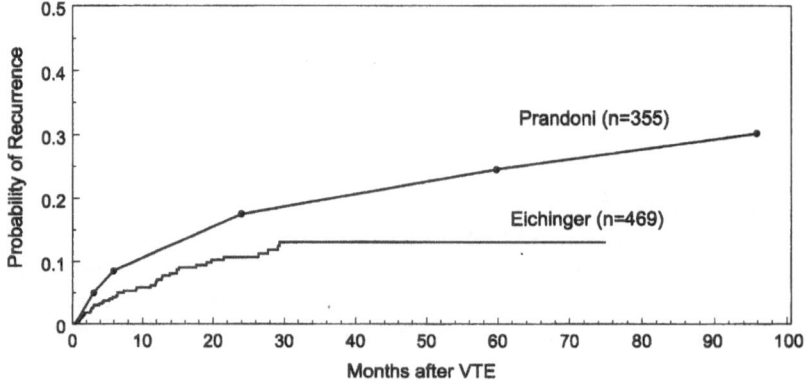

Fig. 1. Cumulative probability of recurrent venous thromboembolism in two different studies.

Table 1. Patient characteristics at study entry in two different studies on the risk of recurrent venous thromboembolism (VTE)

Author	Prandoni et al. (ref. 12)	Eichinger et al. (ref. 4 and unpublished data)
Patient number (n)	355	469
Age (mean)	63 years	51 years
Male gender	55 %	45 %
Proximal vein thrombosis	32.9 %	41.1 %
Spontaneous VTE	59 %	65 %
Previous recurrent VTE	0 %	9.4 %
Cancer	16.3 %	0 % (excluded)
Inhibitor deficiency	13 %	0 % (excluded)
OAC for > 3 months	14.9 %	79.9 %

Identification of patients with high and low risk of recurrence after the first venous thromboembolic event

Patients with a high or a low risk of recurrence may be identified by evaluation of clinical and/or laboratory findings. Among the clinical factors which influence the risk of recurrent thrombosis, the presence of a malignant disease is the most important. The recurrence rate in patients with cancer is almost twice as high as in patients without a malignancy [12]. There is no evidence that other clinical factors, such as sex, age, site and extent of thrombosis, pulmonary embolism, or family history of thrombosis, have an impact on the recurrence rate.

Several inherited or acquired thrombophilic states have been identified which increase the risk of a first thromboembolic event [3, 8]. It appears likely and has often been assumed that carriers of such abnormalities are also at an increased risk of recurrent thrombosis. However, only recently this hypothesis has been tested for some of these conditions.

The most impressive example of a thrombophilic state, which is associated with an increased risk of recurrence, is the APLA-syndrome. Khamashta et al. [6] have shown that affected patients have a high risk of early recurrence after discontinuation of oral anticoagulants with an eventual recurrence rate of almost 90 %. Two third of the recurrences occurred in the venous, one third in the arterial system.

Patients with inherited inhibitor deficiencies, such as antithrombin-, protein C-, or protein S-deficiency have a high risk of venous thrombosis already at a young age. Whether such patients have an increased risk of recurrence after the first thrombosis has not been prospectively evaluated. In a retrospective analysis, Pabinger et al. [10] have shown that patients with inhibitor deficiencies indeed have a higher risk of recurrence than patients without the defect. In a cohort study, Prandoni et al. [12] found a 40 % higher recurrence rate among patients with inhibitor deficiencies. Thus, it is likely – though not definitely proven – that the presence of an inherited inhibitor deficiency is also associated with a higher risk of recurrence. However, the risk may be varying in individual patients depending on the type and severity of the deficiency and, in particular, on the presence or absence of other common thrombotic risk factors, such as factor V Leiden.

Factor V Leiden, a mutation in the factor V gene which renders the factor V protein less sensitive to inactivation by protein C, is associated with an increased risk of a first venous thromboembolic event [1]. Since this defect is rather common (approximately 4 % of the general population in Europe and 20 to 30 % of patients with venous thromboembolism),

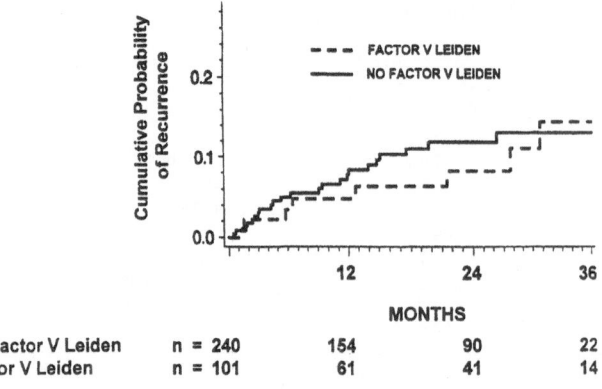

Fig. 2. Cumulative probability of recurrent venous thromboembolism in patients with and without factor V Leiden.

		MONTHS		
		12	24	36
No Factor V Leiden	n = 240	154	90	22
Factor V Leiden	n = 101	61	41	14

it was possible to test the impact of the mutation on the incidence of recurrent venous thrombotic events. In the Physician's Health Study, Ridker et al. [14] found a 2-fold higher risk of recurrence in male physicians with factor V Leiden, but the number of patients in this study was small. In a prospective study, Simioni et al. [17] described a significantly higher risk of recurrence in patients with factor V Leiden after a first venous thrombo-embolic event. The risk was particularly high during the first two years after the initial event. In contrast, we [Eichinger et al. [4]] were not able to confirm the data of Simioni. We conducted a large prospective trial and no difference in the incidence of recurrence between patients with or without factor V Leiden was seen during the first years after the initial event. However, it can be presumed that in the long run (after 5 to 10 years) the cumulative probability of recurrence will be higher in carriers of factor V Leiden than in those without the mutation (Fig. 2).

Hyperhomocysteinemia (HHc) has been known as a risk factor of arterial and venous thrombosis for many years. Recently, even moderate increases of plasma homocysteine levels (mild HHc) have been associated with an increased thrombotic risk [2]. Thus, we were interested in whether mild HHc is also a risk factor of recurrent venous thrombosis. In a prospective study, we demonstrated that patients with mild HHc have a significantly (2-fold) increased risk of recurrence which is particularly evident during the first two years after the initial event [5].

Recently, a new risk factor of venous thrombosis, the G to A transition at position 20210 in the prothrombin gene was discovered [11]. The impact of this genetic variant on the recurrence rate is presently unknown.

On the basis of these data, patients who had a first venous thromboembolic event can be assigned to a high and a low risk group of recurrence (Table 2). This should be helpful to decide whether to continue or discontinue oral anticoagulants.

Table 2. Stratification of patients according to the risk of recurrent venous thromboembolism

High risk	APLA-syndrome Cancer/chemotherapy Inherited inhibitor deficiencies Hyperhomocysteinemia
Controversial/unknown risk	Factor V Leiden G20210A prothrombin variant
Low risk	None of the above

Prediction of recurrent thrombosis by monitoring activation markers of coagulation and fibrinolysis

In patients with an acute venous thromboembolic event, an activation of coagulation and fibrinolysis occurs which can easily be documented by measuring the plasma concentrations of markers of coagulation activation, such as thrombin-antithrombin complexes (TAT), prothrombin fragment F1 + 2 (F1 + 2), and of fibrinolysis, such as D-Dimer, a split product of fibrin. We have speculated that a permanent activation of the clotting system may be present in some patients which may predispose them to recurrent thrombosis. Serial measurement of activation markers in patients who are off anticoagulants after a venous thromboembolic event could, therefore, be useful to predict recurrent thrombosis. In a prospective cohort study, we (Kyrle et al. [7]) tested this hypothesis and found that monitoring of activation markers is not helpful for predicting recurrence. The plasma levels of F1 + 2 were identical in patients with and without recurrence and no increased levels of F1 + 2 at the last measurement before clinical diagnosis of recurrence was detectable.

Risk assessment – Implications for treatment

In view of the relatively high recurrence rate after discontinuation of oral anticoagulants at 3 to 6 months, prolonged secondary thromboprophylaxis might be considered. However, even at low intensity (INR 2.0–3.0) and under optimal supervision, treatment with oral anticoagulants is associated with a definite risk of bleeding (2 to 3 % of major and 0.2 % of fatal bleedings per year) [17]. In the majority of the patients, the bleeding risk may outweigh the benefit (in terms of prevention of recurrence) of prolonged secondary thrombophylaxis, and it is therefore common practice to discontinue oral anticoagulants after 6 months. As outlined above, some patients have an increased risk of recurrence and for this high risk population the benefit/risk ratio may be in favor of prolonged oral anticoagulant therapy. However, the benefits and risks of prolonged oral anticoagulant prophylaxis in various groups of patients at increased risk of recurrence have not been compared in randomized trials. In the absence of these data we suggest that after a first or a second thromboembolic event patients with the highest risk of recurrence, i.e., patients with cancer, with an APLA-syndrome, patients with type I antithrombin deficiency, combined deficiencies, and probably also patients with HHc are candidates for prolonged secondary thromboprophylaxis. In our opinion the presence of factor V Leiden alone does not justify thromboprophylaxis beyond 6 months. It remains to be seen whether the presence of the prothrombin variant is associated with an increased risk of recurrence.

If one has decided – for any of the above reasons – to continue oral anticoagulants beyond 6 months the following questions will arise (1). How long? Will the incidence of recurrence decline after one or two years of oral anticoagulants or will life-long thromboprophylaxis be necessary? (2) How intensive? Should it be possible to reduce the intensity of oral anticoagulant therapy (for example to INR 1.5–2.0) without loss of efficacy? (3) Are there alternatives to oral anticoagulants? Could the risk of recurrence be reduced by vitamin supplementation in patients with HHc?

These issues will have to be addressed in ongoing and future randomized trials.

References

1. Dahlbäck B (1995) Inherited thrombophilia: resistance to activated protein C as a pathogenetic factor of venous thrombosis. Blood 85: 607–614
2. d'Angelo A, Selhub J (1997) Homocysteine and thrombotic disease. Blood 90: 1–11
3. de Stefano V, Finazzi G, Mannucci PM (1996) Inherited thrombophilia: pathogenesis, clinical syndromes and management. Blood 87: 3531–3544
4. Eichinger S, Pabinger I, Stümpflen A, Hirschl M, Bialonczyk C, Schneider B, Mannhalter C, Minar E, Lechner K, Kyrle PA (1997) The risk of recurrent venous thromboembolism in patients with and without factor V Leiden. Thromb Haemost 77: 624–628
5. Eichinger S, Stümpflen A, Hirschl M, Bialonczyk C, Pabinger I, Herkner K, Schneider B, Lechner K, Kyrle PA (1997) Hyperhomocysteinemia is a risk factor of recurrent venous thromboembolism in male patients. Thromb Haemost (Suppl): 184
6. Khamashta MA, Cuadrado MJ, Mujic F, Taub NA, Hunt BJ, Hughes GRV (1995) The management of thrombosis in the antiphospholipid-antibody syndrome. N Engl J Med 332: 993–997
7. Kyrle PA, Eichinger S, Pabinger I, Stümpflen A, Hirschl M, Bialonczyk C, Schneider B, Mannhalter C, Melichart M, Traxler G, Weltermann A, Speiser W, Lechner K (1997) Prothrombin fragment F1 + 2 is not predictive for recurrent venous thromboembolism. Thromb Haemost 77: 829–833
8. Lane DA, Mannucci PM, Bauer KA, Bertina RM, Bochkov NP, Boulyjenkov V, Chandy M, Dahlbäck B, Ginter EK, Miletich JP, Rosendaal FR, Seligsohn U (1996) Inherited thrombophilia: Part 1. Thromb Haemost 76: 651–662
9. Levine MN, Hirsh J, Landefeld S, Raskob G (1992) Hemorrhagic complications of anticoagulant treatment. Chest 102 (Suppl): 352–363
10. Pabinger I, Brücker S, Kyrle PA, Schneider B, Korninger HC, Niessner H, Lechner K (1992) Hereditary deficiency of antithrombin III, protein C and protein S: Prevalence in patients with a history of venous thrombosis and criteria for rational patient screening. Blood Coagul Fibrinolysis 3: 547–553
11. Poort SR, Rosendaal FR, Reitsma PH, Bertina RM (1996) A common genetic variation in the 3'-translated region of the prothrombin gene is associated with elevated plasma prothrombin levels and an increase in venous thrombosis. Blood 88: 3698–3703
12. Prandoni P, Lensing AWA, Cogo A, Cuppini S, Villalta S, Carta M, Cattelan AM, Polistena P, Bernardi E, Prins MH (1996) The long-term clinical course of acute deep venous thrombosis. Ann Intern Med 125: 1–7
13. Research Committee of the British Thoracic Society (1992) Optimum duration of anticoagulation for deep-vein thrombosis and pulmonary embolism. Lancet 340: 783–876
14. Ridker PM, Miletich JP, Stampfer MJ, Goldhaber SZ, Lindpaintner K, Hennekens CH (1995) Factor V Leiden and risks of recurrent idiopathic venous thromboembolism. Circulation 92: 2800–2802
15. Sarasin FP, Bounameaux H (1994) Duration of oral anticoagulant therapy after proximal deep vein thrombosis: A decision analysis. Thromb Haemost 71: 286–291
16. Schulman S, Rhedin AS, Lindmarker P, Carlsson A, Lärfars G, Nicol P, Loogna E, Svensson E, Ljungberg B, Walter H, Viering S, Nordlander S, Leijd B, Kjell-Ake J, Hjorth M, Linder O, Boberg J, and the Duration of Anticoagulation Trial Study Group (1995) A comparison of six weeks with six months of oral anticoagulant therapy after a first episode of venous thromboembolism. N Engl J Med 332: 1661–1665
17. Simioni P, Prandoni P, Lensing AWA, Scudeller A, Sardella C, Prins MH, Villalta S, Dazzi F, Girolami A (1997) The risk of recurrent venous thromboembolism in patients with an $Arg^{506} \rightarrow$ Gln mutation in the gene for factor V (factor V Leiden). N Engl J Med 336: 399–403

S. Eichinger · P. A. Kyrle · I. Pabinger · K. Lechner (✉)
Division of Haematology and Haemostaseology
Department of Medicine I
Währinger Gürtel 18-20
A-1090 Wien, Austria

A randomized trial of the effect of low molecular weight heparin vs. warfarin on mortality in the long-term treatment of proximal vein thrombosis

R. D. Hull, G. F. Pineo, R. F. Brant

Summary It has been shown that several different low molecular weight (LMW) heparins, given by a once- or twice-daily subcutaneous injection without laboratory monitoring, are as effective or even more effective than continuous intravenous, unfractionated heparin monitored by the activated partial thromboplastin time (APTT). One such study demonstrated a statistically significant decrease in mortality over the 3 month follow-up study. This was particularly striking in patients with cancer. Based on these findings, a multicentre, randomized clinical trial has been designed to compare the effect of long-term, once-daily LMW heparin with standard treatment using heparin and warfarin to ensure that equal numbers of cancer patients are in both groups. This will demonstrate whether or not the long-term use of LMW heparin can have a significant impact on mortality in patients who have proximal venous thrombosis with or without cancer.

Introduction

To treat a first episode of proximal deep-vein thrombosis, it is conventional to continuously infuse standard heparin intravenously for 5 days; warfarin sodium is also started on day 1 and continued for 3 months [22, 43]. A heparin nomogram can be used to ensure that adequate heparin is delivered throughout the treatment period [43, 44, 60]. The incidence of recurrent thromboembolism and of major bleeding are both in the range of 5–6 % using the combined treatment of heparin and warfarin [40, 42, 43]. We will review data from clinical trials which support subcutaneous injection of low molecular weight (LMW) heparin for the initial treatment of proximal venous thrombosis and we will describe a clinical trial comparing the long-term use of LMW heparin with standard treatment in patients with an initial episode of proximal deep-vein thrombosis.

Background and rationale

Initial continuous intravenous heparin [40, 63, 68] followed by long-term oral anticoagulant therapy is the accepted treatment for acute deep-vein thrombosis (DVT) [22, 32, 33, 43]. Due to improvements in the methods of clinical trials and the use of accurate objective tests to detect venous thromboembolism [20, 31, 39, 59, 67], it is now possible to perform a series of randomized trials to evaluate various treatments of venous thrombosis. These clinical trials have resolved most of the uncertainties which confront clinicians in deciding upon an appropriate course of anticoagulant therapy [8, 11, 22, 32, 33, 36, 40, 43, 44, 63, 68]. Adequate initial heparin treatment, determined by the activated partial thromboplastin time (APTT) response, is necessary if unacceptably high rates of recurrent venous thromboembolism are to be prevented [11, 33, 40, 60]. It is common clinical practice to adjust the heparin dose to maintain the APTT within a defined therapeutic range (that is, between 1.5 and 2.5 times control). Data from clinical trials support the use of an APTT ratio of 1.5 as the lower limit of the therapeutic range [40, 43, 44]. The relative risk of recurrence of venous thromboembolism was 15 to 1 for patients given inadequate initial heparin treatment (that is, an APTT ratio less than 1.5) [40].

A more recent randomized trial compared intravenous heparin and oral anticoagulants with oral anticoagulants alone for the initial treatment of proximal venous thrombosis [11]. It strongly supported these findings. Recurrent venous thromboembolism occurred in 20 % of patients treated with oral anticoagulants alone compared with 6 % in those who received initial intravenous heparin adjusted to maintain the APTT above 1.5 times control. Most of the symptomatic recurrences occurred after the first month of treatment.

The use of a heparin protocol assures that virtually all patients (98–99 %] will achieve the therapeutic range for the APTT. This decreases the likelihood of recurrent venous thromboembolism and does not increase the risk of bleeding complication [44, 60]. When the bleeding complications associated with this trial were reviewed, it was found that major bleeding occurred most frequently in patients with underlying causes for bleeding such as recent surgery, peptic ulcer disease, and cancer. They did not occur as a result of an elevated APTT [44]. These findings show that there was no association between the supratherapeutic APTT result (a ratio of 2.5 or more) and the risk of clinically important bleeding complications. Recently, trials have demonstrated that the length of initial heparin therapy can be shortened from 10–14 days to approximately 5 days [22, 43]. In an era of fiscal constraint, short-course heparin allows for effective treatment without detracting from patient care and, by shortening the in-hospital stay, offers a significant financial benefit [61].

Although continuous intravenous heparin therapy is highly effective as well as relatively safe, it requires patient hospitalization and, therefore, cannot be given on an outpatient basis. If initial treatment of proximal-vein thrombosis could be developed which would be given on an outpatient basis and would not require laboratory monitoring, it would markedly simplify treatment and improve cost-effectiveness. A conservative estimate of the number of hospital days that would be saved by an outpatient approach to initial therapy is 5–6 days. Such a decrease in the duration of hospitalization could result in savings to the Canadian health care system of at least $ 50 million annually ($ 500 million annually in the United States) [61].

In the past, several randomized trials have compared the effectiveness and safety of heparin given by the subcutaneous route with that given by the continuous intravenous route. One overview concluded that subcutaneous heparin was as effective and safe as intravenous heparin [29]. However, this meta-analysis was criticised on the basis of the studies selected for review and for the lack of data on APTT values in patients receiving subcutaneous heparin [55]. In view of the well-established need to achieve a lower limit for the APTT therapeutic range, heparin given by the subcutaneous route cannot be recommended in the initial treatment of proximal venous thrombosis.

In recent years, LMW derivatives of commercial heparin have been prepared. These LMW heparins have a mean molecular weight of 4,000–5,000 Daltons in contrast to unfractionated heparin which has a mean molecular weight of 12,000–16,000 Daltons [62, 66]. Pharmacokinetic studies [7, 9, 15, 21, 26, 54] as well as recent small clinical trials in selected patients [3, 6, 13, 19, 27] indicate that the bioavailability of the LMW heparin fractions following subcutaneous injection is very high. For example, Bratt et al. reported that the bioavailability of LMW heparin after a subcutaneous injection of 120 factor Xa units per kg to healthy volunteers was approximately 90 % of an equivalent intravenous dose. Two properties of LMW heparin suggest that it may be possible to develop an effective regimen for initial treatment with LMW heparin using a once-daily subcutaneous injection: its excellent bioavailability and its longer half-life (antifactor Xa activity) [2, 7, 9, 15, 54] than unfractionated heparin. The anticoagulant response (factor Xa units/ml) observed using a given dose of LMW heparin correlates highly with body weight [54], suggesting that LMW heparin can be effective when given in standard doses (factor Xa units/kg) without laboratory monitoring. Animal and human experiments indicate LMW heparin has a reduced tendency to cause bleeding for the same antithrombotic effect [16, 17, 18, 28, 56].

Limited venographic data are available for LMW heparin compared with unfractionated heparin for the treatment of DVT [1, 4, 12, 14, 24, 25, 27, 30, 51, 58, 64]. These data suggest that LMW heparin administered subcutaneously twice daily is as effective and safe as continuous intravenous heparin. These findings [1, 4, 12, 14, 24, 25, 27, 30, 51, 58, 64] are largely based on venographic observations rather than clinical outcome.

Two recent studies [42, 57] of fixed-dose subcutaneous LMW heparin therapy in patients with venous thrombosis firmly conclude that certain LMW heparins are as effective and safe as monitored continuous intravenous heparin therapy.

Prandoni et al. [57] performed a randomized trial in consecutive symptomatic patients with proximal-vein thrombosis. They compared the relative effectiveness and risk of bleeding of fixed-dose LMW heparin (CY216 Fraxiparine) with adjusted-dose intravenous unfractionated heparin for 10 days followed by oral warfarin sodium for 3 months. Patients in the LMW heparin groups received subcutaneous injections every 12 hours according to body weight (12,500 anti-Xa ICU for patients < 55 kg; 15,000 anti-Xa ICU for patients 55–80 kg; and 17,500 anti-Xa ICU for patients > 80 kg). Patients in the adjusted-dose intravenous heparin group were continuously infused to maintain the APTT within 1.5–2.0 times the mean normal control value. All patients had baseline perfusion lung scans and chest X-rays. Contrast venography was repeated on day 10 or earlier if new symptoms developed. The principal end-point for assessing efficacy was symptomatic recurrent venous thrombosis or symptomatic pulmonary embolism. Secondary end-points for assessing efficacy were changes between day 0 and day 10 in the venograms and perfusion lung scans. The frequency of objectively diagnosed recurrent venous thromboembolisms between the unfractionated heparin and the LMW heparin groups was not significantly different [12 (14 %) versus 6 (7 %); 95 % CI = –3 to +15 %; p = 0.13]. There was no significant difference in clinically evident bleeding between the 2 groups (3.5 % for unfractionated heparin vs. 1.1 % for LMW heparin; p > 0.2). In the 6 month followup period there were 12 deaths in the unfractionated heparin group versus 6 in the CY216 group; this difference was largely due to cancer deaths (8 of 18 in the unfractionated heparin group versus 1 of 15 in the LMW heparin group).

Hull et al. [42] compared fixed-dose subcutaneous LMW heparin (Logiparin™; 175 factor Xa IU/kg) with intravenous heparin a larger multicenter double-blind clinical trial. Continuous infusion of heparin was adjusted to maintain an APTT of 1.5–2.5 times the mean normal control value. All patients had venographically proven proximal-vein thrombosis and at the time of entry. Outcome events included objectively documented venous thromboembolism (recurrence or extension of DVT or pulmonary embolism), major or minor bleeding, thrombocytopenia, and death. New episodes of venous thromboembolism were seen in 6 of 213 patients receiving LMW heparin (2.8 %) and in 15 of 219 patients receiving intravenous unfractionated heparin (6.9 %; p = 0.07; 95 % CI for the difference = 0.02 to + 8.1 %]. Major bleeding associated with initial therapy was seen in 1 patient receiving LMW heparin (0.5 %) and in 11 patients receiving intravenous unfractionated heparin (5.0 %); the reduction in risk was 95 % (p = 0.006). During long-term warfarin therapy, major hemorrhage was seen in 5 patients who had received LMW heparin (2.3 %) and in none of those receiving intravenous heparin (p = 0.028). Ten patients who received LMW heparin (4.7 %) died compared to 21 patients who received intravenous unfractionated heparin (9.6 %); the risk reduction was 51 % (p = 0.049). The most striking difference was in abrupt deaths in patients with metastatic carcinoma. The majority of these deaths occurred within the first 3 weeks. Long-term use of LMW heparin rather than warfarin sodium may have a greater impact on recurrent thromboembolic events, bleeding, and death, particularly in patients with metastatic carcinoma.

The studies by Prandoni et al. [57] and by Hull et al. [42] provide strong evidence that LMW heparin given subcutaneously is as effective and as safe as unfractionated heparin in the initial treatment of proximal-vein thrombosis. The decreased mortality rate, which was particularly striking in patients with metastatic carcinoma, requires confirmation in further prospective randomized trials [23].

Low molecular weight heparin was compared with intravenous, unfractionated heparin for the initial treatment of proximal venous thrombosis in hospitalised patients [50, 65]. These studies showed that low molecular weight heparin was at least as effective and safe as unfractionated heparin in this setting. An overview concluded that low molecular weight heparin resulted in decreased recurrent venous thromboembolism, major bleeding and mortality with compared with continuous intravenous heparin for the treatment of proximal venous thrombosis [48]. More recently, low molecular weight heparin given primarily out-of-hospital was compared with continuous intravenous heparin given in-hospital for the initial management of proximal vein thrombosis [47, 49]. Both studies showed that out-of-hospital low molecular weight heparin was as effective and as safe as continuous intravenous heparin in-hospital.

The most common defect predisposing to venous thrombosis is activated Protein C (APACE) resistance [19, 69]. It is important to determine the incidence of this defect in patients with deep-vein thrombosis, particularly when there is no precipitating event such as surgery or trauma [69, 70].

Protocol

The *general objective* of the study is to assess and compare the long-term treatment of patients with proximal venous thrombosis using subcutaneous LMW heparin with standard care using intravenous heparin followed by oral warfarin sodium.

The *specific objectives of the study* are

- To determine if LMW heparin, given subcutaneously once daily without laboratory monitoring, is more effective than adjusted oral warfarin sodium in reducing mortality rate.
- To determine if LMW heparin therapy is more cost-effective than present standard care methods, and
- To determine the incidence of activated Protein C resistance.

Eligibility criteria

Patients having a first or recurrent episode of acute proximal-vein thrombosis (thrombosis of the popliteal or more proximal deep veins of the leg) documented by venography *or* B-mode venous ultrasound (compression ultrasonography) are eligible. Patients presenting with documented pulmonary embolism are eligible for the study, providing they have objectively-proven proximal venous thrombosis.

Criteria for ineligibility

Ineligibility criteria include:

- Age < 18 years.
- The presence of familial bleeding diathesis or of active bleeding contraindicating anticoagulant therapy.
- Receiving therapeutic heparin or therapeutic low-molecular-weight heparin for more than 48 hours at the time of referral or who have already been on warfarin for more than two days for the treatment of their proximal deep vein thrombosis.
- Receiving long term warfarin treatment, i.e., treatment for atrial fibrillation, myocardial infarction, or cardiomyopathy. If long-term warfarin treatment is interrupted in these patients or in patients on long-term warfarin for the treatment of venous thromboembolism, and the patient subsequently developed proximal venous thrombosis, they will be eligible for the study.
- Female patients who are pregnant. Female patients of child-bearing potential will be eligible provided that
  (a) a pregnancy test has been performed and is negative;
  (b) the patient is informed that the risk of LMW heparin in pregnancy is unknown, and;
  (c) the patient is counselled not to become pregnant during the course of the study.
- The presence of known allergy to heparin, warfarin sodium, or bisulfites (the stabilizer contained in LMW heparin).
- A history of heparin-associated thrombocytopenia.
- Patients with severe malignant hypertension (blood pressure ⩾250 mm Hg systolic and ⩾130 mm Hg diastolic).
- Patients with hepatic encephalopathy.
- Patients with severe renal failure (dialysis patients).
- Patients who are unable to attend follow-up due to geographic inaccessibility.
- Patients who are unable or refuse to give signed informed consent.

All ineligible patients will be documented and their clinical characteristics recorded. The clinical characteristics of all patients (including the ineligible patients) are recorded to describe the overall population from which the study population is selected.

Baseline assessment

For all patients a clinical history will be taken and a physical examination performed before entry into the study. The findings of the initial history and physical examination, the past medical history, and the demographic characteristics will be documented on the study intake data form. Additionally, a single blood sample (4.5 ml) will be drawn from each patient for analysis of activated Protein C resistance at a central laboratory in Calgary (note: non-iced samples are acceptable).

The performance of ventilation/perfusion lung scans is strongly encouraged, although not mandatory. Baseline lung scans are extremely helpful in assessing recurrent thrombo-embolic events.

Treatment allocation

Consecutive eligible patients who give signed informed consent will be randomly allo-cated (using a predetermined randomized treatment schedule derived by computer) to receive one of the following long-term treatment regimens (patients must be randomized within 48 hours of beginning intravenous heparin therapy).

* Continue with intravenous infusion of unfractionated heparin which is monitored using the heparin protocol to ensure a therapeutic APTT followed by long-term oral warfarin sodium adjusted to maintain the INR between 2.0 and 3.0.
* Subcutaneous low molecular weight heparin (using a LMW heparin which has been proven to be effective) given in a fixed dose (175 F X_a units/kg) once daily for both the initial and long-term therapy.

The randomisation will be stratified according to
* the study center,
* the presence or absence of clinical risk factors for bleeding complications ("high risk for bleeding" or "low risk for bleeding"), and
* cancer

The following patients will be considered to be "high risk for bleeding":
* patients who have had surgery or trauma within the previous 14 days
* patients with a history of peptic ulcer disease, gastrointestinal bleeding, or genitouri-nary bleeding
* patients who have had a recent stroke (that is, thrombotic stroke within the previous 14 days)
* patients with a platelet count of 150×10^6/L, or below the lower level of the platelet count for the study center
* patients with miscellaneous reasons for being at high risk for bleeding (for example, hepatic failure)

All remaining patients will be assigned to the "low risk for bleeding" stratum. Randomi-sation will be balanced in blocks of 2 and 4 selected in random order within each stratum.

Treatment regimens

Anticoagulant therapy will be started in all patients as soon as possible after objective documentation of proximal-vein thrombosis is completed.

Group I: Continuous intravenous heparin followed by oral warfarin sodium

This is the current standard treatment in North America and this group is the control group for the clinical trial. Heparin administration will follow a prescriptive heparin protocol which ensures that intravenous heparin therapy is given adequately [31].

If heparin has not already been started, it will be given as an initial intravenous bolus of 5,000 units. Continuous intravenous heparin infusion will commence at a dose of 40,000 units/24 hours in "low risk for bleeding" patients, and at approximately 30,000 units (29,760 units) in "high risk for bleeding" patients. (Table 1). A standard concentration of unfractionated heparin will be used for continuous intravenous infusion: 20,000 USP units in 500 ml of diluent. The diluent should be either normal saline or a mixture of saline, 5 % dextrose and water (for example, 1/2 : 1/2 or 2/3 : 1/3 of dextrose/saline). The intravenous infusion will begin at 42 ml per hour in "low risk for bleeding" patients, and at 31 ml per hour in "high risk for bleeding" patients. The heparin infusion dose will be adjusted according to the results of laboratory monitoring of the APTT (Table 1). The daily heparin dose will be adjusted to maintain the APTT between 1.5 and 2.5 times the control value. The APTT will be performed in all patients 4 hours after heparin therapy is started and the dose adjusted accordingly. The APTT will then be repeated 3 times at 4 to 6 hour intervals as indicated. Thereafter, the APTT will be measured once daily unless the result is subtherapeutic (< 1.5 times control), in which case the APTT will be repeated 4 hours after the infusion rate is increased.

As an alternative, the weight-based nomogram described by Raschke et al. [60] may be used. In the weight-adjusted nomogram, patients will receive a bolus of 80 units per kg, followed by intravenous infusion of 18 units/kg/h (Table 2). The APTT is monitored every six hours and the heparin dose adjustments are made according to the nomogram (Table 2). The APTT is repeated four hours after any change in infusion rate. When the infusion rate is stabilized, the APTT is repeated once daily. As with the previous protocol, the daily

Table 1. Intravenous heparin dose titration nomogram for APTT using organon thromboplastin reagent; IV infusion

Action APTT (secs)	Rate change (mL/hr)	Dose change (U/24 hrs)*	Additional
≤ 45	+ 6	+ 5,760	Repeat APTT** in 4–6 hrs
46–54	+ 3	+ 2,880	Repeat APTT in 4–6 hrs
55–85	0	0	None**
86–110	3	2,880	Stop Heparin for 1 hr Repeat APTT 4–6 hrs after restarting heparin
> 110	– 6	– 5,760	Stop Heparin for 1 hr Repeat APTT 4–6 hrs after restarting Heparin

* Heparin concentration 20,000 units in 500 mL = 40 units/mL; ** Using Organon Thromboplastin Reagent

Table 2. Weight-Based Nomogram

Initial Dose	80 u/kg bolus, then 18 u/kg/hr
APTT* > 35s (> 1.2 × control)	80 u/kg bolus, then 4 u/kg/hr
APTT, 35–45s, (1.2–1.5 × control)	40 u/kg bolus, then 2 u/kg/hr
APTT, 46–70s (1.5–2.3 × control)	No change
APTT, 71–90s (2.3–3.0 × control)	Decrease infusion rate by 2 u/kg/hr
APTT > 90s (> 3.0 × control)	Hold infusion 1 hour, then decrease infusion rate by 3 u/kg/hr

*APTT = Activated partial thromboplastin time; (Reproduced with permission from Raschke RA, Reilly BM, Guidry JR et al. (1993) The weight-based heparin dosing nomogram compared with "a standard care" nomogram. Ann Int Med 119: 874–881

Table 3. Warfarin protocol

International normalized ratio (INR)	Warfarin dose
0.9	
1.1	10.0 mg
1.3	
1.5	7.5 mg
1.8	
2.0	5.0 mg
2.3	
2.5	2.5 mg
2.8	0

Organon Teknika ISI = 1.89

heparin dose is adjusted to maintain the APTT equivalent to a heparin blood level of 0.2 to 0.4 units/mL using the protamine sulphate titration assay. Each participating laboratory must determine the APTT in seconds equivalent to the therapeutic heparin blood levels using their own thromboplastin reagents and their own laboratory equipment.

Warfarin sodium will be started within 24 hours of randomisation and the initial heparin will be discontinued on the sixth day providing the prothrombin time is prolonged into the prescribed therapeutic range. Warfarin sodium will be given in a dose of 10 mg per day for the first 2 days, and the warfarin dose will then be adjusted by the attending physician daily according to the results of laboratory monitoring of the prothrombin time. The therapeutic range for warfarin sodium will be standardised using the International Normalized Ratio (INR) in all the participating hospitals. The warfarin dose will be adjusted to maintain the INR between 2.0–3.0 (Table 3). This level of anticoagulant intensity corresponds to a prothrombin time of 1.3–1.5 times control using insensitive rabbit brain thromboplastin preparations such as Simplastin or Dade-C. After the sixth day, the prothrombin time will be measured daily until the patient's warfarin dose and prothrombin time response are stabilised. Thereafter, the prothrombin time will be measured every one to two weeks for the duration of long-term treatment (12 weeks).

The daily oral dose during long-term therapy will be prescribed by the primary physician. All patients will visit the laboratory at least once per week to have blood drawn for prothrombin time monitoring (or more frequently if prescribed by the primary physician). It will not be necessary for the patient to visit a central laboratory since the warfarin dose will be prescribed according to the INR. Before the patient is discharged from hospital, the laboratory which the patient wishes to visit for prothrombin time monitoring will be determined. This laboratory will be contacted by the study nurse who will instruct the laboratory about the pertinent details of the protocol.

At the time the individual laboratory is contacted, pertinent details will be collected: the name of the thromboplastin reagent used, its International Sensitivity Index (ISI), and the equipment used to measure the prothrombin time. It was decided that laboratory monitoring of longterm therapy should not be centralised for 2 reasons: first, it will be more representative of routine clinical practice and thus enhance the generalizability of the study findings; secondly, since a number of patients may live in rural areas, the inconvenience of travelling to a central laboratory on a regular basis could decrease patient acceptance of the protocol.

Group II: Low molecular weight heparin

LMW heparin (Innohep™ from Leo Pharmaceutical Products Ltd, A/S, Denmark) will be given subcutaneously in a fixed dose of 175 F X_a units/kg once daily. The second LMW heparin dose will be given between 18 and 24 hours after the first dose. By making the timing of the second LMW heparin dose flexible, the need to give injections at awkward times (such as the middle of the night) will be avoided. After the second dose, all subsequent doses of LMW heparin will be given once every 24 hours.

In order to assess the adverse effect of heparin-associated thrombocytopenia, platelets will be measured on day 5 after the low molecular weight heparin injections are started or on the day of discharge, if that is sooner. The platelet count will be repeated in the follow-up procedure on day 14 ± 2 and day 21 ± 2.

While the patients are hospitalised for the initial therapy they will be taught to self-administer the subcutaneous injections. In the case of the occasional patient who is unable to self-administer the injections, a family member will be taught to do this, or arrangements will be made for a visiting nurse to do it. Unless there are medical reasons for continued hospitalization (for example, co-morbid illness), patients will be discharged on day 2 or day 3 to continue their LMW heparin therapy at home. LMW heparin will be continued for a full 3 months (12 weeks).

Surveillance and follow-up

All patients will be reviewed daily during initial therapy by the consultant physician and/or the study nurse. They will be assessed for symptoms or signs of recurrent venous thrombosis, pulmonary embolism, or bleeding. At the time of discharge, all patients will be instructed to come to the hospital immediately if symptoms or signs of recurrent deep-vein thrombosis, pulmonary embolism, or bleeding develop. All patients will then be followed for a total of 12 weeks after entry. All patients will attend a routine clinic 12 weeks after entry. Additionally, all patients who present with symptoms or signs of recurrent venous thromboembolism will undergo objective testing. At one year after entry, all patients (or their primary physicians) will be contacted by telephone or mail to determine long-term mortality and/or history of recurrent venous thromboembolism. Documentation of recurrent deep vein thrombosis or pulmonary embolism will be reviewed centrally.

Effectiveness

Outcome Measures (during the initial treatment or during the 12 week follow-up period) will be

* Death
* Objectively documented symptomatic recurrent venous thromboembolism
* Bleeding complications

The objective criteria for recurrent deep-vein thrombosis will be
(a) venography demonstrating a constant intraluminal filling defect (or a vessel cut-off) in the deep veins that was not present on the baseline venogram or

(b) a repeat venogram that is difficult to interpret (because of the presence of collateral veins, persistent intraluminal filling defects, or non-filled venous segments); in this case recurrent deep-vein thrombosis will be diagnosed by impedance plethysmography or compression ultrasound if the results have changed from negative to positive (in the absence of clinical conditions known to produce false-positive findings). The management of patients that develop objectively documented recurrent venous thromboembolism will be determined by each patient's attending physician.

The objective criteria for recurrent pulmonary embolism will be
- pulmonary angiography demonstrating a constant intraluminal filling defect or cut-off of a vessel > 2.5 mm in diameter or
- pulmonary embolism found at autopsy.

Safety

Bleeding complications

Bleeding will be defined as major if it is clinically overt and (a) is associated with a fall in hemoglobin of 20 Grams/L or more, (b) leads to the transfusion of 2 or more units of blood, or [3] is retroperitoneal, intracranial, or occurs into a major prosthetic joint. Bleeding will be defined as minor if it is clinically overt but does not meet the other criteria for major bleeding. These criteria were used successfully in previous studies [32, 33, 36, 40, 42, 43].

Activated protein C resistance

Positive results will be reported to the patient's family physician.

Adverse effects

Heparin-associated thrombocytopenia may occur. It will be defined as a decline in platelet count to $< 150 \times 10^9$/L, or less than the established normal range at the investigator site in patients with normal platelet counts at entry. Heparin-associated thrombosis will be defined as arterial thrombotic events or recurrent venous thromboembolism in association with thrombocytopenia.

Cost-effectiveness analysis

A formal economic evaluation will be undertaken using previously described methods [34, 35, 37, 38, 41, 45, 46] to compare the cost-effectiveness of LMW heparin with heparin and warfarin in both Canada and the United States. An analysis will be made of the benefits of early discharge from hospital and of possible continued protection against major bleeding when LMW heparin is used. Finally, incremental cost analysis will be performed if reduced mortality is demonstrated to assess quality lifeyears saved.

Avoidance of bias, contamination, and co-intervention

ASA-containing drugs, sulfinpyrazone, dipyridamole, and nonsteroidal anti-inflammatory agents will be prohibited during the study, unless the patient requires treatment with these medications for other concurrent illnesses. All patients will be questioned at regular intervals during follow-up about the use of these agents. The outcome measures of effectiveness and safety will be interpreted by a central Adjudicating Committee which is unaware of the patient's treatment group. The objective test results will be interpreted independently and without knowledge of other interpretations, the patient's clinical findings, or the patient's treatment group.

Calculation of sample size

There will be 455 patients in each treatment group (a total of 910 patients). The observed frequencies of recurrent venous thromboembolism and bleeding complications between the treatment groups will be compared using Fisher's Exact Test and 95 % confidence intervals for the mortality difference will be calculated using a normal approximation. Four hundred patients in each group will have the power to detect a 50 % reduction in mortality in favour of LMW heparin (n = 455 per group, a = 0.05 2-sided, β = 0.20). The anticipated mortality from the previous treatment trial is 9.6 %.

Significance

This study promises to be highly significant, and has the potential of verifying that the use of LMW heparin as opposed to warfarin sodium for the long-term treatment of proximal-vein thrombosis can produce a significant reduction in mortality. No other long-term treatment trial using LMW heparin is being performed. The adoption of a LMW heparin therapy may bring about significant improvement in the cost-effectiveness of treatment, potentially saving many millions of dollars every year.

Concluding remarks

This clinical trial is currently underway in more than 25 centres in Canada, with 15 more centres undergoing IRB review. Funding is being provided by Leo Pharmaceuticals Ltd, A/S, Denmark, and by a University-Industry grant from the Medical Research Council of Canada.

References

1. A Collaborative European Multicentre Study (1991) A randomised trial of subcutaneous low molecular weight heparin (CY 216) compared with intravenous unfractionated heparin in the treatment of deep vein thrombosis. Thromb Haemostasis 65: 251

2. Aiach M, Michaud A, Balian JL, Lefebvre M, Woler M, Fourtillan J (1983) A new low molecular weight heparin derivative, in vitro and in vivo studies. Thrombosis Res 31: 611
3. Albada J, Neuwenhuis HK, Sixma JJ. Comparison of intravenous standard heparin and Fragmin in the treatment of venous thromboembolism: A randomized double-blind study. Thrombosis Res. Suppl VI: (abstract), 1987.
4. Albada J, Nieuwenhuis HK, Sixma JJ (1989) Treatment of acute venous thromboembolism with low molecular weight heparin (Fragmin). Results of a double-blind randomized study. Circulation 80: 935
5. Arnesen H, Heilo A, Jakobsen E, Ly B, Skaga E (1978) A prospective study of streptokinase and heparin in the treatment of deep vein thrombosis. Acta Med Scand 203: 457
6. Arneson KE, Handeland GF, Abildgaard U, Holm HA (1987) What is the optimal dosage of LMW heparin in the subcutaneous treatment of deep vein thrombosis? Thromb Hemostasis 58: 214 (abstract 794)
7. Bara L, Billaud E, Gramond G, Kher A, Sammama M (1985) Comparative pharmacokinetics of a low molecular weight heparin and unfractionated heparin after intravenous and subcutaneous administration. Thrombosis Res 39: 631
8. Basu D, Gallus A, Hirsh J, Cade J (1972) A prospective study of the value of monitoring heparin treatment with the activated partial thromboplastin time. N Engl J Med 287: 324
9. Bergqvist D, Hedner U, Sjorin E, Holmer E (1983) Anticoagulant effects of two types of low molecular weight heparin administered subcutaneously. Thrombosis Res 32: 381
10. Bertina RM, Koeleman BPC, Koster T, Rosendaal FR, Dirven RJ, de Ronde H, van der Velden PA, Reitsma PH (1994) Mutation in blood coagulation factor V associated with resistance to activated protein C. Nature 369: 64–67
11. Brandjes DPM, Heijboer H, Büller HR, de Rijk M, Jagt H, ten Cate JW (1992) Acenocoumarol and heparin compared with acenocoumarol alone in the initial treatment of proximal-vein thrombosis. N Engl J Med 327: 1485
12. Bratt G, Aberg W, Johansson M, Törnebohm E, Granqvist S, Lockner D (1990) Two daily subcutaneous injections of Fragmin as compared with intravenous standard heparin in the treatment of deep venous thrombosis (DVT). Thromb Haemostasis 64: 506
13. Bratt G, Aberg W, Tornebohm E, Henriksson P, Lockner D (1987) Subcutaneous KABI 2165 in the treatment of deep venous thrombosis of the leg. Thrombosis Res Suppl VII: 24 (abstract)
14. Bratt G, Tornebohm E, Granqvist S, Aberg W, Lockner D (1985) A comparison between low molecular weight heparin (KABI 2165) and standard heparin in the intravenous treatment of deep venous thrombosis. Thromb Haemostasis 54: 813
15. Bratt G, Tornebohm E, Widlund L, Lockner D (1986) Low molecular weight heparin (Kabi 2165; Fragmin): pharmacokinetics after intravenous and subcutaneous administration in human volunteers. Thrombosis Res 42: 613
16. Cade JF, Buchanan MR, Boneau B et al. (1984) A comparison of the antithrombotic and haemorrhagic effects of low molecular weight heparin fractions: The influence of the method of preparation. Thrombosis Res 35: 613
17. Carter CJ, Kelton JG, Hirsh J, Cerskus A, Santos AV, Gent M (1982) The relationship between the hemorrhagic and antithrombotic properties of low molecular weight heparin in rabbits. Blood 59: 1239
18. Carter CJ, Kelton JF, Hirsh J, Gent M (1981) Relationship between the antithrombotic and anticoagulant effects of low molecular weight heparin. Thrombosis Res 21: 169
19. Dahlback B, Carlsson M, Svensson PJ (1993) Familial thrombophilia due to a previously unrecognized mechanism characterized by poor anticoagulant response to activated protein C: Prediction of a cofactor to activated protein C. Proc Natl Acad Sci USA 90: 1–8
20. Dalen JE, Brooks HL, Johnson LW, Meister SG, Szucs MM, Dexter L (1971) Pulmonary angiography in acute pulmonary embolism: indications, techniques, and results in 367 patients. Am Heart J 81: 175
21. Frydman AM, Bara L, LeRoux Y, Woler M, Chauliac F, Samama MM (1988) The antithrombotic activity and pharmacokinetics of enoxaparine, a low molecular weight heparin, in humans given single subcutaneous doses of 20 to 80 mg. J Clin Pharmacol 28: 609
22. Gallus AS, Jackaman J, Tillett J, Mills W, Wycherley A (1986) Safety and efficacy of warfarin started early after submassive venous thrombosis or pulmonary embolism. Lancet 2: 1293
23. Green D, Hull RD, Brant R, Pineo GF (1992) Lower mortality in cancer patients treated with low-molecular-weight versus standard heparin. Lancet 339: 1476
24. Handeland GF, Abildgaard U, Holm HA, Arnesen KE (1990) Dose adjusted heparin treatment of deep venous thrombosis: A comparison of unfractionated and low molecular weight heparin. Eur J Clin Pharmacol 39: 107
25. Harenberg J, Huck K, Bratsch H, Stehle G, Dempfle CE, Mall K, Blauth M, Usadel KH, Heene DL (1990) Therapeutic application of subcutaneous low-molecular-weight heparin in acute venous thrombosis. Haemostasis 20 (Suppl 1): 205
26. Harenberg J, Wurzner B, Zimmermann R, Schettler G (1986) Bioavailability and antagonization of the low molecular weight heparin CY216 in man. Thrombosis Res 44: 549
27. Holm HA, Ly B, Handeland GF (1986) Subcutaneous heparin treatment of deep venous thrombosis: a comparison of unfractionated and low molecular weight heparin. Haemostasis 16: 30
28. Holmer E, Mattsson C, Nilsson S (1982) Anticoagulant and antithrombotic effects of heparin and low molecular weight heparin fragments in rabbits. Thrombosis Res 25: 475

29. Hommes DW, Bura A, Mazzolai L, Büller HR, ten Cate JW (1992) Subcutaneous heparin compared with continuous intravenous heparin administration in the initial treatment of deep vein thrombosis. Ann Intern Med 116: 279
30. Huet Y, Janvier G, Bendriss PH, Winnock S, Dugrais G, Freyburger G, Boisseras P (1990) Treatment of established venous thromboembolism with Enoxaparin: Preliminary report. Acta Chir Scand Suppl 556: 116
31. Hull RD, Carter CJ, Jay RM, Ockelford PA, Hirsch J, Turpie AG, Zielinsky A, Gent M, Powers PJ (1983) The diagnosis of acute, recurrent, deep-vein thrombosis: a diagnostic challenge. Circulation 67: 901
32. Hull R, Delmore T, Carter C, Hirsh J, Genton E, Gent M, Turpie G, McLaughlin D (1982) Adjusted subcutaneous heparin versus warfarin sodium in the long-term treatment of venous thrombosis. N Engl J Med 306: 189
33. Hull R, Delmore T, Genton E, Hirsh J, Gent M, Sackett D, McLoughlin D, Armstrong P (1979) Warfarin sodium versus low dose heparin in the long-term treatment of venous thrombosis. N Engl J Med 301: 855
34. Hull RD, Feldstein W, Pineo GF, Raskob GE (1995) Cost-effectiveness of diagnosis of deep vein thrombosis in symptomatic patients. Thromb Haemost 74 (1): 189
35. Hull RD, Feldstein W, Stein PD, Pineo GF (1996) Cost-effectiveness of pulmonary embolism diagnosis. Arch Int Med 156: 68–72
36. Hull R, Hirsh J, Jay R et al. (1982) Different intensities of oral anticoagulant therapy in the treatment of proximal-vein thrombosis. N Engl J Med 307: 1676
37. Hull R, Hirsh J, Sackett DL, Stoddart G (1981) Cost-effectiveness of clinical diagnosis, venography and non-invasive testing in patients with symptomatic deep-vein thrombosis. N Engl J Med 304: 1561
38. Hull R, Hirsh J, Sackett DL, Stoddart GL (1982) Cost-effectiveness of primary and secondary prevention of fatal pulmonary embolism in high-risk surgical patients. Can Med Ass J 127: 990
39. Hull R, Hirsh J, Sackett DL, Powers P, Turpie AG, Walker I (1977) Combined use of leg scanning and impedance plethysmography in suspected venous thrombosis: An alternative to venography. N Engl J Med 296: 1497
40. Hull RD, Raskob GE, Hirsh J, Jay RM, Leclerc JR, Geerts WH, Rosenbloom D, Sackett DL, Anderson C, Harrison L et al. (1986) Continuous intravenous heparin compared with intermittent subcutaneous heparin in the initial treatment of proximal vein thrombosis. N Engl J Med 315: 1109
41. Hull R, Raskob G, Hirsh J, Sackett DL (1984) A cost-effectiveness analysis of alternative approaches for long-term treatment of proximal venous thrombosis. J Am Med Ass 252 (2): 235
42. Hull RD, Raskob GE, Pineo GF, Green D, Trowbridge AA, Elliott CG, Lerner RG, Hall J, Sparling T, Brettell HR et al. (1992) Subcutaneous low-molecular weight heparin compared with continuous intravenous heparin in the treatment of proximal-vein thrombosis. N Eng J Med 326: 975
43. Hull RD, Raskob GE, Rosenbloom D, Panju AA, Brill-Edwards P, Ginsberg JS, Hirsh J, Martin GJ, Green D (1990) Heparin for 5 days as compared with 10 days in the initial treatment of proximal venous thrombosis. N Engl J Med 322: 1260
44. Hull RD, Raskob GE, Rosenbloom D, Lemaire J, Pineo GF, Baylis B, Ginsberg JS, Panju AA, Brill-Edwards P, Brant R (1992) Optimal therapeutic levels of heparin therapy in patients with venous thrombosis. Arch Int Med 152: 1589
45. Hull RD, Raskob GE, Rosenbloom D, Pineo GF, Feldstein W, Rosenbloom D, Gafni A, Green D, Feinglass J, Trowbridge AA, Elliott CG (1997) Subcutaneous low-molecular-weight heparin vs. warfarin for prophylaxis of deep vein thrombosis after hip or knee implantation: an economic perspective. Arch Intern Med 157: 298–303
46. Hull RD, Raskob GE, Rosenblom D, Pineo GF, Lerner RG, Gafni A, Trowbridge AA, Elliott CG, Green D, Feinglass J (1997) Treatment of proximal vein thrombosis with subcutaneous low-molecular-weight heparin vs intravenous heparin: an economic perspective. Arch Intern Med 157: 289–294
47. Koopman MMW, Prandoni P, Piovella F, Ockelford PA, Brandjes DP, van der Meer J, Gallus AS, Simonneau G, Chesterman CH, Prins MH (1996) Treatment of venous thrombosis with intravenous unfractionated heparin administered in the hospital as compared with subcutaneous low-molecular-weight heparin administered at home. N Engl J Med 334: 682–687
48. Lensing AW, Prins MH, Davidson BL, Hirsh J (1995) Treatment of deep venous thrombosis with low-molecular-weight heparins. Arch Intern Med 155: 601–607
49. Levine M, Gent M, Hirsh J, Leclerc J, Anderson D, Weitz J, Ginsberg J, Turpie AG, Demers C, Kovacs M (1996) A comparison of low-molecular-weight heparin administered primarily at home with unfractionated heparin administered in the hospital for proximal deep-vein thrombosis. N Engl J Med 334: 677–681
50. Lindmarker P, Holmstrom M, Granqvist S, Johnsson H, Lockner D (1994) Comparison of once-daily subcutaneous Fragmin with continuous intravenous unfractionated heparin in the treatment of deep venous thrombosis. Thromb Haemost 72: 186–190
51. Lockner D, Bratt G, Tornebohm E, Aberg W, Granqvist S (1986) Intravenous and subcutaneous administration of Fragmin in deep venous thrombosis. Haemostasis 16: 25
52. Lopaciuk S, Meissner AJ, Filipecki S, Zawilska K, Sowier J, Ciesielski L, Bielawiec M, Glowinski S, Czestochowska E (1992) Subcutaneous low-molecularweight heparin versus subcutaneous unfractionated heparin in the treatment of deep vein thrombosis: a Polish multicentre trial. Thromb Haemost 68: 14–18
53. Marder VJ, Soulen RL, Atchartakarn V, Budzynski AZ, Parulekar S, Kim JR, Edward N, Zahavi J, Algazy KM (1977) Quantitative venographic assessment of deep vein thrombosis in the evaluation of streptokinase and heparin therapy. J Lab Clin Med 89 (5): 1018

54. Matzsch T, Bergqvist D, Hedner U, Ostergaard P (1987) Effects of an enzymatically depolymerized heparin as compared with conventional heparin in healthy volunteers. Thromb Haemostasis 57: 97
55. Moser KM, Fedullo PF (1992) Subcutaneous compared with intravenous heparin for deep vein thrombosis. Ann Int Med 117: 265
56. Nurmohamed MT, Rosendaal FR, Buller HR, Dekker E, Hommes DW, Vandenbroucke JP, Briet E (1992) Low molecular weight heparin in the prophylaxis of venous thrombosis: a meta-analysis. Lancet 340: 152
57. Prandoni P, Lensing AW, Buller HR, Carta M, Cogo A, Vigo M, Casara D, Ruol A, ten Cate JW (1992) Comparison of subcutaneous low-molecular-weight heparin with intravenous standard heparin in proximal deep-vein thrombosis. Lancet 339: 441
58. Prandoni P, Vigo M, Cattelan AM, Ruol A (1990) Treatment of deep venous thrombosis by fixed doses of a low-molecular-weight heparin (CY216). Haemostasis 20 (Suppl 1): 220
59. Rabinov K, Paulin S (1972) Roentgen diagnosis of venous thrombosis in the leg. Arch Surg 104: 134
60. Raschke RA, Reilly BM, Guidry JR, Fontana JR, Srinivas S (1993) The weight-based heparin dosing nomogram compared with a "standard care" nomogram. Ann Int Med 119: 874
61. Rooke TW, Osmundson PJ (1986) Heparin and the in-hospital management of deep-venous thrombosis: Cost considerations. Mayo Clin Proc 61: 198
62. Salzman EW (1986) Low molecular weight heparin. Is small beautiful? N Engl J Med 315: 957
63. Salzman EW, Deykin D, Shapiro RM, Rosenberg R (1975) Management of heparin therapy: controlled prospective trial. N Engl J Med 292: 1046
64. Siegbahn A, Y-Hassan S, Boberg J, Bylund H, Neerstrand HS, Ostergaard P, Hedner U (1989) Subcutaneous treatment of deep venous thrombosis with low molecular weight heparin. A dose finding study with LMWH-Novo. Thromb Res 55: 767
65. Simonneau G, Charbonnier B, Decousus H, Planchon B, Ninet J, Sie P, Silsiguen M, Combe S (1993) Subcutaneous low-molecular-weight heparin compared with continuous intravenous unfractionated heparin in the treatment of proximal deep vein thrombosis. Arch Intern Med 153: 1541–1546
66. Verstraete M (1990) Pharmacotherapeutic aspects of unfractionated and low molecular weight heparin. Drugs 40: 498
67. Wheeler HB, O'Donnell JA, Anderson FA Jr, Benedict KJ (1974) Occlusive impedance phlebography: a diagnostic procedure for venous thrombosis and pulmonary embolism. Prog Cardiovasc Dis 17: 199
68. Wilson JR, Lampman J (1979) Heparin therapy: A randomized prospective study. Am Heat J 97: 155
69. Zoller B, Hillarp A, Berntorp E, Dahlback B (1997) Activated protein C resistance due to a common factor V gene mutation is a major risk factor for venous thrombosis. Ann Rev Med 48: 45–58
70. Zoller B, Dahlback B (1994) Linkage between inherited resistance to activated protein C and factor V gene mutation in venous thrombosis. Lancet 343: 1536–1538

R. D. Hull · G. F. Pineo (✉) · R. F. Brant
601 South Tower
Foothills Hospital
1403 – 29th St., NW
Calgary, Alberta T2N 2T9
Canada

Thrombolytic therapy in pulmonary embolism. Which patients should be treated, which regimen should be used?

G. Meyer, H. Sors

Summary The indications of thrombolytic therapy in the management of pulmonary embolism remain unclear. Thrombolysis is a lifesaving procedure in patients with major embolism and cardiogenic shock, but in patients with normal blood pressure, randomized studies did not show a decrease in mortality in patients receiving thrombolysis. Recent data however suggest that this therapy may be beneficial in patients with major pulmonary embolism and evidence of right ventricular afterload.

Several controlled studies have compared different thrombolytic regimen in patients with pulmonary embolism and indicate that a 2-h infusion of rtPA or urokinase is more rapidly effective than a 12 to 24-h infusion of either streptokinase or urokinase and that a 0.6 mg/kg bolus injection of rtPA is as effective and safe as the 2-h 100 mg regimen.

Key words Pulmonary embolism – fibrinolysis – treatment

Introduction

Most patients with pulmonary embolism have a favorable clinical outcome under anticoagulant therapy. As a part of a multicenter diagnostic study, Carson et al. evaluated the in-hospital and one-year mortality of 399 patients with objectively confirmed pulmonary embolism, most of them receiving intravenous heparin followed by oral anticoagulants [1]. The mortality rate was 9.5 % during hospitalization and 24 % after one year follow-up, but only about 10 % of these deaths were related to pulmonary embolism suggesting that additional therapeutic interventions such as thrombolytic treatment may have a small role in managing most of these patients. On the other hand, the results of a small randomized trial suggest that thrombolysis may be a lifesaving procedure for pulmonary embolism patients in cardiogenic shock [9]. The optimal management of patients with massive pulmonary embolism and normal arterial pressure is less clear. In these patients, thrombolytic treatment has been shown to produce a rapid decrease in pulmonary vascular obstruction and a rapid improvement in pulmonary hemodynamics and right ventricular function [2, 6]. However, the consequences of these hemodynamic changes on the clinical outcome remain to be established. In several randomized studies comparing thrombolytic therapy with heparin in patients without systemic hypotension, the mortality rate was not significantly lower in the thrombolytic group, whereas major bleedings occured less frequently in the heparin group [2, 6, 13, 25]. The results of two recent studies however suggest that thrombolytic therapy may be of value in a subgroup of these "clinically stable" patients with major embolism or echocardiographic evidence of right ventricular dysfunction [6, 12].

The thrombolytic regimens described in the early seventies for the treatment of pulmonary embolism consisted of prolonged infusions of either streptokinase (SK) or urokinase (UK) given over 10 to 72 h. Subsequent studies compared recombinant tissue-type plasminogen activator (rtPA) with several UK regimen and reached conflicting conclusions. More recently, investigators aimed to confirm laboratory and animal data suggesting that a higher efficacy of thrombolytic therapy may be obtained with a shorter administration. This hypothesis has been supported in part by the results of the clinical trials undertaken to resolve this issue.

Is there a place for thrombolysis in the treatment of pulmonary embolism?

Hemodynamic effects of thrombolytic therapy as compared to heparin

The Urokinase Pulmonary Embolism Trial (UPET) published in 1973, compared heparin and UK in 160 patients with acute pulmonary embolism [25]. Hemodynamic data were available before and 24 hours after the beginning of therapy in 143 of these patients; 80 were considered as having massive pulmonary embolism and 63 submassive pulmonary embolism. At 24 h, the mean pulmonary arterial mean pressure (PAPm) did not change significantly in the heparin group (25 mmHg at 24 h versus 26.2 mmHg before treatment) whereas it decreased significantly from 26.2 to 20 mmHg in the UK group. The preinfusion cardiac index (CI) value was in the normal range in both groups and did not vary at 24 h [25]. Tibbutt et al. compared heparin with SK in a smaller group of 30 patients with more severe disease [23]. These authors observed a significant difference in favor of SK as regards the decrease in PAPm at 72 h. Cardiac index rose from 1.5 to 2.2 l/mn m^2 in the SK group and remained unchanged (2.5 at 72 h versus 2.6 l/mn · m^2 before inclusion) in the patients receiving heparin but this difference in CI improvement did not reach statistical significance [23]. Italian investigators compared rtPA in 36 patients with massive pulmonary embolism and normal systolic blood pressure [2]. Two hours after the beginning of therapy, PAPm decreased from 30.2 ± 7.8 mmHg to 21 ± 6.7 mmHg in the rtPA group ($p < 0.01$) whereas it increased from 22.3 ± 10.5 mmHg to 24.8 ± 11.2 mmHg in the heparin group. In that study, CI increased from 2.1 ± 0.5 to 2.4 ± 0.5 l/mn · m^2 ($p < 0.01$) in the rtPA group and remained unchanged (2.9 ± 1.01/mn m^2 before and 2 h after treatment institution) in the heparin group.

A multicenter American trial compared the effects of rtPA and heparin on right ventricular function assessed by echocardiography performed before treatment and repeated 3 and 24 h thereafter in 101 patients with acute pulmonary embolism. In the 89 patients with sets of 3 echocardiograms that were technically adequate, there was a significant decrease in right ventricular end-diastolic area during the 24 h after randomization, whereas this value did not change significantly in the patients allocated to heparin alone. Most of the change observed in the rtPA group occurred during the first 3 hours after thrombolytic therapy was given [6].

Angiographic and scintigraphic evolution

In the study by Tibbutt et al., the mean angiographic score of pulmonary vascular obstruction (assessed by Miller index [17]) decreased from 18.6 ± 5.7 to 15.8 ± 7.0 in the heparin group and from 21.9 ± 6.1 to 8.6 ± 5.9 in the SK group ($p < 0.001$) [23]. In the PAIMS 2 study, the Miller index decreased from 28.3 ± 2.9 to 24.8 ± 5.2 at 2 hours ($p < 0.01$) in the alteplase group and remained unchanged in the heparin group [2].

In the study by Goldhaber et al., the lung scan severity score decreased from 0.43 ± 0.20 to 0.28 ± 0.16 at 24 h in the alteplase group and from 0.36 ± 0.21 to 0.34 ± 0.20 in the heparin group ($p < 0.0001$) [6]. Two randomized studies have focused on the subsequent evolution of pulmonary vascular obstruction assessed by perfusion lung scan performed several days or weeks after inclusion. In the UPET study, although absolute improvement in lung scan perfusion defect was significantly higher in the UK group (6.2 %) than in the heparin group (2.5 %) on the lung scans taken at 24 h, the treatment differences in resolution were less marked in the following days, and by the seventh day, the mean lung scan improvement was almost identical in the two treatment groups [25]. These findings were confirmed in the PAIMS 2 study where the scintigraphic scores of obstruction were 12.0 (day 0), 7.0 (day 7), and 5.5 (day 30) in the rtPA allocated patients and 8.5 (day 0), 5.3 (day 7) and 2.7 (day 30) in the heparin group [2]. These data indicate that UK, SK, and rtPA significantly accelerate the dissolution of pulmonary emboli when compared to heparin alone. On the other hand, the difference in resolution rate observed during the first 24 hours is no more apparent on and after the seventh day.

Hemorrhagic complications

Bleeding represents the main limitation of thrombolytic therapy. It has recently been estimated that severe bleeding occurs in about 14 % of the patients with pulmonary embolism who receive thrombolytic therapy after an invasive diagnostic procedure and that intracranial hemorrhage occurs in about 1.9 % of such patients [10, 22].

The major hemorrhagic complication rates reported in the eight randomized studies comparing thrombolytic therapy and heparin in patients with pulmonary embolism are given in Table 1. The large difference in major bleeding rate between heparin and thrombolytic therapy observed in the UPET study may be related to several grounds. First, all patients included in that study underwent pulmonary angiography before and 24 h after inclusion; as a result, 36 % of major bleeds occurred at cutdown site for pulmonary angiography [25]. In addition, several patients had conditions such as stroke, yet considered as major contraindication to thrombolysis. Finally, the high UK dosage used (about 50,000 IU/kg) may also explain the high bleeding rate observed in the UK group. Such an increase in bleeding rate was, however, not observed in the recent studies where most of the patients were included after a non-invasive diagnostic procedure [2, 6, 13].

Table 1. Major bleeding complications in the randomized studies comparing thrombolytic therapy and heparin in patients with pulmonary embolism. UK: urokinase; SK: streptokinase; rtPA: recombinant tissue plasminogen activator; *: major bleeding rate as reported by the authors using definitions which vary widely from one study to another

Study (reference)	Thrombolytic treatment				Heparin		
	Drug	n	Major bleedings*		n	Major bleedings*	
			n	(%)		n	(%)
UPET [25]	UK	82	22	(26)	78	11	(14)
Tibbutt [23]	SK	13	0	(0)	17	0	(0)
Ly [14]	SK	14	4	(28)	11	2	(18)
PIOPED [18]	rtPA	9	1	(11)	4	0	(0)
Levine [13]	rtPA	33	0	(0)	25	0	(0)
Dalla Volta [2]	rtPA	20	3	(15)	16	2	(12)
Goldhaber [6]	rtPA	46	0	(0)	55	1	(2)
Jerjes-Sanchez [9]	SK	4	0	(0)	4	0	(0)

Mortality

Among the eight randomized studies comparing thrombolytic therapy with heparin in patients with pulmonary embolism, only one found a significant reduction in death rate in favor of thrombolysis. In that study, Jerjes-Sanchez et al. randomized patients with massive pulmonary embolism hypotension and shock to anticoagulant plus SK or heparin alone [9]. Because of ethical considerations resulting from a clear survival benefit in the SK group, the study was stopped after 8 patients were enrolled. All 4 patients who received SK survived whereas all 4 patients allocated to heparin alone died of right heart failure (p < 0.02). Such a survival benefit was not observed in other studies. In the UPET study, the 2-week mortality was 7 % in the UK group and 9 % in the heparin group. However, 70 of the 160 patients included in this study had submassive embolism on angiography, the initial mean cardiac index was in the normal range in both groups and most patients were clinically stable with only 11 patients being in cardiogenic shock at inclusion [25]. In the study by Levine et al., 58 patients were allocated to receive a 2-minute infusion of rtPA at a dose of 0.6 mg/kg followed by heparin (n = 33) or heparin alone (n = 25). One death was observed in the rtPA group and none in the heparin group. Patients with massive pulmonary embolism who were hypotensive or hemodynamically unstable were considered ineligible; as a result, the baseline perfusion defect was 27.4 ± 3.6 % and 21.3 ± 3.7 % in the rtPA and heparin groups, respectively, suggesting that most patients had submassive embolism [13].

In the PAIMS 2 study, 2 of the 20 patients receiving alteplase died from hemorrhage and one of the 16 patients allocated to heparin died of recurrent pulmonary embolism. Although massive embolism was confirmed by angiography in all patients, none had systolic blood pressure less than 90 mmHg at inclusion and mean baseline CI in the heparin group was in the normal range (2.9 ± 0.1) indicating moderate hemodynamic disturbance [2].

Ly et al. allocated 24 patients with massive embolism to heparin (n = 11) or SK 250,000 IU as a loading dose given over 20 minutes followed by a maintenance dose of 100,000 IU/h for 72 hours (n = 14) [14]. Only one patient in each group had systolic blood pressure below 90 mmHg. Two patients allocated to heparin died as a result of pulmonary embolism; one had initial systolic blood pressure below 90 mmHg and the second was "moderately hypotensive". In the SK group, one patient died 3 weeks after enrolment from phlegmasia coerulae dolens.

Tibbutt et al. allocated randomly 30 patients with "lifethreatening" pulmonary embolism to either heparin (n = 12) or SK with a loading dose of 600,000 IU given over 30 minutes followed by an hourly infusion of 100,000 IU for 72 hours (n = 18) [23]. Most patients had angiographically confirmed massive pulmonary embolism on admission and significant hemodynamic disturbances assessed by a low mean CI value before treatment and elevated mean initial PAPm in both groups. In addition, 15 patients (9 in the heparin group and 6 in the SK group) had initial systolic blood pressure below 100 mmHg. One patient allocated to heparin died of recurrent pulmonary embolism 18 hours after starting therapy. Four other heparin receiving patients were withdrawn from the trial because their clinical condition deteriorated and alternative treatment was instituted, 3 underwent pulmonary embolectomy, and another was subsequently treated with SK. In the SK group, 2 patients deteriorated despite thrombolysis and underwent pulmonary embolectomy with satisfactory recovery. Interestingly, all patients with treatment failure had initial systolic blood pressure less than 100 mmHg.

In the study by Goldhaber et al., 2 out of the 55 patients allocated to heparin died of recurrent pulmonary embolism whereas no fatalities were observed among the 46 patients randomized to rt-PA [6]. The 101 patients enrolled in this study were hemo-dynamically stable, none had systolic blood pressure less than 90 mmHg, and most of them had normal right ventricular function at baseline.

Although thrombolytic therapy may be a life saving procedure in patients with massive pulmonary embolism and cardiogenic shock, the results of the randomized studies comparing this treatment with heparin in clinically stable patients did not demonstrate any benefit of thrombolysis with regard to mortality. However, none of these studies had enough power to detect potentially important differences in clinical outcome between the two treatments. As a result, the indications of thrombolytic therapy in clinically stable patients with anatomically massive pulmonary embolism (i.e. vascular obstruction > 50 %) remains an area of controversy [3]. Recent data however suggest that this group of patients may be further categorized in subgroups with different clinical outcomes [6, 11, 12].

In the multicenter American trial by Goldhaber et al., the outcome of patients allocated to heparin was influenced by the echocardiographic findings [6]. Five out of the 18 patients with right ventricular hypokinesis on initial echocardiogram had symptomatic recurrent pulmonary embolism (2 fatal) during the 14 days after randomization. This finding contrasts with the uneventful outcome of the 32 heparin treated patients with normal right ventricular wall movement on initial echocardiogram. A more recent study by Kasper et al. also suggests that in patients with clinically suspected pulmonary embolism, the presence of right ventricular afterload stress detected by echocardio-graphy is a major determinant of short term prognosis [11]. Konstantinides et al. carefully analyzed 719 consecutive patients with major pulmonary embolism without clinical evidence of cardiogenic shock included in a large multicenter German registry [12]. These authors found that the overall 30-day mortality rate was significantly lower in patients who received thrombolytic therapy (4.7 % vs 11.1 %, p = 0.016). In addition, syncope, arterial hypotension, dilatation of the right ventricle on echocardiography, history of congestive heart failure, and chronic pulmonary disease were all associated with a high death rate. However, multivariate analysis indicated that only primary thrombolysis was independently associated with survival (Odds Ratio for in-hospital death: 0.46; 95 % CI: 0.21 to 1.00). The benefit of thrombolytic therapy may have been even more pronounced in patients under 65 years of age (3 % death rate in those receiving thrombolysis vs 9.2 % in those treated with heparin) and in patients presenting with syncope or systolic blood pressure < 90 mmHg. In patients with right ventricular enlargement on echocardio-graphy, the mortality rate was 4.7 % and 11.1 % in those receiving thrombolysis and anticoagulant therapy, respectively. These data arise from an observational study where the patients were not randomly assigned to the two treatment regimens. As a result, selection bias may have occurred as suggested by the older age of the patients receiving heparin and the greater incidence of pre-existing cardiac or pulmonary disease in that group. However, the results presented suggest that the early use of thrombolysis is associated with a survival benefit in clinically stable patients with major pulmonary embolism. As the authors suggest, these findings emphasize the need for a large randomized study comparing thrombolytic therapy and heparin in these patients [12].

Which thrombolytic regimen should be used?

A number of studies have evaluated different thrombolytic regimens for the treatment of pulmonary embolism. Most reports consist of uncontrolled cases series with different efficacy and safety end-points; their results are therefore difficult to compare and were previously reviewed [15]. The present analysis will focus on the main controlled studies which compared two different thrombolytic drugs or dosages.

In the Urokinase-Streptokinase pulmonary embolism trial, SK given as a 250,000 IU 20-min bolus injection followed by a 100,000 IU hourly infusion for 24 h was compared to UK given as a 30 min 4,400 IU/kg bolus injection followed by a 4,400 IU/kg hourly infusion for 12 to 24 h. These 3 regimens produced comparable hemodynamic and angiographic improvements and no significant difference in bleeding and mortality rates was observed [26].

A multicenter European trial compared UK given as an hourly dose of 2,000 IU/kg for 24 h and UK given as a 4,400 IU/kg hourly dose for 12 hours. These two UK regimen produce similar angiographic and hemodynamic improvements and similar bleeding rates [24].

Goldhaber et al. compared the USPET 24 h UK regimen (4,400 IU/kg as a bolus followed by 4,400 IU/kg h for 24 h) and a 100 mg dose of rtPA given over 2 hours [7]. Hemodynamic and angiographic results were compared 2 h after initiating treatment. At this time, PAPm felt from 31 ± 14 mmHg to 24 ± 6.8 mmHg in the rtPA group and remained unchanged in the UK group. Patients treated with rtPA had a 22.6 % improvement in the angiographic score at 2 h as compared to 8.3 % among those assigned to UK (p = 0.003). By contrast, the improvement in lung scan perfusion at 24 h was identical in the two treatment groups. No difference was observed in bleeding complication rate and 2 patients died in each group. This study was criticized because the two treatment regimens were compared at a time when only 12 % of the total dose of UK had been administered, thus, favoring rtPA in the angiographic and hemodynamic evaluation [20]. It has also been emphasized that the UK dosage was twice the dose recommended by the manufacturer [20].

The same rtPA regimen was subsequently compared to the UPET UK dosage (4,400 IU/kg as a bolus followed by 4,400 IU/kg h for 12 h) in 63 patients with angiographically confirmed massive pulmonary embolism in a multicenter European randomized study [16]. Two hours after the beginning of treatment, total pulmonary resistance decreased by 18 ± 22 % in the UK group and by 36 ± 17 % in the rtPA group (p = 0.009). Continuous monitoring of cardiac index and PAPm over the initial 12 h revealed that hemodynamic status improved faster in the rtPA group with a significant intergroup difference from 30 min up to 4 h. At 12 h, the decrease in total pulmonary resistance was 53 ± 19 % in the UK group and 48 ± 17 % in the rtPA group (p = 0.14) and the angiographic severity score (assessed by the method of Miller et al. [17]) decreased by 7.5 ± 6.2 in the UK group and 5.9 ± 4.3 in the rtPA treated patients (p = 0.25). Major bleeding occurred in 8 patients (28 %) allocated to UK and 7 (21 %) of the rtPA treated patients (p = 0.56). Four patients (3 belonging to rtPA group and 1 in the UK group) died within the 14-day study period.

Goldhaber et al. later compared the 100 mg rtPA dosage with a novel 3 million IU dose of UK given over 2 h in 90 patients with acute pulmonary embolism [8]. At 2 h, the angiographic score decreased from 6.04 ± 2.23 to 4.69 ± 2.15 in the patients receiving rtPA and from 6.43 ± 2.05 to 5.29 ± 2.21 in the patients allocated to UK (difference nonsignificant). Surprisingly, PAPm did not change significantly at 2 h in either group. Major bleeding rate was similar in both groups and 3 patients (2 in the rtPA group and 1 in the UK group) died within the 14-day study period.

The results of animal experiments suggest that rtPA may be more effective in improving pulmonary hemodynamics when given as a short infusion [19]. A 0.6 mg/kg short infusion has been proven safe and effective in patients with acute pulmonary embolism

[13]. These results prompted American and European investigators to compare this new dosage with the 100 mg reference rtPA dosage in two parallel randomized studies [4, 21]. Fifty three patients with acute massive pulmonary embolism were included in the European trial and 90 in the American study. Continuous hemodynamic monitoring revealed a significant improvement in total pulmonary resistance over the 12 h study period with a faster decrease in the 2-h group over the first hour [21]. Perfusion lung scans obtained in both trials at baseline and at 24 h did not show any difference in the absolute improvement in the perfusion lung scan score between the two treatment groups [5]. Safety factors including death rate (5 % in the bolus group vs 2 % in the 2-h group, $p = 0.67$) and major bleeding (11 % in the bolus group vs 20 % in the 2-h group) did not differ significantly between the groups [5].

The current available data indicate that a 2-h 100 mg infusion of rtPA acts more rapidly and may induce less bleeding than the 12–24 h high dosage of UK previously described for the treatment of pulmonary embolism. A 0.6 mg/kg bolus injection of rtPA is as effective and at least as safe as the 2-h 100 mg regimen and allows a 60 % reduction in the total dose of rtPA. However, according to its lower cost, a short infusion of SK merits to be compared with this latter rtPA dosage in an adequate randomized trial. Although the search for an ideal thrombolytic drug or dosage remains an important clinical issue in treating patients with pulmonary embolism, efforts of investigators have to focus on a better definition of the indications of this therapy in patients with massive pulmonary embolism.

References

1. Carson JL, Kelley MA, Duff A, Weg JG, Fulkerson WJ, Palevsky HI, Schwartz JS, Thompson BT, Popovich J, Hobbins TE, Spera MA, Alavi A, Terrin ML (1992) The clinical course of pulmonary embolism. N Engl J Med 326: 1240–5
2. Dalla-Volta S, Palla A, Santolicandro A, Giuntini C, Pengo V, Visioli O, Zonzin P, Zanuttini D, Barbaresi F, Agnelli G, Morpugo M, Marini MG, Visani L (1992) Paims 2: alteplase combined with heparin versus heparin in the treatment of acute pulmonary embolism. Plasminogen activator italian multicenter study 2. J Am Coll Cardiol 20: 520–526
3. Goldhaber SZ (1997) Pulmonary embolism thrombolysis. Broadening the paradigm for its administration. Circulation 96: 716–718
4. Goldhaber SZ, Agnelli G, Levine MN (1994) Reduced dose bolus alteplase vs conventional alteplase infusion for pulmonary embolism thrombolysis. An international multicenter randomized trial. Chest 106: 718–724
5. Goldhaber SZ, Feldstein ML, Sors H (1994) Two trials of reduced bolus alteplase in the treatment of pulmonary embolism. Chest 106: 725–726
6. Goldhaber SZ, Haire WD, Feldstein ML, Miller M, Toltzis R, Smith JL, Taveira Da Silva AM, Come PC, Lee RT, Parker JA, Mogtader A, McDonough TJ, Braunwald E (1993) Alteplase versus heparin in acute pulmonary embolism: Randomised trial assessing right-ventricular function and pulmonary perfusion. Lancet 341: 507–511
7. Goldhaber SZ, Heit J, Sharma GVRK, Nagel JS, Kim D, Parker JA, Drum D, Reagan K, Anderson J, Kessler CM, Markis J, Dawley D, Meyerovitz M, Vaughan DE, Tumeh SS, Loscalzo J, Selwyn AP, Braunwald E (1988) Randomised controlled trial of recombinant tissue plasminogen activator versus urokinase in the treatment of acute pulmonary embolism. Lancet 2: 293–298
8. Goldhaber SZ, Kessler CM, Heit JA, Elliot CG, Friedenberg WR, Heiselman DE, Wilson DB, Parker JA, Bennet D, Feldstein ML, Selwyn AP, Kim D, Sharma GVRK, Nagel JS, Meyerovitz MF (1992) Recombinant tissue-type plasminogen activator versus a novel dosing regimen of urokinase in acute pulmonary embolism: a randomized controlled multicenter trial. J Am Coll Cardiol 20: 24–30
9. Jerjes-Sanchez C, Ramirez-Rivera A, De Lourdes Garcia M, Arriaga-Nava R, Valencia S, Rosado-Buzzo A, Pierzo A, Rosas E (1995) Streptokinase and heparin versus heparin alone in massive pulmonary embolism: A randomized controlled trail. J Thromb Thrombolys 2: 227–229
10. Kanter DS, Mikkola KM, Patel SR, Parker JA, Goldhaber SZ (1997) Thrombolytic therapy for pulmonary embolism. Frequency of intracranial hemorrhage and associated risk factors. Chest 111: 1241–1245
11. Kasper W, Konstantinides S, Geibel A, Tiede N, Krause T, Just H (1997) Prognostic significance of right ventricular afterload stress detected by echocardiography in patients with clinically suspected pulmonary embolism. Heart 77: 346–349

12. Konstantinides S, Geibel A, Olschewski M, Heinrich F, Grosser K, Rauber K, Iversen S, Redecker M, Kienast J, Just H, Kasper W (1997) Association between thrombolytic treatment and the prognosis of hemodynamically stable patients with major pulmonary embolism. Circulation 96: 882–888
13. Levine M, Hirsh J, Weitz J, Cruickshank M, Neemeh J, Turpie AG, Gent M (1990) A randomized trial of a single bolus dosage regimen of recombinant tissue plasminogen activator in patients with acute pulmonary embolism. Chest 98: 1473–79
14. Ly B, Arnesen H, Eie H, Hol R (1978) A controlled clinical trial of streptokinase and heparin in the treatment of major pulmonary embolism. Acta Med Scand 203: 465–470
15. Meyer G, Charbonnier B, Stern M, Brochier M, Sors H (1989) Thrombolysis in acute pulmonary embolism. In: Julian DG, Kubler W, Norris RM, Swan HJ, Collen D, Verstraeta M (eds) Thrombolysis in Cardiovascular Disease. New-York, Marcel Dekker, pp. 337–60
16. Meyer G, Sors H, Charbonnier B, Kasper W, Bassand JP, Kerr IH, Lesaffre E, Vanhove P, Verstraete M (1992) Effects of intravenous urokinase versus alteplase on total pulmonary resistance in acute massive pulmonary embolism: A european multicenter double-blind trial. J. Am Coll Cardiol 19: 239–245
17. Miller GAH, Sutton GC, Kerr IH, Gibson RV, Honey M (1971) Comparison of streptokinase and heparin in treatment of isolated acute massive pulmonary embolism. Br Med J 2: 681
18. The PIOPED Investigators (1990) Tissue plasminogen activator for the treatment of acute pulmonary embolism. Chest 97: 528–533
19. Prewitt RM (1991) Principles of thrombolysis in pulmonary embolism. Chest 99: 157S–164S
20. Sasahara AA, Henkin J, Janicki RS (1988) Urokinase versus tissue plasminogen activator in pulmonary embolism. Lancet 2: 691
21. Sors H, Pacouret G, Azarian R, Meyer G, Charbonnier B, Bassand JP, Simonneau G (1994) Hemodynamic effects of bolus versus two hour infusion of alteplase in acute massive pulmonary embolism. A randomized controlled multicenter trial. Chest 106: 712–717
22. Stein PD, Hull RD, Raskob G (1994) Risks for major bleeding from thrombolytic therapy in patients with acute pulmonary embolism. Ann Intern Med 121: 313–317
23. Tibbutt DA, Davies JA, Anderson JA, Fletcher EWL, Hamill J, Holt JM, Lea Thomas M, De J. Lee G, Miller GAH, Sharp AA, Sutton GC (1974) Comparison by controlled clinical trial of streptokinase and heparin in treatment of life-threatening pulmonary embolism. Br Med J 1: 343–347
24. The UKEP study: multicentre clinical trial on two local regimens of urokinase in massive pulmonary embolism. Eur Heart J (1987) 8: 2–10
25. The Urokinase Pulmonary Embolism Trial (1973) A national cooperative study. Circulation 47 (suppl. II): 1–108
26. Urokinase-Streptokinase Embolism Trial, a cooperative study. Phase 2 results. JAMA (1974) 229: 1606–1613

G. Meyer · H. Sors (✉)
Respiratory and Intensive Care
Hôpital Laennec
42 rue de Sévres
75007 Paris, France

Thrombolytic treatment of pulmonary embolism: Life-saving option or unacceptable risk?

S. Konstantinides, A. Geibel, W. Kasper

Summary Thrombolytic agents have been consistently demonstrated to dissolve pulmonary thrombi much more rapidly and effectively than heparin alone. Rapid resolution of pulmonary embolism (PE) is accompanied by a significant decrease in pulmonary artery pressure and an improvement in right ventricular function. However, it is no longer than 7 days until the findings of patients treated with heparin improve to a similar extent. Previous studies were not designed to determine whether this short-lasting difference in favor of thrombolysis can indeed affect the prognosis of patients with PE and, thus, justify the 1 % (or even higher) risk of cerebral or fatal bleeding. Recently, two large registries demonstrated the importance of right ventricular dysfunction assessed by echocardiography as an independent predictor of mortality. Thrombolytic treatment was shown in one of these studies to be associated with a 50 % reduction of death risk in clinically stable patients with right ventricular enlargement. It was, thus, possible to identify a group of patients with massive PE who are most likely to benefit from early thrombolysis. These findings now have to be confirmed by a prospective randomized trial which will compare thrombolysis with heparin alone in this high-risk patient population, focusing on clinical end points such as overall and event-free survival in the acute phase of PE.

Key words Pulmonary embolism – thrombolysis – prognosis – mortality

Introduction

Three decades have passed since the earliest reports on the use of thrombolytic agents in acute pulmonary embolism (PE) [16, 34]. During this time, a number of well-designed trials assessed various thrombolytic regimens, comparing their effects on hemodynamic, angiographic or scintigraphic parameters with those of conventional heparin anticoagulation. Based on the results of these investigations, it was repeatedly attempted to establish guidelines or recommendations in order to optimize the therapeutic approach to venous thromboembolic disease [1, 3, 10, 18]. However, efforts to reach a consensus on the indications for thrombolytic treatment [37] proved far less successful in PE than in the setting of acute myocardial infarction [40]. Consequently, the debate between supporters and opponents of thrombolysis seems at present as hard as ever to resolve. In an excellent review of the literature published a year ago, it was concluded that "there is no evidence that thrombolytic therapy reduces mortality or reduces the rate of recurrent PE compared with heparin therapy." Furthermore, the authors expressed their concern about the risk of serious bleeding complications and the costs of thrombolytic agents and advocated their use only in patients with hemodynamic instability and arterial hypotension [8]. Since that time, however, the results of recent studies elucidated several important clinical issues including the determinants of outcome in PE and the identification of high-risk patients requiring prompt resolution of occlusive thrombus. We thus feel that it is again warranted to review our current state of knowledge regarding the impact of the type of treatment on the prognosis of patients with submassive or massive PE.

The hemodynamic benefits of thrombolysis: Undisputed but short-lasting

In a landmark study of 23 patients with massive PE, Miller et al. showed as early as 1971 that streptokinase infusion over 72 h resulted in a significant reduction of systolic pulmonary artery pressure, total pulmonary resistance and the angiographic index of severity (the so-called Miller score) [34]. Heparin anticoagulation, on the other hand, seemed to have no significant effect on these parameters during this period of time. Of note, common characteristics of this and other [13, 16, 41] non-randomized trials in the early years of thrombolysis were persistence on angiographic confirmation of PE for patient inclusion, definition of severity ("massive" or "major" PE) on the basis of angio-graphic rather than clinical or hemodynamic criteria, and focusing on hemodynamic or angiographic (rather than clinical) end points to determine efficacy of treatment. Confirmation of Miller's results during the 70s and 80s led to FDA approval of strepto-kinase for PE in 1977, urokinase in 1978, and alteplase in 1990. However, randomized trials of thrombolytic agents and, in particular, alteplase versus heparin alone, were not conducted until the early 90s. Angiographic diagnosis and assessment of severity (Miller Score) again dominated the inclusion criteria in the Prospective Investigation of Pulmonary Embolism Diagnosis (PIOPED) [35], the study of Levine et al. (58 patients) [31], and the Plasminogen Activator Italian Multicenter Study (PAIMS-2; 36 patients) [9]. Two of these studies demonstrated significant favorable effects of alteplase on the angio-graphic, hemodynamic, and scintigraphic findings within the first 24 hours [9, 31], whereas the difference between the two treatment groups did not reach statistical significance in the third trial [35], probably due to the smaller number of patients (13) and the somewhat lower dose of the thrombolytic agent (40 to 80 mg over 40 to 90 min). On the other hand, none of the three trials could show any difference in the findings of lung scans performed 7 days after treatment [9, 31]. Goldhaber's prospective study [12] included 101 patients and was unique in applying previously described [6] echocardio-graphic criteria to detect right ventricular pressure overload and dysfunction. However, pathognomonic ultrasound findings were reported in no more than 54 % of their patients since the study did not focus on major or massive PE. The authors pointed out the rapid improvement of right ventricular function in the alteplase group as assessed by 24-h echocardiographic follow-up.

In another prospective study, our group directly compared the hemodynamic effects of alteplase treatment with those of heparin alone in 40 consecutive patients with acute *major* PE confirmed by pulmonary angiography and/or lung scan [29]. Repeat invasive measurements of pulmonary artery pressure were performed 12 h after initiation of treatment, whereas echocardiographic follow-up was available for one week. Significant reduction of pulmonary artery pressure and total pulmonary resistance together with an increase in cardiac output was observed within 12 h in the alteplase group, confirming the results of previous studies. Furthermore, patients given alteplase had more pro-nounced changes in the dimensions of the right and the left ventricle during this period as assessed by echocardiography. By the end of the first week, however, no difference existed between the two treatment groups regarding the overall change in right or left

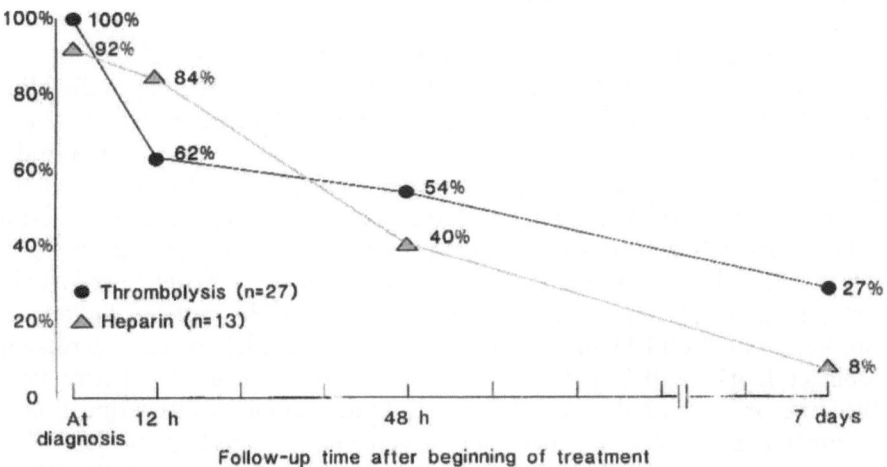

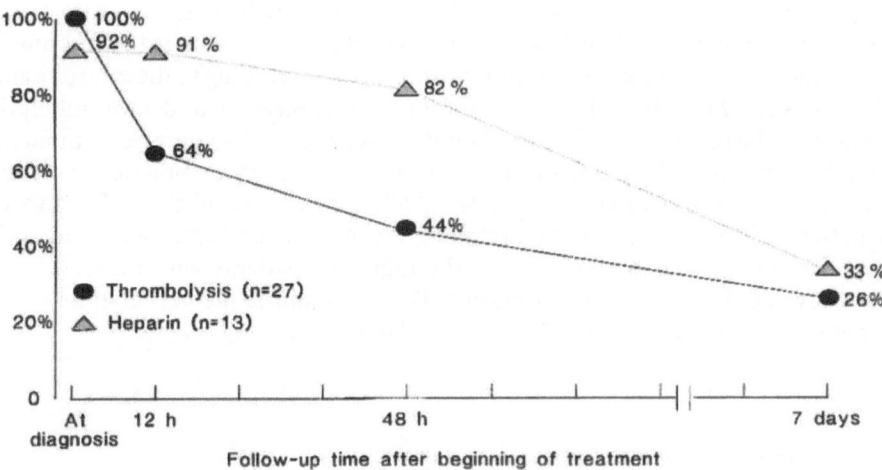

Fig. 1. Incidence of right ventricular enlargement (Fig. 1a) and paradoxical septal wall motion (Fig. 1b) in 40 consecutive patients with major pulmonary embolism: 7-day echocardiographic follow-up in the alteplase and heparin treatment groups (shown by circles and triangles, respectively).

heart chamber dimensions, or the incidence of right ventricular dilation (Fig. 1a) and paradoxical septal wall motion (Fig. 1b). It was concluded that, in patients with major PE treated with heparin alone, recovery of right ventricular function occurs within one week and thus earlier than previously assumed [7, 19]. In fact, one of the echocardiographic parameters, right ventricular free wall motion, was found to improve even before that time, returning to normal in the majority of our patients within 12 h [29]. The question that now remains to be answered is, therefore, whether the undisputed but short-lasting benefits of thrombolysis on hemodynamics and right ventricular function can affect the patients' prognosis substantially enough to justify the potential risks of that treatment.

Major bleeding complications: What is the price of rapid clot lysis?

The hemodynamic benefits of thrombolytic agents discussed above will be clinically relevant only if they are not offset by an unacceptable risk of life-threatening or disabling hemorrhage. By analyzing the data from 14 clinical trials published between 1987 and 1996, Dalen et al. found a 2.1 % rate of intracranial hemorrhage or a total of 12 episodes in 559 patients treated with alteplase [8]. The outcome was fatal in 9 of these cases. Relatively high rates (2.2 % incidence of fatal hemorrhage) had also been reported by Levine in an earlier review [30], whereas Kanter et al., observed an 1.9 % overall incidence of cerebral bleeding and found arterial diastolic hypertension and age over 55 years to be important risk factors [21]. In the Management Strategy and Prognosis of Pulmonary Embolism Registry (MAPPET), major hemorrhagic episodes (defined as a decrease in hemoglobin levels of ≥ 2 g/dL, requirement for a blood transfusion of ≥ 2 units, retroperitoneal bleeding, or bleeding that required surgical intervention or discontinuation of thrombolytic treatment) occurred in 22 % of the patients [27]. This high incidence is in accordance with the findings of the Urokinase in Pulmonary Embolism Trial (UPET) [38]. On the other hand, hemorrhagic stroke was diagnosed in 1.2 % of the patients in MAPPET and fatal hemorrhage occurred in 1 out of 169 treated patients (0.6 %). These are relatively low rates considering the fact that, in some cases, the clinicians proceeded to thrombolysis despite the presence of formal contraindications [23]. According to these results and the estimations of other authors [4, 10], the risk of cerebral bleeding under thrombolytic therapy seems to be in the range of 1 % und might thus be lower than previously thought. However, this conclusion by no means obscures the fact that thrombolytic agents are potentially dangerous drugs. In fact, the results of all studies underline the importance of proper patient selection, not only by excluding those with contraindications to such treatment but also by reliably identifying the high-risk patients with PE who most urgently need rapid resolution of thrombus. This selection is the cornerstone of an effective and efficient approach to PE as discussed in the following chapter.

Risk stratification of patients with acute pulmonary embolism: Who is expected to benefit from thrombolytic treatment?

A review of the literature reveals that many issues regarding the clinical course of acute PE are still poorly understood. One-year mortality was reported to be as low as 1 % in a multicenter study performed by the British Thoracic Society to find out the optimal duration of anticoagulation for venous thromboembolism [36]. On the other hand, 18 % of patients with massive PE died in the series of Hall et al. [15] and death rates approached [14] or exceeded 30 % [2] in patients presenting with cardiogenic shock due to right heart failure. In PIOPED, overall in-hospital mortality was 9.5 % but death was directly related to the thromboembolic event in only 10 patients (2.5 % of the study population) [5]. Twenty years earlier, UPET had come to similar conclusions [38, 39]. The authors of PIOPED further reported that age and underlying disease were important prognostic indicators in their patients and argued that "pulmonary embolism is an unusual cause of death" [15]. The aforementioned randomized studies of alteplase versus heparin alone seemed to provide further support to this thesis. In the latter trials [9, 12, 31, 35], only 3 % of patients treated with conventional heparin anticoagulation died in the acute phase, and alteplase did not result in a further reduction of mortality. It cannot be overemphasized, however, that the strict scintigraphic and angiographic criteria required to confirm PE in all of those series virtually precluded the study of severely compromised, high-risk patients and the low death rates observed are thus hardly surprising. In fact, the Management Strategy and Prognosis of Pulmonary Embolism Registry [23] found that patients with definite confirmation of PE by pulmonary angiography or lung scan had a much lower death rate than patients in whom the diagnosis was based on clinical, ECG, and echocardiographic findings alone. Apparently, the extent of diagnostic work-up was influenced by the severity of clinical instability at presentation. Therefore, the results of trials addressing a specific patient (sub)population cannot be simply translated into

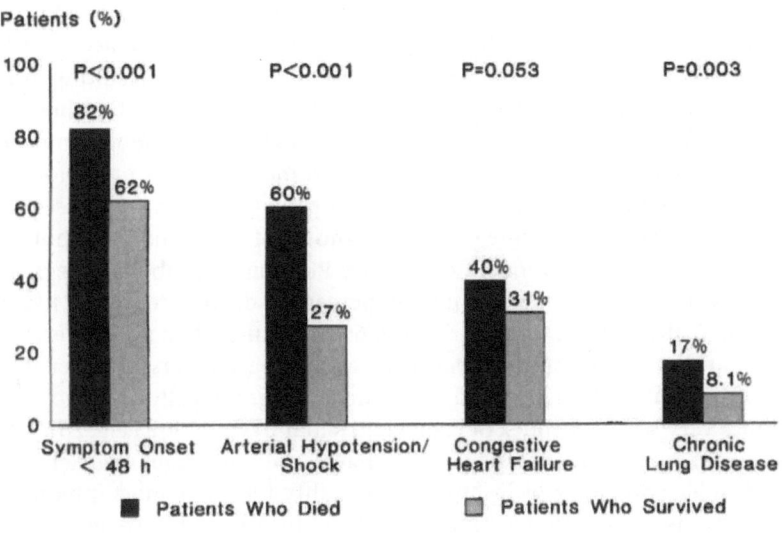

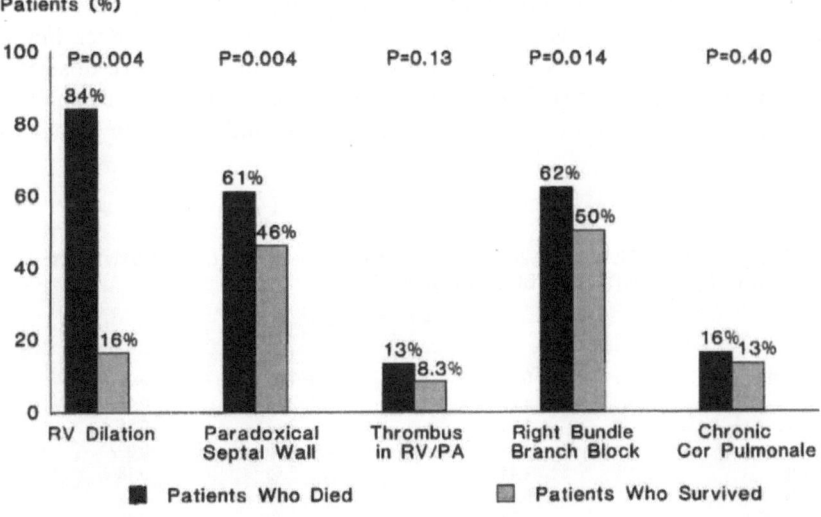

Fig. 2. Association between mortality and baseline clinical (Fig. 2a) and echocardiographic parameters (Fig. 2b) in 1001 consecutive patients with acute pulmonary embolism; data from the Management Strategy and Prognosis of Pulmonary Embolism Registry. RV: right ventricle, PA: pulmonary artery.

arguments against thrombolysis in PE. Conflicting reports in the literature all provide "true" data and simply demonstrate that patients with acute PE comprise a heterogeneous population whose prognosis and clinical course should be stratified rather than globally determined.

The extent of pulmonary artery obstruction determines the pathophysiology of acute PE [33]. Other important factors include the severity of pre-existing cardiopulmonary dysfunction and the peripheral venous clot burden which signifies the potential of recurrent thromboembolic events [17, 25]. The interactions of these factors result in the development of pulmonary artery hypertension and right ventricular pressure overload. The abrupt or progressive increase in afterload leads, in turn, to enlargement and dysfunction (hypokinesis) of the right ventricle. It was recently demonstrated that the presence of right ventricular dilation, which can be rapidly and reliably diagnosed by bedside echocardiography [22, 25, 26], is associated with increased in-hospital mortality in patients presenting with clinically suspected PE [24]. These findings are in accordance with current theories which emphasize that death due to acute PE is death resulting from right heart failure [32]. To confirm this thesis, however, it was important to show in large numbers of patients that clinical, echocardiographic or hemodynamic findings indicating overt or impending right heart failure are indeed the most relevant predictors of outcome in the setting of acute PE [4]. This evidence was provided during the past year by the results of the Management Strategy and Prognosis of Pulmonary Embolism Registry [23] as well as by the International Cooperative Pulmonary Embolism Registry (ICOPER) [11]. In MAPPET, there was a substantial increase in death rate from 8.1 % in patients who were clinically stable at presentation to 65 % in unstable patients necessitating cardiopulmonary resuscitation [23]. Apart from clinical parameters, however (Fig. 2a), mortality was also significantly associated with echocardiographically detected right ventricular dilation, a very sensitive index of right ventricular dysfunction (Fig. 2b) [22]. In fact, multiple logistic regression analysis showed that an enlarged right ventricle was the strongest independent predictor of in-hospital mortality [28]. The most important finding was that early thrombolytic treatment of 719 clinically stable patients with echocardiographic evidence of *impending* right heart failure was independently associated with an almost 50 % reduction in the risk of in-hospital death (Table 1) [27]. Frequent bleeding complications were the price paid for this beneficial effect, but, as discussed above, no excessive rates of intracranial or fatal bleeding were observed. Patients in cardiogenic shock or circulatory collapse were not included in this analysis, since there is consensus that their extremely poor prognosis under heparin alone [23]

Table 1. Predictors of 30-day mortality* in 719 patients with right ventricular pressure overload and clinical stability at presentation (The Management Strategy and Prognosis of Pulmonary Embolism Registry)

Characteristic	Odds ratio	95% CI	P value
Thrombolytic treatment	0.46	0.21–1.00	0.05
Age over 65 years	1.25	0.71–2.20	0.43
Acute symptom onset	1.19	0.67–2.11	0.55
Syncope	1.61	0.93–2.80	0.092
Arterial hypotension	1.44	0.85–2.46	0.18
Recent major surgery	0.76	0.40–1.43	0.39
History of venous thrombosis	0.78	0.43–1.40	0.40
Congestive heart failure	1.37	0.77–2.45	0.28
Chronic pulmonary disease	1.60	0.77–3.32	0.21

*Values shown were derived by a logistic regression analysis. CI: confidence interval warrants some form of "aggressive" treatment notwithstanding the bleeding or surgical risks [14, 20]. Although MAPPET was not a randomized trial, its findings in a large patient population provide a first link between the hemodynamic benefits of thrombolysis and a favorable impact on the patients' prognosis. This multicenter registry also identified a group of high-risk patients who are most likely to benefit from rapid clot lysis before the increase in pulmonary vascular resistance leads to right ventricular decompensation and cardiogenic shock.

Conclusions

The hemodynamic benefits of thrombolysis have been consistently demonstrated during the past 30 years. Compared with heparin alone, thrombolysis rapidly reduces the pulmonary clot burden (verified by angiographic and scintigraphic studies), thereby significantly decreasing pulmonary artery pressure and pulmonary vascular resistance and improving right ventricular function. However, it is no longer than 7 d until patients treated with heparin improve to a similar extent. The clinical importance of this short-lasting difference in the resolution rates of PE remains, at present, a controversial issue while awaiting the results of a randomized trial which will prospectively compare alteplase with heparin alone focusing on patients with major PE and addressing clinical end points. Such a multicenter trial is currently underway in Germany. In the meantime, the results of recently published registries reveal the importance of right ventricular dysfunction as a predictor of increased death risk. Recognizing the importance of risk stratification in PE helps optimize (and simplify) diagnostic strategies by placing emphasis on noninvasive, rapidly available echocardiographic studies. It may also prove to be an important step in defining the indications for thrombolytic treatment and may thus help develop a more effective therapeutic approach to patients with pulmonary embolism.

References

1. ACCP Consensus Committee on Pulmonary Embolism (1996) Opinions regarding the diagnosis and management of venous thromboembolic disease. Chest 109: 233–237
2. Alpert JS, Smith R, Carlson J, Ockene IS, Dexter L, Dalen JE (1976) Mortality in patients treated for pulmonary embolism. JAMA 236: 1477–1480
3. British Thoracic Society, Standards of Care Committee (1997) Suspected acute pulmonary embolism: A practical approach. Thorax 52 (Suppl 4): S1–S24
4. Cannon CP, Goldhaber SZ (1996) Cardiovascular risk stratification of pulmonary embolism. Am J Cardiol 78: 1149–1151
5. Carson JL, Kelley MA, Duff A, Weg JG, Fulkerson WJ, Palevsky HI, Schwartz S, Thompson BT, Popovich J, Hobbins TE, Spera MA, Alavi MA, Terrin ML (1992) The clinical course of pulmonary embolism. N Engl J Med 326: 1240–1245
6. Come PC, Kim D, Parker JA, Goldhaber SZ, Braunwald E, Markis JE (1987) Early reversal of right ventricular dysfunction in patients with acute pulmonary embolism after treatment with intravenous tissue plasminogen activator. J Am Coll Cardiol 10: 971–978
7. Dalen JE, Banas JS, Brooks HL, Evans GL, Paraskos JA, Dexter L (1969) Resolution rate of acute pulmonary embolism in man. N Engl J Med 280: 1194–99
8. Dalen JE, Alpert JS (1997) Thrombolytic therapy for pulmonary embolism: Is it effective? Is it safe? When is it indicated? Arch Intern Med 157: 2550–2556
9. Dalla-Volta S, Palla A, Santolicandro A, Giuntini C, Pengo V, Visioli O, Zonzin P, Zanuttini D, Barbaresi F, Agnelli G, Morpurgo M, Marini MG, Visani L (1992) PAIMS 2: Alteplase combined with heparin versus heparin in the treatment of acute pulmonary embolism. Plasminogen Activator Italian Multicenter Study 2. J Am Coll Cardiol 20: 520–526

10. Goldhaber SZ (1995) Contemporary pulmonary embolism thrombolysis. Chest 107: 45S–51S
11. Goldhaber SZ, De Rosa M, Visani L (1997) International Cooperative Pulmonary Embolism Registry detects high mortality rate. Circulation 96: Suppl 1: 1–159. Abstract
12. Goldhaber SZ, Haire WD, Feldstein ML, Miller M, Toltzis R, Smith JL, Taveira da Silva AM, Come PC, Lee RT, Parker JA, Mogtader A, McDonough TJ, Braunwald E (1993) Alteplase versus heparin in acute pulmonary embolism: randomised trial assessing right-ventricular function and pulmonary perfusion. Lancet 341: 507–511
13. Goldhaber SZ, Vaughan DE, Markis JE, Selwyn AP, Meyerowitz MF, Loscalzo, J, Kim DS, Kessler CM, Dawley DL, Sharma GVRK, Sasahara A, Grossbard EB, Braunwald E (1986) Acute pulmonary embolism treated with tissue plasminogen activator. Lancet 2: 886–889
14. Gulba DC, Schmid C, Borst HG, Lichtlen P, Dietz R, Luft FC (1994) Medical compared with surgical treatment for massive pulmonary embolism. Lancet 343: 576–577
15. Hall RJC, Sutton GC, Kerr IH (1997) Long-term prognosis of treated acute masssive pulmonary embolism. Br Heart J 39: 1128–1134
16. Hirsh J, Gale GS, McDonald IG, McCarthy RA, Pitt A (1968) Streptokinase therapy in acute major pulmonary embolism: effectiveness and problems. Br Med J 4: 729–734
17. Hull RD, Raskob GE, Coates G, Panju AA, Gill GJ (1989) A new noninvasive management strategy for patients with suspected pulmonary embolism. Arch Intern Med 149: 2549–2555
18. Hyers TM, Hull RD, Weg JG (1995) Antithrombotic therapy for venous thromboembolic disease. Chest 108: 335S–351S
19. Jardin F, Dubourg O, Guéret P, Delorme G, Bourdarias JP (1987) Quantitative two-dimensional echocardiography in massive pulmonary embolism: Emphasis on ventricular interdependence and leftward septal displacement. J Am Coll Cardiol 10: 1201–06
20. Jerjes-Sanchez C, Ramírez-Rivera A, de Lourdes Garcia M, Arriaga-Nava R, Valencia S, Rosado-Buzzo A, Pierzo JA, Rosas E (1995) Streptokinase and heparin versus heparin alone in massive pulmonary embolism: a randomized controlled trial. J Thromb Thrombolys 2: 227–229
21. Kanter DS, Mikkola KM, Patel SR, Parker JA, Goldhaber SZ (1997) Thrombolytic therapy for pulmonary embolism. Frequency of intracranial hemorrhage and associated risk factors. Chest 111: 1241–1245
22. Kasper W, Geibel A, Tiede N, Bassenge D, Kauder E, Konstantinides S, Meinertz T, Just H (1993) Distinguishing between acute and subacute massive pulmonary embolism by conventional and Doppler echocardiography. Br Heart J 70: 352–356
23. Kasper W, Konstantinides S, Geibel A, Olschewski M, Heinrich F, Grosser KD, Rauber K, Iversen S, Redecker M, Kienast J (1997) Management strategies and determinants of outcome in acute major pulmonary embolism: Results of a multicenter registry. J Am Coll Cardiol 30: 1165–1171
24. Kasper W, Konstantinides S, Geibel A, Tiede N, Krause T, Just H (1997) Prognostic significance of right ventricular afterload stress detected by echocardiography in patients with clinically suspected pulmonary embolism. Heart 77: 346–349
25. Kasper W, Meinertz T, Henkel, B, Eissner D, Hahn K, Hofmann T, Zeiher A, Just H (1986) Echocardiographic findings in patients with proven pulmonary embolism. Am Heart J 112: 1284–1290
26. Konstantinides S, Geibel A, Kasper W (1996) Role of cardiac ultrasound in the detection of pulmonary embolism. Semin Respir Crit Care Med 17: 39–49
27. Konstantinides S, Geibel A, Olschewski M, Heinrich F, Grosser KD, Rauber K, Iversen S, Redecker M, Kienast J, Just H, Kasper W (1997) Association between thrombolytic treatment and the prognosis of hemodynamically stable patients with major pulmonary embolism: Results of a multicenter registry. Circulation 96: 882–888
28. Konstantinides S, Geibel A, Olschewski M, Kasper W, Just H (1997) Acute pulmonary embolism: the value of echocardiography for identification of high-risk patients. Circulation 96: Suppl 1: 1–25. Abstract
29. Konstantinides S, Tiede N, Geibel A, Olschewski M, Just H, Kasper W (1998) Comparison of alteplase-vs-heparin for resolution of major pulmonary embolism. Am J Cardiol 82: 966–970
30. Levine M (1995) Thrombolytic therapy for venous thromboembolism. Clin Chest Med 16: 321–328
31. Levine M, Hirsh J, Weitz J, Cruickshank M, Neemeh J, Turpie AJ, Gent M (1990) A randomized trial of a single bolus dosage regimen of recombinant tissue plasminogen activator in patients with acute pulmonary embolism. Chest 98: 1473–1479
32. Lualdi JC, Goldhaber SZ (1995) Right ventricular dysfunction after acute pulmonary embolism: pathophysiologic factors, detection, and therapeutic implications. Am Heart J 130: 1276–1282
33. McIntyre KM, Sasahara AA (1974) Hemodynamic and ventricular response to pulmonary embolism. Progr Cardiovasc Dis 17: 175–78
34. Miller AH, Sutton GC, Kerr IH, Gibson RV, Honey M (1971) Comparison of streptokinase and heparin in treatment of isolated acute massive pulmonary embolism. Br Med J 2: 681–684
35. PIOPED Investigators (1990) Tissue plasminogen activator for the treatment of acute pulmonary embolism. Chest 97: 528–533
36. Research Committee of the British Thoracic Society (1992) Optimum duration of anticoagulation for deep-vein thrombosis and pulmonary embolism. Lancet 340: 873–876
37. Stein PD, Hull RD, Raskob G (1994) Risks for major bleeding from thrombolytic therapy in patients with acute pulmonary embolism. Ann Intern Med 121: 313–317
38. Urokinase in Pulmonary Embolism Trial: (1970) Phase 1 results: A cooperative study. JAMA 214: 2163–2172
39. Urokinase in Pulmonary Embolism Trial: (1974) Phase 2 results: A cooperative study. JAMA 229: 1606–1613

40. Verstraete M (1995) Thrombolytic treatment. Br Med J 311: 582–583
41. Verstraete M, Miller GAH, Bounameaux H, Charbonnier B, Colle JP, Lecorf G, Marbet GA, Mombaerts P, Olsson CG (1988) Intravenous and intrapulmonary recombinant tissue-type plasminogen activator in the treatment of acute massive pulmonary embolism. Circulation 77: 353–360

Stavros Konstantinides, M.D. (✉)
Klinikum der Georg-August-Universität
Zentrum Innere Medizin
Abteilung Kardiologie und Pneumonologie
Robert-Koch-Str. 40
D-37075 Göttingen, Germany

A. Geibel
Abteilung Innere Medizin III, Kardiologie
Hugstetter Str. 55
Universitätsklinik Freiburg
79106 Freiburg, Germany

W. Kasper
St. Josefs-Hospital
Medizinische Klinik
Solmsstr. 15
65189 Wiesbaden, Germany

Surgical treatment of acute pulmonary embolism

C. Schlensak, T. Doenst, F. Beyersdorf

Summary Pulmonary embolism is a common event in hospitalized patients. In most cases, pulmonary embolism is asymptomatic and undergoes spontaneous resolution. Pulmonary embolectomy is required when refractory hypotension persists, despite all resuscitative efforts, and a thrombus has clearly been documented by angiography, computed tomography or magnetic resonance angiography. Embolectomy for massive embolism is performed through median sternotomy with the use of cardiopulmonary bypass. Usually the common pulmonary artery is incised and the emboli are extracted using forceps, suction or Fogarty catheters. For chronic embolisation or if no cardiopulmonary bypass is available, a lateral thoracotomy may be performed. The embolus may be removed after proximal occlusion of the pulmonary artery while normal circulation continues in the opposite lung. In patients with high risk of recurrence, the vena cava inferior may be interrupted or a vena cava filter may be implanted. Postoperatively, systemic anticoagulation should be administered for 3 months or longer depending on the patient's risk profile. Interventional approaches for the treatment of pulmonary embolism are currently under investigation. Their benefit over surgical embolectomy remains to be established.

Key words Emergency surgery – pulmonary embolectomy – vena cava filter

Introduction

Pulmonary embolism is a potentially fatal disorder. It is one of the most common acute causes of death in Europe and in the USA [5]. In the majority of cases pulmonary embolism is a complication of deep venous thrombosis, which in turn may be associated with long immobilization periods (e.g., postoperative recovery period) or other pathological conditions such as AT III, protein C or S deficiency, different types of cancer, or trauma [3, 23]. Postoperatively, asymptomatic pulmonary embolism is a common event. Although the natural history of pulmonary embolism in most patients is spontaneous resolution, pulmonary embolism is the cause of death in an estimated 10,000–20,000 patients in Germany [19] and 50,000 patients in the US each year [2].

Fig. 1 illustrates that most cases of acute pulmonary embolism are clinically unrecognized (70 %) and become evident only during autopsy. Up to 60 % of autopsies performed on patients above the age of 40 show evidence of varying degrees of blood clots in the pulmonary bed [5]. A reason for the large amount of undetected pulmonary embolisms may be the heterogeneous presentation of the disease. The classical triad dyspnea, chest pain, and hemoptysis is only present in 14 % of the patients with pulmonary embolism and is not specific for this particular condition [18]. In general, the symptoms are vague and often consistent with an underlying disease process. For instance, dyspnea is present in up to 73 % of the patients with pulmonary embolism [9, 22]. Many of those patients also suffer from ischemic heart disease or chronic obstructive lung disease.

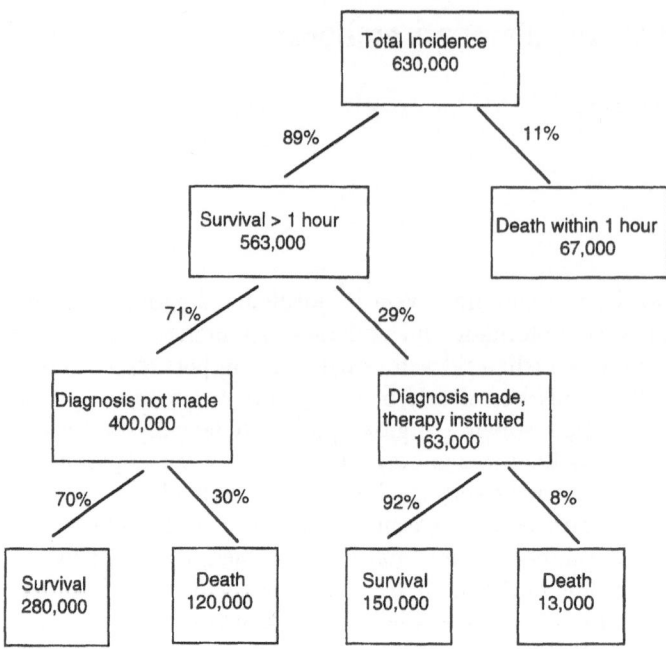

Fig. 1. Incidence of pulmonary embolism in the United States showing the subsequent course of this complication with deaths and survivors.

In addition, it is important to be aware of the extent of embolization of the pulmonary arteries necessary to produce clinical symptoms. A 50 % reduction of pulmonary artery does not usually cause changes in pulmonary perfusion pressures or impairment of contractile function of the heart [1].

If pulmonary embolism is undiagnosed, which is true for the majority of the cases, 30 % of the patients die acutely. If diagnosis is made and therapy is initiated immediately, mortality decreases to 8 % (Fig. 1). However, the later diagnosis is made, the higher the mortality [5]. Thus, establishing the diagnosis early is crucial for the clinical outcome. This conclusion is supported by the report that only 55 % of patients with symptomatic pulmonary embolism who were previously in good condition survive the first two hours after diagnosis [7].

The usual treatment for pulmonary embolism is intravenous application of heparin. Some authors advocate the use of fibrinolytic agents. A clear benefit of these agents over conventional treatment with heparin has not yet been demonstrated [8]. Although the majority of patients with pulmonary embolism recovers either spontaneously or with heparin treatment, a small portion of patients present with symptomatic pulmonary embolism that is refractory to conventional treatment and require surgical intervention.

Historical aspects

In a manuscript on the diagnosis of diseases of the lung and the heart from 1819, Laennec described pulmonary embolism as "pulmonary apoplexy" [12]. Soon after this description, Cruveilhier found blood clots in the pulmonary artery to be the pathological substrate for this clinical picture [4]. Virchow finally demonstrated the "embolic concept" as pathomechanism. He provided evidence that blood clots which can be formed in the periphery end up in the pulmonary arteries once they are released into the venous blood stream [26]. Virchow also suggested the presence of bronchial collateral circulation because only selected patients would suffer from pulmonary infarction during pulmonary embolism. It was not until 1964 that these collaterals were demonstrated angiographically [15].

The first pulmonary embolectomy was performed by Trendelenburg in 1908. Trendelenburg performed an emergency thoracotomy and removed the emboli from the pulmonary arteries in three patients. None of them survived longer than 2 days. Others also began to perform this procedure but the postoperative prognosis was grim. Occasionally, long term survival was reported [11]. Most patients suffered varying degrees of brain damage due to intraoperative hypoxia. The advent of cardiopulmonary bypass finally provided a safe tool for the removal of emboli from the pulmonary arteries [20].

Indications for surgery

Pulmonary embolectomy is indicated when refractory hypotension persists despite maximal resuscitation in patients where pulmonary embolism has been documented clearly with pulmonary angiography or recently with gadolinium-enhanced magnetic resonance angiography (MRI) [16]. Heparin treatment should be taken in an attempt to restore acceptable cardiopulmonary function. If the approach results in the maintenance of a systolic blood pressure above 80 mmHg, by continuous intraarterial monitoring, and cerebral and renal function is unimpaired, embolectomy may be deferred [18].

Operative procedure

Embolectomy for massive embolism is performed through median sternotomy [14, 20]. This approach provides excellent exposure of the pulmonary arteries. After the pericardium is opened cardiopulmonary bypass (CPB) is established immediately by cannulating both vena cava and the ascending aorta. In extremely critical cases extracorporal circulation may be established through the femoral artery and vein before opening the pericardium to avoid right heart decompensation. Mild cooling (32 °C) is used with the heart beating. Once extracorporal circulation is established, the common pulmonary artery is exposed and incised. The emboli are usually located in the left and right pulmonary arteries, while the common artery is free or only partially occluded. Using forceps and suction catheters, the emboli are removed as far as visible. Subsequently, a Fogarty catheter is passed into the branches of the pulmonary artery for the removal of smaller emboli. In some cases the lungs are gently massaged after opening of the parietal pleura to mobilize peripheral clots. The pulmonary artery is closed using 6-0 monofilament continuous sutures, cardiopulmonary function reestablished, and bypass discontinued.

Recently Jacob et al. reported a modified surgical strategy for fulminant pulmonary embolism [10] which includes a selective embolectomy of the main pulmonary arteries. After initiation of CPB, a hockeystick-like incision is made from branches, so that all lobar and segmental artery ostia become accessible. Clots are extracted using forceps and suction devices with tip sizes down to 2 mm. For right-sided embolectomy, the superior vena cava is mobilized and the right main pulmonary artery is incised between the aorta

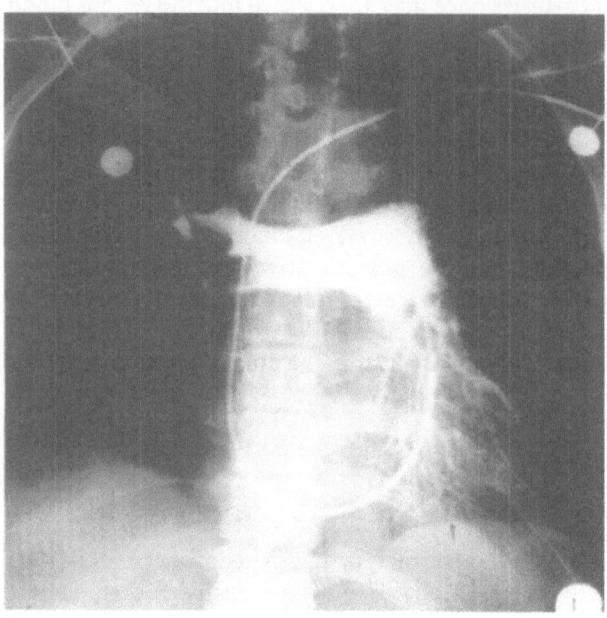

Fig. 2. Preoperative pulmonary angiography of a 44 year old patient, who suffered from postsurgical deep vein thrombosis.

and the superior vena cava for selective embolectomy. Thereafter, the right atrium is opened for atrial and ventricular inspection and the inferior caval vein cannula removed allowing for free flooding of all inferior body venous blood into the pericardial cavity. To mobilize fresh thromboses from the major leg veins, the legs are massaged centripetally [10].

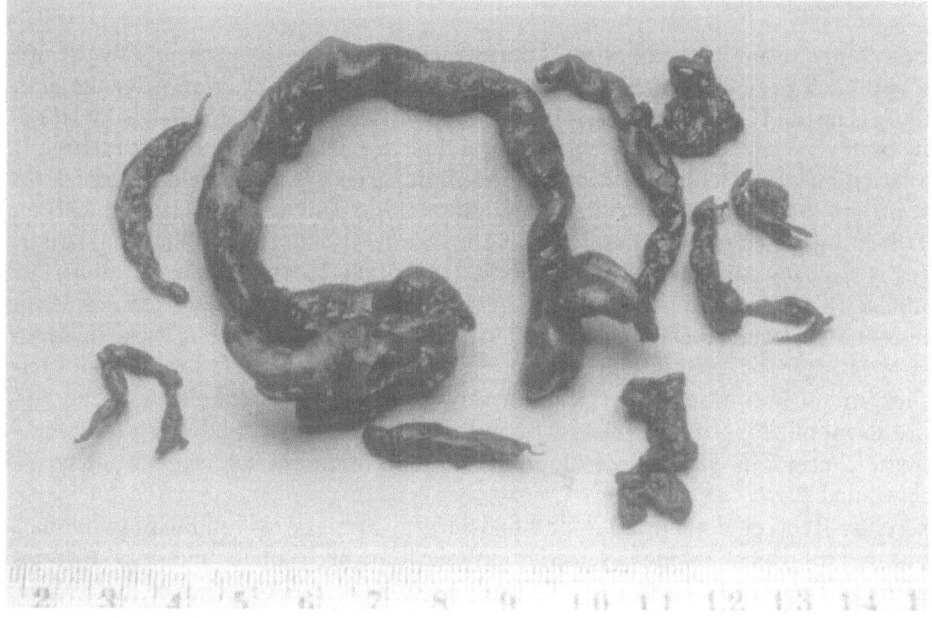

Fig. 3. Embolic material removed from the pulmonary arteries of a 44 year old patient, who suffered from postsurgical deep vein thrombosis.

If extracorporal circulation is not available or in case of chronic embolization, a lateral thoracotomy may be performed at the side of the most severely affected artery. An anterior thoracotomy in the third interspace is appropriate for exposure of the right or left pulmonary artery. The embolus may be removed after proximal occlusion of the pulmonary artery, while normal circulation continues in the opposite lung. Reflow of blood from the distal branches of the proximally occluded pulmonary artery can be used as an indicator for patency of the vessels [18].

Fig. 2 shows the preoperative pulmonary angiography and Fig. 3 the corresponding embolic material removed from the pulmonary artery bed of a patient with massive pulmonary embolism which occurred while the patient was recovering from abdominal surgery.

Postoperative management

The postoperative management of patients after pulmonary embolectomy is directed at the prevention of recurrence of pulmonary embolism or venous thrombosis or both. Early mobilization, pressure stockings, and physical therapy (e.g., with phenprocoumon coumadine) should be administered for at least three months. This time period may have to be extended dependent on the risk profile. In patients with a high risk profile (e.g., AT III deficiency, protein C or S deficiency), the placement of a vena cava filter, intraoperatively or after the procedure interventionally, should be considered and anticoagulation should be maintained as long as the risk factors are present [6].

Prognosis of patients undergoing embolectomy

Between 1980 and 1996 we performed pulmonary embolectomy after massive pulmonary embolism with the use of CPB on 10 patients. The operative mortality was 30 %. Two patients died due to right heart failure, 1 due to lung reperfusion injury.

Other investigators report an operative mortality of 23 % in a study of 17 patients [25] and 46 % in a study of 50 patients [24].

Alternative treatments

Recently, attempts have been made to remove pulmonary emboli with percutaneus endo-luminal techniques [17, 27]. The destruction of the emboli in situ or the aspiration with suction catheters have been described. Although the results are encouraging, the procedures are difficult to initiate, little experimented in humans, or still at the experimental stage in animals [17]. The clinical benefit over surgical embolectomy remains to be established in a prospective, randomized trial.

Once venous thromboembolism is detected, it may be tempting to directly remove the thrombi. However, this procedure cannot be recommended because of the high incidence of recurrent postoperative thrombosis. The only occasion which necessitates the removal of venous thrombi is the rare condition of phlegmasia coerulea dolens with secondary arterial spasm. Even though venous thromboembolism may recur after thrombectomy, patency of the venous lumen may persist sufficiently long to relieve the arterial spasm and may prevent the development of a gangrenous limb [17].

Preventative treatment

The interruption of the inferior vena cava in selected patients has been recommended as a preventative measure for recurrence of pulmonary embolism [8, 27]. The routine use of this procedure after pulmonary embolectomy is controversial [27]. The controversy is mainly based on the observation that 20 % of the patients show signs of recurrent pulmonary embolism after ligation [21]. Thus, clinicians have resorted to other measures for the prevention of recurrence, such as vena cava filters or long-term anticoagulation, or both.

The central goal of implantation of filters into the vena cava is to avoid pulmonary vascular obstruction in case of massive embolism originating in the lower part of the body. There are three established indications for filter placement [6]. First, protection against pulmonary embolism in patients with acute venous thromboembolism in whom conventional coagulation is contraindicated. Secondly, protection against pulmonary embolism in patients with acute venous thromboembolism in whom conventional coagulation has proven ineffective. Third, protection of an already compromised vascular bed from further thromboembolic risk. It is unclear whether anticoagulant therapy should follow the placement of a vena cava filter [6], even though the filter itself may give rise to thrombogenesis.

Complications

Occasionally following pulmonary embolectomy, massive endobronchial hemorrhage occurs. The complication may be treated successfully with an endotracheal tube obstructing the affected bronchial system [15].

The re-establishment of blood flow to underperfused pulmonary areas may give rise to the development of pulmonary edema. This reperfusion pulmonary edema may necessitate prolonged mechanical ventilation.

If the natural history or the treatment of pulmonary embolism does not resolve the embolic material in the pulmonary arteries, chronic pulmonary embolism may develop, which occurs in 0.5 to 4 % of patients with acute pulmonary embolism [13]. Usually, recurrent embolizations lead to the gradual obstruction of the pulmonary vascular bed. When obstruction exceeds the compensatory mechanisms of the pulmonary vasculature pulmonary perfusion pressure increases, giving rise to the development of pulmonary hypertension and cor pulmonale. Since the thrombi in the arteries become organized with time the operative procedure is different from acute pulmonary embolectomy. A thrombendarterectomy has to be performed [13].

Conclusions

Pulmonary embolism is a common condition in hospitalized patients. It is diagnosed only in the minority of patients and rarely requires surgical intervention. However, when systemic circulatory function is impaired and shock is developing or present, it is imperative to verify the presence and localize the site of embolization by pulmonary angiography, CT or MRI, and immediately proceed to the operating room. Pulmonary embolectomy is a potentially curative procedure but the time period from diagnosis to surgery is inversely related to survival.

References

1. Brofman BL, Charms BL, Kohn PM, Elder J, Newman R, Rizika M (1957) Unilateral pulmonary artery occlusion in man. J Thorac Surg 34: 206
2. Coon WW (1984) Venous thromboembolism: Prevalence, risk factors, and prevention. Clin Chest Med 5: 391
3. Coon WW, Coller FA (1959) Some epidemiologic considerations of thromboembolism. Surg Gynecol Obstet 109: 487
4. Cruveilhier J (1829) Anatomie pathologique de corps humain. Paris: Bailliere, J B; pp 42
5. Dalen JE, Alpert JS (1975) Natural history of pulmonary embolism. Prog Cardiovasc Dis 17: 259
6. Fedullo PF, Moser KM (1997) Advances in acute pulmonary embolism and chronic pulmonary hypertension. Adv Int Med 42: 67
7. Flemma RJ, Young WG Jr, Wallace A et al. (1964) Feasibility of pulmonary embolectomy. Circulation 30: 234
8. Gulba DC, Schmid C, Borst HG, Lichtlen P, Dietz R, Luft FC (1994) Medical compared with surgical treatment for massive pulmonary embolism. Lancet 343: 576
9. The PIOPED investigators. Value of ventilation/perfusion scan in acute pulmonary embolism: Results of the prospective investigation of pulmonary embolism diagnosis (PIOPED) (1990) JAMA 263: 2753
10. Jakob H, Vahl C, Lange R et al. (1995) Modified surgical concept for fulminant pulmonary embolism. Eur J Cardio-Thorac Surg 9: 557
11. Kirschner M (1924) Ein durch die trendelenburgsche Operation geheilter Fall von Embolie der Arteria pulmonalis. Arch Klin Chir 133: 312
12. Laennec RTH (1819) De l'auscultation mediate. Paris: Brossen et Chaude
13. Long J, Cohenca N, Rivera-Camilon MS (1994) Pulmonary Thromboendarterectomy. Clinical profile, surgical treatment. AORN Journal 59: 801
14. Luciano N, Gaudin M, Possati G (1996) Surgical treatment of massive pulmonary embolism. Rays 21: 432
15. Lyerly HK, Reves JG, Sabiston DC Jr (1986) Management of primary sarcomas of the pulmonary artery and reperfusion of intrabronchial haemorrhage. Surg Gynecol Obstet 163: 291
16. Meaney JF, Weg JG, Chenevert TL, Statford-Johnson D, Hamilton BH, Prince MR (1997) Diagnosis of pulmonary embolism with magnetic resonance angiography. N Engl J Med 336: 1422
17. Meyer G, Diehl JL, Philippe B, Reynaund P, Sors H (1995) Pulmonary embolectomy in pulmonary embolism: Surgery and endoluminal techniques. Arch Mal Coeur Vaiss 88: 1770
18. Sabiston DC Jr (1997) Pulmonary Embolism. In: Sabiston, 4th (ed.) pp 1502–1512
19. Schulte HD (1979) Lungenarterienembolie. Dt Ärztebl 2: 85
20. Sharp EH (1962) Pulmonary embolectomy: Successful removal of a massive pulmonary embolus with the support of cardiopulmonary bypass: A case report. Ann Surg 156: 1
21. Silver D, Sabiston DC Jr (1975) The role of vena cava interruption in the management of pulmonary embolism. Surgery 77: 1
22. Stein PD, Terrin ML, Hales CA, Palevsky HI, Saltzman HA, Thompson BT, Weg JG (1991) Clinical, laboratory, roentgenographic, and electrocardiographic findings in patients with acute pulmonary embolism and no preexisting cardiac or pulmonary disease. Chest 100: 598
23. Storti S, Crucitti P, Cina G (1996) Risk factors and prevention of venous thromboembolism. Rays 21: 439
24. Stulz P, Schläpfer R, Feer R, Habicht J, Gradel E (1994) Decision making in the surgical treatment of massive pulmonary embolism. Eur J Cardio-Thorac Surg 8: 188
25. Tschirkov A, Krause E, Elert O et al. (1978) Surgical management of massive pulmonary embolism. J Thorac Cardiovasc Surg 75: 730
26. Virchow R (1858) Die Zellularpathologie und ihre Begründung auf physiologische und pathologische Gewebelehre. Berlin: Hirschwald, A
27. Wakefield TW, Greenfield LJ (1993) Diagnostic approaches and surgical treatment of deep venous thrombosis and pulmonary embolism. Hematology/Oncology 7: 1251

C. Schlensak · T. Doenst · F. Beyersdorf (✉)
Abteilung für Herz- und Gefäßchirurgie
Universität Freiburg
Hugstetter Str. 55
79106 Freiburg, Germany